Tantra

ALSO BY
GEORG FEUERSTEIN

The Yoga Tradition (forthcoming)
Teachings of Yoga (1997)*
The Shambhala Encyclopedia of Yoga (1997)*
Lucid Waking (1997)
The Shambhala Guide to Yoga (1996)*
In Search of the Cradle of Civilization,
    coauthored with Subhash Kak and David Frawley (1995)
The Mystery of Light (1994)
Voices on the Threshold of Tomorrow,
    coedited with Trisha Lamb Feuerstein (1993)
Sacred Sexuality (1993)
Living Yoga, coedited with Stephan Bodian (1993)
Wholeness or Transcendence? (1992)
Sacred Paths (1991)
The Yoga-Sutra of Patanjali (1990)
The Bhagavad-Gita: Its Philosophy and Cultural Setting (1983)
The Essence of Yoga (1976)

*Published by Shambhala Publications

Tantra

THE PATH
OF ECSTASY

Georg Feuerstein

SHAMBHALA

Boston & London   *1998*

Shambhala Publications, Inc.
Horticultural Hall
300 Massachusetts Avenue
Boston, Massachusetts 02115
www.shambhala.com

The author thanks Princeton University Press for permission to quote from
Religions of India in Practice, D. S. Lopez, Jr., ed., copyright 1995 by Princeton
University Press.

9   8   7   6   5   4   3

Printed in the United States of America

♾ This edition is printed on acid-free paper that meets the
American National Standards Institute z39.48 Standard.

Distributed in the United States by Random House, Inc.,
and in Canada by Random House of Canada Ltd

Library of Congress Cataloging-in-Publication Data

Feuerstein, Georg.
    Tantra: the path of ecstasy: an introduction to Hindu tantrism /
by Georg Feuerstein.
        p.   cm.
    Includes bibliographical references and index.
    ISBN 1-57062-304-X (pbk.)
        1. Tantrism.   I. Title.
BL1283.84.F47   1998   97-29983
294.5'514—dc21   CIP

This book is dedicated to my kalyāna-mitra Lama
Segyu Choepel, who opened my eyes to the reality
behind Tantra in the form of Vajrayāna Buddhism,
and to the memory of the great masters of the Tantric
tradition whose potent liberation teachings have, for century
after century to the present time, been a bright lamp illumin-
ing the steps of seekers in the trouble-filled Age of Darkness.
May modern seekers, pure in intent, walk safely and
swiftly on the path of self-transformation and discover
the unsurpassable bliss of Reality, free from all concern,
in their own hearts and in the hearts of all others.

—⁂—

Contents

Preface   ix

Introduction: Tantra, the Great Spiritual Synthesis of India   1

1   Samsāra: Cyclic Existence   20

2   Time, Bondage, and the Goddess Kālī   32

3   This Is the Other World: Samsāra Equals Nirvāna   42

4   The Secret of Embodiment: As Above, So Below   52

5   The Divine Play of Shiva and Shakti   70

6   The Guru Principle: Shiva Incarnate   85

7   Initiation: Bringing Down the Light   95

8   Discipleship: The Ordeal of Self-Transformation   110

9   The Tantric Path: Ritual and Spontaneity   120

10   The Subtle Body and Its Environment   139

11   Awakening the Serpent Power   165

12   Mantra: The Potency of Sound   184

13   Creating Sacred Space: Nyāsa, Mudrā, Yantra   201

14   The Transmutation of Desire   224

15   Enlightenment and the Hidden Powers of the Mind   250

Epilogue: Tantra Yesterday, Today, and Tomorrow   268

Notes   275

Select Bibliography   295

Index   301

About the Author   315

Preface

I worship in my heart the Goddess
whose body is awash with ambrosia,
beautiful like lightning, who, going from her abode
to Shiva's royal palace, opens the lotuses
of the lovely axial channel (*sushumnā*).
—*Bhairavī-Stotra* (12)

"Tantra" has become a household word in certain circles in the West. But, as is often the case with household words, popularity does not necessarily imply understanding. Frequently we hear words like "consciousness," "holistic," "creativity," or "imagination," but how many people could give an intelligent explanation of any of these? Similarly, Tantra has captured the fascination of a good many Westerners, but few of them actually know what it stands for, including some of those who profess to practice, teach, or write about it.

Tantra, or Tantrism, is an exceptionally ramified and complex esoteric tradition of Indic origin. It made its appearance around 500

CE, though some of its proponents claim a far longer history. Tantra-like ideas and practices can indeed be found in traditions and teach-ings of a much earlier era. As a full-fledged movement or cultural style extending over both Hinduism and Buddhism, however, Tantra seems to have originated around the middle of the first millennium CE. It reached maturity around 1000 CE in the philosophical school of Abhinava Gupta. It profoundly influenced the outlook and practices of many non-Tantric traditions, such as Vedānta. Often practitioners of those traditions have been unaware of that influence and might even be offended at the suggestion that they engage in typically Tantric practices.

The reason for this is that within the fold of Hinduism, Tantra gradually fell into disrepute because of the radical antinomian prac-tices of some of its adherents. During the Victorian colonization of India, puritanism drove Tantric practitioners underground. Today Tantra survives mainly in the conservative (*samaya*) molds of the Shrī-Vidyā tradition of South India and the Buddhist tradition of Tibet, though both heritages also have their more radical practitioners who understandably prefer to stay out of the public limelight. Particularly Tibetan Vajrayāna has become increasingly popular in the West, and it is relatively easy to receive initiation and instruction in this form of Tantra.

From the beginning, Tantra understood itself as a "new age" teaching especially tailored for the needs of the *kali-yuga,* the era of spiritual decline that is still in progress today. According to Herbert V. Guenther, a renowned scholar of Buddhism, the *Tantras*—the scrip-tures of Tantrism—"contain a very sound and healthy view of life."[1] His implied point, that the Tantric view is valid and pertinent even today, matches the appraisal of other Western scholars and students of Tantra. Robert Beer, a color-blind British painter of beautiful, richly colored *thankas,* remarked that the psychological core of the numerous Tantric legends "has a universal appeal and application that transcends culture, religion, and race."[2] I would go further and say that many facets of Tantric psychology and practice are relevant to all who seek to cultivate self-understanding and are sincerely engaged in the noble task of spiritual self-transformation.

From the outset, Tantra has straddled both Hinduism and Buddhism, and Tantra-style teachings can be found even in the Indic minority religion of Jainism. Hindu Tantra, which I will somewhat arbitrarily call "Tantra Yoga" to distinguish it from the Buddhist and Jaina varieties, was introduced to the Western world through the writings of Sir John Woodroffe. His English rendering of the famous *Mahānirvāna-Tantra* was published in 1913 and was followed a few years later by his books *Shakti and Shākta* and *The Serpent Power.*[3] At that time it was still considered odious for a scholar to study the Tantric tradition, which was deemed the most decadent manifestation of Hindu culture. Woodroffe, a high-court judge in Calcutta, broke all the rules when he put on Indian garb and sat at the feet of Hindu pundits well versed in Tantra. As he once said:

> I have often been asked why I had undertaken the study of the Tantra Śāstra, and in some English (as opposed to Continental) quarters it has been suggested that my time and labour might be more worthily employed. One answer is this: Following the track of unmeasured abuse I have always found something good. The present case is no exception. I protest and have always protested against unjust aspersions upon the Civilization of India and its peoples. . . . I found that the Śāstra was of high importance in the history of Indian religion. The Tantra Śāstra or Āgama is not, as some seem to suppose, a petty Śāstra of no account; one, and an unimportant sample, of the multitudinous manifestations of religion in a country which swarms with every form of religious sect. It is on the contrary with Veda, Smṛti and Purāna one of the foremost important Śāstras in India, governing, in various degrees and ways, the temple and household ritual of the whole of India today and for centuries past. . . . Over and above the fact that the Śāstra is an historical fact, it possesses, in some respects, an intrinsic value which justifies its study. Thus it is the storehouse of Indian occultism. This occult side of the Tantras is of scientific importance, the more particularly having regard to the present revived interest in occultist study in the West.[4]

These words, written eight decades ago, are relevant today for the same reasons.[5] In the succeeding years a few other Western scholars, for the most part still feeling apologetic about their research, have followed in the footsteps of this intrepid pioneer. Even today, however, Hindu Tantra Yoga is only poorly researched, and most of its high teachings, which require direct experience or at least the explanations of an initiate, remain unlocked.

The situation is strikingly different with the teachings of Buddhist Tantra, in the form of the Tibetan tradition of Vajrayāna (Diamond Vehicle). Ever since the Chinese invasion of Tibet in 1950 and particularly since the escape of His Holiness the Dalai Lama in 1959, Tibetan *lamas* have been generously teaching and initiating Western practitioners into all schools and levels of Vajrayāna Buddhism. To preserve their teachings in exile, many high *lamas* have consented to work closely with Western scholars on accurate translations of the Tibetan *Tantras* and on explanatory monographs. Today, therefore, the Buddhist branch of Tantrism is not only more widely disseminated than the Hindu branch but also better understood in the West than its Hindu counterpart.

The many excellent books on Buddhist Tantra give one a real appreciation of the tremendous sophistication of this tradition.[6] Good works on Hindu Tantra Yoga, however, are few, and the books by Woodroffe, though dated and incorrect in places, are still exemplary in many respects. The Hindus never had the kind of extensive monastic tradition of learning and practice that characterizes the Buddhists, particularly the Tibetan Gelugpa school. It is difficult (though not impossible) to find a Hindu Tantric adept who not only has mastered the practical dimension of Tantra Yoga but also can talk knowledgeably about the theoretical aspects. Western scholars are therefore naturally drawn to the study of Buddhist Tantra. A notable exception was the late Swami Lakshmanjoo (1907–94), an adept and master expounder of the Kaula tradition of Kashmir, who inspired many Western scholars and Hindu pundits.[7] Many of Swami Lakshmanjoo's disciples think of him as the reincarnation of the famous tenth-century adept and scholar Abhinava Gupta.

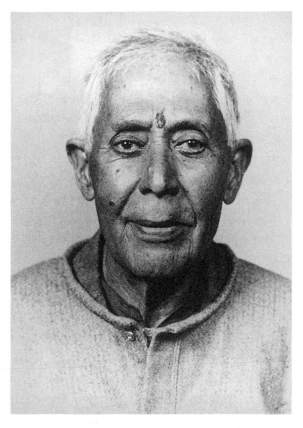

Swami Lakshmanjoo (1907–94), a master of both the theoretical and practical dimensions of Hindu Tantra.
(PHOTOGRAPH BY JOHN HUGHES © COPYRIGHT KASHMIR SHAIVISM FELLOWSHIP)

The paucity of research and publications on the Tantric heritage of Hinduism has in recent years made room for a whole crop of ill-informed popular books on what I have called "Neo-Tantrism."[8] Their reductionism is so extreme that a true initiate would barely recognize the Tantric heritage in these writings. The most common distortion is to present Tantra Yoga as a mere discipline of ritualized or sacred sex. In the popular mind, Tantra has become equivalent to sex. Nothing could be farther from the truth!

I have looked at a number of these popular books on what one well-known Tibetan *lama* once jokingly referred to as "California Tantra." One time I even sat through half of a thoroughly uninspiring and essentially pornographic video presentation on Neo-Tantrism. In each case I was left with the overwhelming impression that these Neo-Tantric publications are based on a profound misunderstanding of the Tantric path. Their main error is to confuse Tantric bliss (*ānanda, mahā-sukha*) with ordinary orgasmic pleasure. Indeed, the words "pleasure" and "fun" are prominent catchphrases in the Neo-Tantric literature. These publications may conceivably be helpful to people looking for a more fulfilling or entertaining sex life, but they are in most cases far removed from the true spirit of Tantra. In this sense they are sadly misleading, for instead of awakening a person's impulse to attain enlightenment for the benefit of all beings, they tend to foster narcissism, self-delusion, and false hopes.

There is a growing need for more faithful portrayals of the philosophy and practice of genuine Hindu Tantra, and the present volume seeks to respond to this need. My presentation is chiefly based on my research into the original scriptures of Hindu Tantra and secondarily on my personal experience with Yoga over a period of thirty-five years. Secondarily, I am basing my presentation on my study and practice of Vajrayāna Buddhism since 1993. My approach is meant to be sympathetic rather than "objective" and detached. In writing about those many areas of which I have no personal experience, I have relied on the testimony of the Tantric scriptures, the available scholarly literature, and the explanations of advanced practitioners.

Although there are many differences between Hindu and Buddhist Tantra, I believe there are also numerous commonalities that help students of one tradition gain understanding of the other. Hence, where necessary or useful, I have freely drawn on my knowledge of Buddhist Tantra to present Hindu Tantra Yoga in a more faithful and interesting way. I have, however, made no attempt in this book to cover Buddhist Tantra or even compare this branch of Tantra with the Hindu variety.

I believe that it is possible to write with adequate fidelity an introductory volume about Tantra without having attained adeptship on the Tantric path. One does not have to be an electronic engineer to accurately describe the parts and functions of a computer to another lay person, providing one has done one's homework. In fact, a lay person may do a much better descriptive job than a professional engineer, who is apt to focus on the arcane details of his or her expertise, or who simply may not be a skillful communicator. When it comes to furnishing accurate instructions for building a computer from scratch, however, much more profound knowledge is required than should be expected from a lay person.

I see my task as being mostly descriptive and occasionally evaluative, but definitely not as being prescriptive. In other words, the present volume is *not* a manual for Tantric practice. The conceptual universe of Tantra is vastly more detailed than can possibly be conveyed in a book such as this, which is intended for the lay reader. I cannot even claim to have covered all the major ideas and practices. For instance, the chapter on subtle anatomy (i.e., the *cakras* and *nādīs*) could easily be expanded into a whole book. Likewise, the section on the serpent power (*kundalinī-shakti*) could just as readily be developed into a hefty volume. Nor have I mentioned all the branches, schools, or approaches of Tantra, partly because many of them are still only poorly understood in themselves and in their relationship to each other and partly because I did not want to burden this introduction with materials more suitable for an academic monograph. Thus I have refrained from going into great detail about Hatha Yoga, which also is a Tantric tradition and which I plan to write about separately. Space constraints also obliged me to confine myself to just a few mythological stories and biographical details about some of the great adepts. I hope that one day, in the not-too-distant future, a comprehensive overview of the philosophy, literature, history, and practice of Tantra will be published, and I am sure this will have to be based on the combined effort of a number of experts on the subject.

In contrast to one widely read book on Neo-Tantrism, I do not claim that this—or indeed any—book on Tantra Yoga, or Yoga in general, could possibly replace the teacher, initiation, and spiritual transmission process. Success on the Tantric path most certainly requires initiation at the hand of a qualified teacher and many years of intensive personal practice. Without guidance, proper initiation, and total commitment, practitioners of Tantra Yoga risk their sanity and health. The numerous warnings in the traditional scriptures are not merely rhetorical, and the dangers they describe are certainly not exaggerated. Tantra Yoga, as not a few scriptures emphasize, is indeed a dangerous path that leads fools into greater bondage and only wise practitioners to freedom and bliss. It is no accident that true Tantric practitioners are called "heroes" (*vīra*), because they must navigate in treacherous waters that demand constant vigilance and great inner strength.

There is no reason why genuine spiritual seekers in the Western hemisphere should not achieve adeptship in Tantra Yoga, and some have in fact done so. But in each case, the fulfillment of the spiritual path is preceded by hard work on oneself. There are no shortcuts, and the quest for quick fixes and weekend enlightenment is merely one of the symptoms of the *kali-yuga*, governed by delusion and greed.

Tantra is a highly complex tradition. Even an introductory book such as the present one will therefore contain much that requires thoughtful reading. This volume is certainly more demanding than its companion, *The Shambhala Guide to Yoga.*[9] For newcomers to Yoga, I recommend reading the latter work first before turning to the more demanding subject of Tantra.

If the present book can help remove the worst popular misconceptions about Tantra Yoga and thus clear the way to fruitful spiritual practice, Tantric or otherwise, it will have fulfilled its purpose.

It remains for me to thank several people who have helped give this book material shape: my publisher Samuel Bercholz and my editor Peter Turner for their vision and commitment to excellence, Larry Hamberlin for his judicious copyediting, Ron Suresha for ably guiding the manuscript through the editorial process, as well as the other helpful spirits at Shambhala Publications for their part in the birthing process; Glen Hayes, Michael Magee, Swami Atmarupananda, and Douglas Renfrew Brooks for readily responding to my questions and requests; David Gordon White and Christopher Chapple for their valuable comments on the manuscript; James Rhea and Margo Gal for allowing me to use some of their drawings; and, last but not least, my wife, Trisha, for applying her keen editorial vision to the manuscript and also for her understanding and continuing support of my work.

Tantra

Tantra, the Great Spiritual Synthesis

The thousands of evils arising from one's
birth can be removed by means of practice.
  —*Matsyendra-Samhitā* (7.20a)

DEFINITIONS

Tantra is a Sanskrit word that, like the term *yoga*, has many distinct but basically related meanings. At the most mundane level, it denotes "web" or "woof." It derives from the verbal root *tan*, meaning "to expand." This root also yields the word *tantu* (thread or cord).[1] Whereas a thread is something that is extensive, a web suggests expansion. *Tantra* can also stand for "system," "ritual," "doctrine," and "compendium." According to esoteric explanations, *tantra* is that which expands *jnāna*, which can mean either "knowledge" or

"wisdom." The late Agehananda Bharati, an Austrian-born professor
of anthropology at Syracuse University and a monk of the Dashanāmi
order, argued that only knowledge can be expanded, not the immuta-
ble wisdom.² But this is not entirely correct. Wisdom, though coes-
sential with Reality and therefore perennial, can be expanded in the
sense of informing the spiritual practitioner more and more. This
process is like placing a sponge in a shallow pool of water. It gradually
soaks up the water and becomes completely suffused with moisture.
Thus while wisdom is always the same, it can also, paradoxically, grow
inside a person. Or, to put it differently, a person can grow to reflect
more and more of the eternal wisdom.

But *tantra* is also the "expansive," all-encompassing Reality revealed by wisdom. As such it stands for "continuum," the seamless
whole that comprises both transcendence and immanence, Reality
and reality, Being and becoming, Consciousness and mental consciousness, Infinity and finitude, Spirit and matter, Transcendence
and immanence, or, in Sanskrit terminology, *nirvāna* and *samsāra*, or
brahman and *jagat*. Here the words *samsāra* and *jagat* stand for the
familiar world of flux that we experience through our senses.

Historically, *tantra* denotes a particular style or genre of spiritual
teachings beginning to achieve prominence in India about fifteen hundred years ago—teachings that affirm the continuity between Spirit
and matter. The word also signifies a scripture in which such teachings are revealed. By extension, the term is often applied to textbooks
or manuals in general. Tradition speaks of 64 *Tantras*, though as with
the 108 *Upanishads* this is an ideal figure that does not reflect historical reality. We know of many more *Tantras*, though few of them have
survived the ravages of time.³

A practitioner of Tantra is called a *sādhaka* (if male) or a *sādhikā*
(if female). Other expressions are *tāntrika* or *tantra-yogin* (if male) and
tantra-yoginī (if female). An adept of the Tantric path is typically
known as a *siddha* ("accomplished one," from *sidh*, meaning "to be
accomplished" or "to attain") or *mahā-siddha* ("greatly accomplished
one," that is, a great adept). The female adept is called *siddha-anganā*
("woman adept," from *anga*, meaning "limb" or "part"). The Tantric

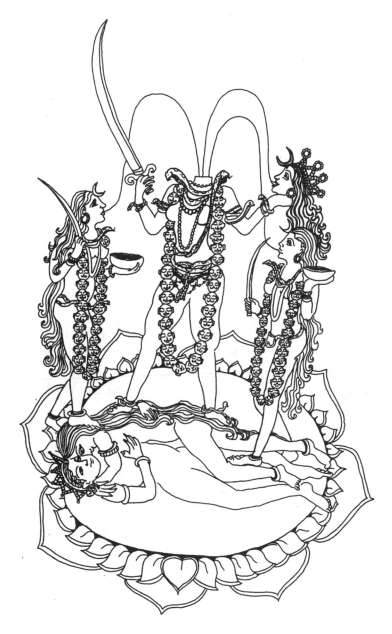

Chinnamastā, whose severed head symbolizes the transcendence of the body through Tantra. (ILLUSTRATION BY MARGO GAL)

path itself is frequently referred to as *sādhana* or *sādhanā* (from the same verbal root as *siddha*), and the spiritual achievement of this path is called *siddhi* (having the dual meaning of "perfection" and "powerful accomplishment"). *Siddhi* can refer either to the spiritual attainment of liberation, or enlightenment, or to the extraordinary powers or paranormal abilities ascribed to Tantric masters as a result of enlightenment or by virtue of mastery of the advanced stages of concentration. A Tantric preceptor, whether he or she is enlightened or not, is called either an *ācārya* ("conductor," which is related to *ācāra*, "way of life") or a *guru* ("weighty one").

TANTRA: *A Teaching for the Dark Age*

Tantra understands itself as a gospel for the "new age" of darkness, the *kali-yuga*. According to the Hindu worldview, history unfolds in a cyclical pattern that proceeds from a golden age to world ages of progressive spiritual decline, and then back to an era of light and plenty. These ages are called *yugas* (yokes), presumably because they fasten beings to the wheel of time (*kāla-cakra*), the flux of conditioned existence. There are four such *yugas*, which repeat themselves over and over again, all the while maturing all beings, but especially human beings. The scriptures speak of this developmental process as "cooking." The four world ages, in order, are:

1. The *satya-yuga*, in which truth (*satya*) reigns supreme, and which is also known as *krita-yuga* because everything in it is well made (*krita*)

2. The *tretā-yuga*, in which truth and virtue are somewhat diminished

3. The *dvāpara-yuga*, in which truth and virtue are further diminished

4. The *kali-yuga*, which is marked by ignorance, delusion, and greed

These correspond to the four ages known in classical Greece and ancient Persia. Significantly, the Sanskrit names of the four world ages derive from dice playing, a favorite pastime of Indic humanity ever since Vedic times. The *Rig-Veda*, which is at least five thousand years old, has a hymn (10.34) that has been dubbed "Gambler's Lament" because its composer talks poetically of his addiction to gambling. Of the dice he says that "handless, they master him who has hands," causing loss, shame, and grief. The Bhārata war, chronicled in the *Mahābhārata* epic, was the ill-gotten fruit of gambling, for Yudhishthira lost his entire kingdom to his wicked cousin Duryodhana with the throw of a die.

Krita signifies the lucky or "well-made" throw, *dvāpara* (deuce) a throw of two points, *tretā* (trey) a throw of three points, and *kali* (from the verbal root *kal*, "to impel") the total loss, indicated by a single point on the die. The word *kali* is not, as is often thought, the same as the name of the well-known goddess Kālī.[4] However, since Kālī symbolizes both time and destruction, it does not seem far-fetched to connect her specifically with the *kali-yuga*, though of course she is deemed to govern all spans and modes of time.

The *Tantras* describe the first, golden age as an era of material and spiritual plenty. According to the *Mahānirvāna-Tantra* (1.20–29), people were wise and virtuous and pleased the deities and forefathers by their practice of Yoga and sacrificial rituals. By means of their study of the *Vedas*, meditation, austerities, mastery of the senses, and charitable deeds, they acquired great fortitude and power. Even though mortal, they were like the deities (*deva*). The rulers were high minded and ever concerned with protecting the people entrusted to them, while among the ordinary people there were no thieves, liars, fools, or gluttons. Nobody was selfish, envious, or lustful. The favorable psychology of the people was reflected outwardly in land producing all kinds of grain in plenty, cows yielding abundant milk, trees laden with fruits, and ample seasonable rains fertilizing all vegetation. There was neither famine nor sickness, nor untimely death. People were good-hearted, happy, beautiful, and prosperous. Society was well ordered and peaceful.

In the next world age, the *tretā-yuga*, people lost their inner peace and became incapable of applying the Vedic rituals properly, yet clung to them anxiously. Out of pity, the god Shiva brought helpful traditions (*smriti*) into the world, by which the ancient teachings could be better understood and practiced.

But humanity was set on a worsening course, which became obvious in the third world age. People abandoned the methods prescribed in the *Smritis,* and thereby only magnified their perplexity and suffering. Their physical and emotional illnesses increased, and as the *Mahānirvāna-Tantra* insists, they lost half of the divinely appointed law (*dharma*). Again Shiva intervened by making the teachings of the *Samhitās* and other religious scriptures available.

With the rise of the fourth world age, the *kali-yuga*, all of the divinely appointed law was lost. Many Hindus believe that the *kali-yuga* was ushered in at the time of the death of the god-man Krishna, who is said to have left this earth in 3102 BCE at the end of the famous Bhārata war. There is no archaeological evidence for this date, and it is probable that Krishna lived much later, but this is relatively unimportant for the present consideration.[5] What matters, however, is that most traditional authorities consider the *kali-yuga* to be still very much in progress.[6] In fact, according to Hindu computations, we are only in the opening phase of this dark world age, which is believed to have a total span of 360,000 years.[7] Thus from a Hindu perspective, the current talk in certain Western circles of a promising new age—the Age of Aquarius—is misguided. At best, this is a mini-cycle of self-deception leading to false optimism and complacency, followed by worsening conditions. This is in fact what some Western critics of the New Age movement have suggested as well. Other critics have argued, conversely, that the Hindu model of cyclical time is unrealistic and outdated.

Whatever the truth of this matter may be, the *Tantras* emphasize that their teachings are designed for spiritual seekers trapped in the dark age, which is in effect today. This is how the *Mahānirvāna-Tantra* (1.36–42), in the prophetic words of the Goddess, describes the current world age:

With the sinful *kali*[-*yuga*] in progress, in which all law is destroyed and which abounds with evil ways and evil phenomena, and gives rise to evil activities,

then the *Vedas* become inefficient, to say nothing of remembering the *Smritis*. And the many *Purānas* containing various stories and showing the many ways [to liberation]

will be destroyed, O Lord. Then people will turn away from virtuous action

and become habitually unrestrained, mad with pride, fond of evil deeds, lustful, confused, cruel, rude, scurrilous, deceitful,

short-lived, dull-witted, troubled by sickness and grief, ugly, weak, vile, attached to vile behavior,

fond of vile company, and stealers of other's money. They become rogues who are intent on blaming, slandering, and injuring others

and who feel no reluctance, sin, or fear in seducing the wife of another. They become destitute, filthy, wretched beggars who are sick from their vagrancy.

The *Mahānirvāna-Tantra* continues its description of the dreariness of the *kali-yuga* by saying that even the brahmins become degenerate and perform their religious practices mainly to dupe the people. Thus the custodians of the law (*dharma*) merely contribute to the destruction of the sacred tradition and the moral order. The *Tantra* next reiterates that Shiva revealed the Tantric teachings to stem the tide of history and correct this tragic situation. The masters of Tantra are profoundly optimistic.

THE RADICAL APPROACH OF TANTRA

The adepts of Tantra believe that it is possible to attain liberation, or enlightenment, even in the worst social and moral conditions. They also believe, however, that the traditional means devised or revealed in previous world ages are no longer useful or optimal, for

those means were designed for people of far greater spiritual and
moral stamina who lived in a more peaceful environment conducive
to inner growth. The present age of darkness has innumerable obstacles that make spiritual maturation exceedingly difficult. Therefore
more drastic measures are needed: the Tantric methodology.

What is so special about the Tantric teachings that they should
serve the spiritual needs of the dark age better than all other approaches? In many ways, the Tantric methods are similar to non-
Tantric practices. What is strikingly different about them is their inclusiveness and the radical attitude with which they are pursued. A
desperate person will grasp for a straw, and seekers in the *kali-yuga*
are, or should be, desperate. From the vantage point of a spiritual
heritage extending over several thousand years, the Tantric masters at
the beginning of the common era realized that the dark age calls for
especially powerful techniques to break through lethargy, resistance,
and attachment to conventional relationships and worldly things, as
well as to deal with the lack of understanding. Looking at the available
means handed down from teacher to student through countless generations, they acknowledged that these required a purity and nobility
of character that people of the dark age no longer possess. To help
humanity in the *kali-yuga*, the Tantric adepts modified the old teachings and created a new repertoire of practices. Their orientation can
be summed up in two words: Anything goes. Or, at least, almost
anything.

The Tantric masters even sanctioned practices that are considered sinful from within a conventional moral and spiritual framework.
This feature of Tantra has been termed antinomianism, which, as
this Greek-derived word implies, consists in going against (*anti*) the
accepted norm or law (*nomos*). The Tantric texts use words like *pratilo-
man* (against the grain) and *parāvritti* (inversion) to describe their
teachings. Some Tantric adepts have made a way of life out of this
principle of reversal, as can be seen in the extremist lifestyle of the
avadhūtas, who walk about naked and live amid heaps of garbage. They
model themselves after the god-man Dattātreya, who supposedly lived
in the *tretā-yuga*. In the Puranic literature he is celebrated as an incar-

nation of the *tri-mūrti* (the Trinity of Hinduism), namely, the deities Brahma (the Creator), Vishnu (the Preserver), and Shiva (the Destroyer).

Such initiates can still be found today, and the twentieth-century adept Rang Avadhoot (Ranga Avadhūta) of Nareshvar in Gujarat was venerated as a form of Dattātreya. This *avadhūta* was a college graduate who translated Tolstoy's works and composed his own books in Sanskrit, yet he lived in utter simplicity and quite unattached to any formal religion. The members of the Aghorī sect are still more extreme in their unconventionality and can be seen near cremation grounds, where, clothed only in the ashes from the funeral pyres, they pursue their solitary meditations.

Tantric antinomianism can be seen at work especially in the notorious left-hand schools of Tantra. Their members avail themselves of "unlawful" practices such as ritualized sexual intercourse (*maithunā*) with a person other than one's marital partner and the consumption of aphrodisiacs, alcohol, and meat (a taboo food in traditional India's vegetarian culture), as well as frequenting burial grounds for necromantic rituals. I will say more about this "left-hand" side of Tantra in chapter 14.

Understandably, the religious orthodoxy of the brahmins has always looked at Tantra and Tantric practitioners with dismay or even disdain. But Hindu society, which is apparently the oldest continuous pluralistic society on earth, has something of a built-in tolerance, which over the millennia has allowed all kinds of religious and spiritual traditions to flourish side by side. Another factor that facilitated the widespread acceptance of Tantra in the span of a few generations was the reputation of Tantric initiates as powerful magicians, be it of the white or the black variety. People feared the curses and spells of *tāntrikas* and did not want to be seen condemning or denigrating them, even if they thought the Tantric views and practices were in error. Even today, the rural population of India both venerates and fears ascetics, particularly those manifesting a Tantric demeanor. *Yogins* and *yoginīs* have always been looked upon as wielders of numinous power. In the case of Tantric initiates, this power is felt to be espe-

cially great because of their often close association with the shadow
side of life, notably the realm of the dead.

At one end of the Tantric spectrum we have highly unorthodox
practices such as black magic that go against the moral grain of Hindu
society (and that of most societies). At the other end we have Tantric
masters who decry all doctrines and all rituals and instead applaud
the ideal of perfect spontaneity (*sahaja*). Most schools fall between
these two poles; they are typically highly ritualistic but infused with
the recognition that liberation springs from wisdom, which is innate
and therefore cannot be produced by any external means. All the
many Tantric techniques merely serve to cleanse the mirror of the
mind so as to faithfully reflect the ever-present Reality, allowing the
native wisdom to shine forth without distortion.

THE HISTORICAL ROOTS OF TANTRA

Tantra, though highly innovative, has from the beginning deemed
itself a continuation of earlier teachings. Thus while Buddhist Tantra
understands itself as an esoteric tradition going back to Gautama the
Buddha himself, Hindu Tantra by and large regards the revelatory
teachings of the *Vedas* as its starting point. Some authorities have associated it particularly with the *Atharva-Veda*, no doubt because of that
Vedic hymnody's magical content with the marginal status it has
within more strictly orthodox Hindu circles. Then again, the *Tantras*
are sometimes referred to as the "fifth *Veda*."

The Tantric claim to a Vedic origin is controversial and disputed
by orthodox brahmins.[8] They not only deny the Vedic origin of Tantra
but consider the Tantric teachings to be corrupt, if not altogether
heretical. Their evaluation lags behind actual social reality, however,
for Tantra has been an integral part of Hindu culture since at least
the turn of the second millennium CE. To be able to understand
Hindu Tantra, we must first understand Hinduism and the Vedic heritage, just as a proper understanding of Buddhist Tantrism (Vajrayāna)
presupposes an understanding of at least Mahāyāna Buddhism.

The *Vedas*, originally a purely oral literature, form the sacred bedrock of Hinduism, and they may well be the oldest literary compositions in any language. In the nineteenth century, Western scholars arbitrarily fixed their date at around 1200–1500 BCE, whereas for India's pundits they are timeless revelation. Recent geological evidence of a great cataclysm that overtook North India around 1900 BCE has forced scholars to reexamine the facts.[9] In this cataclysm, a major tectonic shift followed by far-reaching climatic changes, the Sarasvatī River was reduced to a mere trickle. Because this river is hailed in the *Rig-Veda* as the mightiest of all rivers, this particular hymnody at least must have been composed prior to 1900 BCE, and probably long before then. A growing number of experts now favor the third and even the fourth millennium BCE for the time of the original composition of the bulk of the Rig-Vedic hymns. The other three Vedic collections—the *Yajur-Veda*, the *Sāma-Veda*, and the *Atharva-Veda*—very probably also belong to the precataclysm era. Also some of the *Brāhmanas*—explanatory ritual texts—may have been composed in the third millennium.

The revised date for the *Vedas* makes the Vedic civilization contemporaneous with the so-called Indus civilization, which flourished between c. 3000 BCE and 1700 BCE in what is now Pakistan, in the western portion of Northern India. The parallels between the two civilizations are so striking, in fact, that we must assume they are not separate civilizations but one and the same. This means that, in addition to the testimonial of the Vedic scriptures, we also have archaeological artifacts that can help us better understand this ancient civilization. The stereovision we obtain from the joint images of literary and archaeological evidence is exciting, for the Vedic civilization appears to have been governed by profound spiritual insights and values. It now appears that India is not only the oldest continuous civilization on earth (going back to the seventh millennium BCE) but also the one that harbors the most enduring spiritual heritage. As anyone who has studied the wisdom traditions of India without prejudice will have discovered, the Indic heritage is a gold mine with

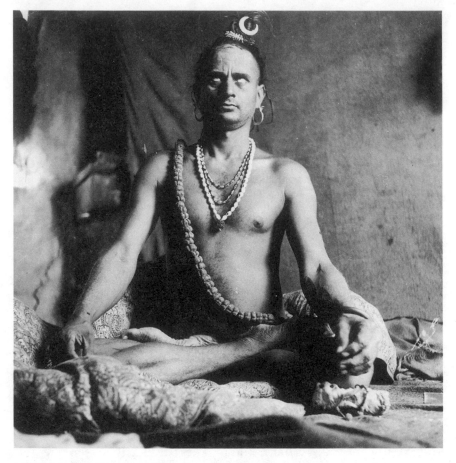

A Tantric adept. (PHOTOGRAPH BY RICHARD LANNOY)

countless boulder-size nuggets. And the Tantric nugget is one of the largest.

Except for the most orthodox pundits, who view Tantra as an abomination, educated traditional Hindus have long looked upon Tantra as running parallel and in close interaction with (rather than merely in opposition to) the Vedic heritage. They distinguish between Vedic and Tantric—*vaidika* and *tāntrika*—currents of Hindu spirituality. This distinction demonstrates the huge success of Tantra as a tradition or cultural movement within Hinduism. In many instances, Tantra has been so influential as to reshape the Vedic stream by infusing it with typically Tantric practices and ideas. For example, the type of ritual called *pūjā* (worship), which involves iconic representations of deities and their employment in ritual worship, has been characterized as Tantric rather than Vedic in nature. Yet brahmins throughout India employ it either in addition to, or instead of, more typically Vedic forms of ritual. To most of these brahmins it would not even occur to them that they are engaging in a practice that may well have originated in Tantric circles.

Many *tāntrikas* themselves regard the *Vedas* as an earlier revelation that, as has already been indicated, has lost efficacy in the present *kali-yuga*. Thus we can read in the *Mahānirvāna-Tantra* (2.14–15):

> In the *kali-yuga*, the *mantras* revealed in the *Tantras* are efficient, yield immediate fruit, and are recommended for all practices, such as recitation, sacrifice, rituals, and so on.

> The Vedic practices are powerless as a snake lacking poison fangs or like a corpse, though in the beginning, in the *satya-yuga*, they were bearing fruit.

We can appreciate the gravity of this pronouncement only when we know that the Vedic heritage is deemed to be a revelation of the Divine. It borders on heresy to say that it is no longer useful. The author of the *Mahānirvāna-Tantra* gets around this difficulty by presenting his own tradition as the direct utterances of the Divine as well. He can make this claim because the Indic civilization has always accepted the possibility of profound knowledge and wisdom arising from higher states of meditation and ecstasy. To attribute teachings to the Divine or a particular deity is both a convenient didactic device and an acknowledgment that the teachings are not merely products of the intellect or the imagination; rather, they are based on the sages' direct realizations of the subtle dimensions and the ultimate Reality. This is what is meant when the *Vedas* are said to be "superhuman" (*atimānusha*).

In any case, the *Mahānirvāna-Tantra* does not reject the Vedic revelation in its entirety but uses it as the foundation for its own, novel brand of esotericism. It is not that the Vedic repertoire of psychospiritual practices is considered worthless in itself, only that people of the *kali-yuga* are incapable of employing them successfully. In the *Kula-Arnava-Tantra* (2.10) Shiva even declares that he extracted its teachings by churning the "ocean of the *Vedas* and *Āgamas* with the staff of wisdom." This is a clear vote of confidence in the Vedic revelation. Yet in the same *Tantra* (2.68) we find this stanza (uttered by Shiva):

> O Beloved, those who are proficient in the four *Vedas* but ignorant of the *kula* are "dog cookers." However, even a low-caste dog cooker who knows the *kula* is superior to a brahmin.

Here the word *kula*, as I will explain in detail later, denotes essential Tantric wisdom, which is the wisdom of divine power (*shakti*). The above stanza contains a concealed criticism of the priestly establishment, which is thought to favor intellectual learning over actual spiritual experience. By contrast, the Tantric practitioners are first and foremost practical theologians. Their sole purpose is to gain mastery over the subtle realms and, finally, to realize the transcendental Reality itself. It is by virtue of their powerful spiritual practice that, as the Tantric authorities affirm, they outrank the brahmins, the hereditary custodians of the Vedic revelation who form the highest social class of Hindu society.

Is there any evidence, as some pundits have claimed, of Tantric ideas and practices in the *Vedas*? According to the pundit Manoranjan Basu, the *Tantras* "are the most ancient scriptures contemporaneous with the *Vedas* if not earlier."[10] Since the *Vedas* have recently been redated to the third and even fourth millennium BCE, this would make the *Tantras* at least five or six thousand years old. This agrees with some Tibetan Buddhist *lamas*, who believe that Tantra (in its Buddhist variety) was first taught thousands of years prior to Gautama the Buddha. They ascribe the original Tantric teachings to another awakened being, the Buddha Tenpa Shenrab, founder of the Tibetan Bon tradition.[11] According to the *Nārāyanīya-Tantra*, a late Hindu work, the *Vedas* originated from the *Tantras*, rather than the reverse. The typical Tantric view, however, is that the *Tantras* are a new revelation replacing that of the *Vedas*. Likewise, most scholars reject the notion that Tantra originated in the era of the *Vedas* or earlier.

What we may safely say is that there is an undeniable continuity between the Vedic revelation and the Tantric revelation. Many important Tantric practices have their Vedic equivalent. Thus, scholars have pointed to the magical ideas and practices of the *Atharva-Veda*, which is especially associated with the very old priestly family of the Angirases, chief custodians of ancient magical lore. Researchers also have seen Tantric overtones in the Vedic gods Shiva and Rudra and the Vedic goddesses Nirriti and Yamī. Furthermore, the Vedic seers used *mantras*, sacrificial formulas, animal sacrifices, magical diagrams (*yantra*), and visualization in their rituals, as do the Tantric initiates. It is generally thought that the Vedic people did not practice worship with the aid of statues and that this was the unique contribution of Tantra. However, the *Rig-Veda* (1.21.2) has the intriguing line "men adorn Indra and Agni" (*indra-agnī shumbhatā narah*), which could be a reference to the practice of *pūjā*. Also, like the *tāntrikas*, the Vedic seers were eager to acquire knowledge about the hidden realms and realities, and not merely the ultimate liberating gnosis. As the eleventh-century *Siddha-Siddhānta-Paddhati* (2.31) states, a *yogin* is someone who truly knows the psychospiritual centers (*cakra*) of the body, the five kinds of inner space, and so on.

There is even a possibility that the Tantric notion of *kundalinī*, the multiply coiled spiritual energy, is present in Vedic times. In one hymn of the *Rig-Veda* (10.136.7) the expression *kunamnamā* is found, which means "she who is badly bent." Some scholars have regarded this as a hidden reference to the *kundalinī-shakti* or serpent power, also called *kubjikā* (crooked one) in some early Tantric schools.

To return to our historical overview: as the ancient Vedic ritualism became more and more complex, the surrounding explanations also became increasingly sophisticated. Before long the brahmins felt the need for interpretive scriptures. These are known as the *Brāhmanas*, the earliest of which were created in the time just before the cataclysm mentioned above. As their name suggests, these works are intended for the brahmins (or *brāhmanas*) and their students, who needed to learn not only how to perform the Vedic rituals but also the cosmology and theology behind them.

If we look for Tantric elements in the *Brāhmanas,* we can readily find them in the idea that sexual union is a form of sacrifice, a notion that builds a bridge to the Tantric *maithunā.* Sexual symbolism is pervasive in the *Brāhmanas,* but can already be amply found in the *Vedas.* Moreover, *bīja-mantras* (seed *mantras*) first appear in the *Brāhmanas,* where they are associated with specific deities. For instance, in the *Shata-Patha-Brāhmana* the *mantra* of the solar deity, Sūrya, is given as *om ghrini sūryāya namah,* or "*Om. Ghrini.* Salutation to Sūrya." The *bīja-mantra "ghrini"* is explained onomatopoeically in the following legend: Once upon a time, Vishnu was resting his head on the end of a bow. Ants ate through the bow string; it snapped and severed Vishnu's head from his body. The head fell, making the sound *ghrin,* and thereupon became transformed into the sun. (I will say more about *bīja-mantras* in chapter 12.) Another idea that bespeaks the continuity between the Vedic and the Tantric heritage is the notion, first expressed in the *Aitareya-Brāhmana,* that during ritual sacrifice all participants are elevated to the status of a brahmin. Some *Tantras* went further, though, by rejecting caste differences outside the ritual context as well. This is, in fact, one of the hallmarks of the Tantric tradition.

Chronologically, the *Brāhmanas* were followed by the *Āranyakas* (scriptures for forest hermits) and the *Upanishads* (gnostic treatises for mystics). The last-mentioned texts afford further comparisons with Tantra. The early *Upanishads* present the concepts of subtle currents of life energy (*prāna* or *vāyu*), psychospiritual vortices (*cakra*), and channels (*nādī*) so typical of the Tantric teachings. These ideas, however, were not altogether new, because already the *Atharva-Veda* mentions the various currents of the life force (15.15.2–9) and the eight "wheels" (*cakra*) of the stronghold (i.e., the body) of the deities (10.2.31).

The early *Upanishads* also continued the sexological considerations of an earlier era. Thus the *Chāndogya-Upanishad* (2.1.13.1–2), through magical analogy, equates the various parts of the Vedic chant (*sāman*) to the various phases of sexual intercourse, which invites comparison with the *maithunā* ritual of the left-hand and Kaula schools of Tantrism. The text even employs the word *mithuna* (intercourse). Also, the phrase *vāma-devya* in this passage, which refers to a particular kind of chant, reminds one of the Tantric expression *vāma*, standing for both "woman" and "left hand."

The *Brihad-Āranyaka-Upanishad* (6.4.3) compares the various female parts to religious objects:

> Her genitals are the sacrificial altar, her hairs the grass offering, her skin the *soma* press, and her two labia the fire in the center. Verily, as great as the world is for him who sacrifices with the *vājapeya* [strength libation] sacrifice, so great is the world for him who, knowing this, practices sexual intercourse. He diverts the good deeds of women to himself. But he who practices sexual intercourse without knowing this—women divert his good deeds to themselves.

The *Brihad-Āranyaka-Upanishad* goes on to say that as soon as the man enters the woman, he should press his mouth on hers, stroke her genitals, and mutter the following incantation:

> You who have arisen from every limb and have been generated from the heart are the essence of the limbs! Distract this woman here in me as if pierced by a poisoned arrow!

This ancient *Upanishad* also describes what ritual steps are to be taken when the man's semen is spilled: "He should take it with ring finger and thumb and rub it on his chest [i.e., the location of the heart *cakra*] or between his eyebrows [i.e., the location of the so-called third eye]." This prescription, by which the man can reclaim his vigor, could come straight out of the Tantric literature. Not surprisingly, one of the more orthodox translators of the *Brihad-Āranyaka-Upanishad* omitted this passage altogether![12]

Despite the similarities between the Vedic and the Tantric heritages, however, Tantra is a distinct tradition, meandering down India's history as a mighty companion to the Vedic stream of spirituality and culture. The interplay between both traditions has been extremely complex and continues to this day, yet the adherents of the Vedic

heritage by and large have looked upon Tantra as a false gospel. They
have often branded Tantric teachings as *nāstika*—from *na*, "not," *asti*,
"it is," and the suffix *ka*, meaning "unorthodox" in the sense of not
affirming the truth of the *Vedas*. As we have seen, the situation is
not so simple, and particularly some later *Tantras* deliberately seek to
construct a bridge to the Vedic heritage of the brahmins.

TANTRA YOGA

Tantra is a profoundly yogic tradition, and the *Tantras* call themselves *sādhanā-shāstras*, or books of spiritual practice. The Sanskrit
word *yoga* means both "discipline" and "union" and can be translated
as "unitive discipline." It stands for what in the West is called spirituality or mysticism. The oft-used compound *tantra-yoga* means simply
"Tantric discipline" and captures the intensely experiential character
of the Tantric heritage, which emphasizes the realization of higher or
subtle states of existence right up to the ultimate Reality itself. Tantra
Yoga is unitive discipline based on the expansion, or intensification,
of wisdom by means of the beliefs and practices promulgated in the
Tantras and the exegetical literature that has crystallized around them.
By "unifying" the mind—that is, by focusing it—Tantra Yoga unifies
the seemingly disparate realities of space-time and the transcendental
Reality. It recaptures the primordial continuum that is apparently lost
in the process of becoming an individuated being.

Tantra Yoga, as understood here, is a relative latecomer in the
long history of Yoga. As we have seen, however, proto-Tantric elements can be detected even in the Vedic era. To be sure, the taproots
of Yoga are to be found in the *Vedas*, composed some five thousand
years ago. In its most archaic form, Yoga was a combination of ritual
worship and meditation, having the purpose of opening the gates to
the celestial realms and beyond. It was closely associated with the
Vedic sacrificial cult, priestly hymn making, the mystery of the sacred
ecstasy-inducing *soma* potion, and visions of the subtle dimensions

with their hierarchy of male and female deities, as well as ancestral and other spirits.

The typical Vedic *yogin* was the *rishi* or "seer," who envisioned or perceived the reality or realities given voice in the sacred words (*mantra*) of the hymns. Crafting the Vedic hymns was a fine yogic art demanding not only extraordinary linguistic skills but also tremendous concentration in their composition and delivery. Here we have the very beginnings both of *mantra-yoga* and meditative visualization, which are fundamental to Tantrism.

The Tantric *esprit* continued to evolve through the period of the *Brāhmanas* and *Upanishads*, as well as the intellectually and spiritually fertile era of the *Mahābhārata*, until it reached its typical form in the *Tantras* of the early centuries of the common era. In the subsequent centuries, Tantric schools proliferated and created a massive literature in Sanskrit and various vernacular languages, which is still scarcely researched. Much of this corpus has been lost and is only known to us from stray quotes and references in the extant manuscripts.

Whatever *Tantra* you may read, you will always discover an emphasis on personal experimentation and experience. Westerners thirsting for a direct encounter with the spiritual dimension of existence relate to such an orientation easily enough. But they may not understand quite so readily the theoretical and practical framework within which the Tantric adepts have pursued their supreme goal of Self-realization, or enlightenment. There are many things in Tantra, however, that will be familiar to students of Yoga. From the larger perspective of the history of India's spirituality, Tantra Yoga is simply another form of Yoga, or spiritual discipline. Yet it also represents a vast synthesis of spiritual knowledge and psychotechnology. Because of its integrative approach, Tantra holds special appeal for modern Western seekers, who have come to appreciate the value of holistic thinking.

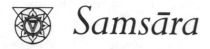 Samsāra

Cyclic Existence

O Arjuna! The Lord abides in the heart region
of all beings, whirling all beings by
his power (*māyā*), [as if they were] mounted on
a machine (*yantra*).
—*Bhagavad-Gītā* (18.61)

Understanding the World We Live In

When we speak of the world, we generally mean all the many
things that make up the stuff of human experience, specifically the
environment and the activities of our earth and our busy species. By
contrast, the cognate words *universe* and *cosmos* have a far more abstract, impersonal ring to them. Few people know that the word *world*
derives from the Old Norse word *verold*, meaning literally "man age"

(*ver* being related to Latin *vir*, meaning "man"), or human era. Thus in its original sense, *world* denotes "world age," that is, a particular phase or cycle within the unfolding story of the cosmos as it relates to humankind. To the ancients, it would have made no sense to contemplate the world apart from its relevance to human existence. "The world" meant "the world as humanity's dwelling place."

The traditional idea of world ages served the ancients as a convenient device for understanding large cultural contexts from a spiritual perspective. As I explained in the introduction, the Indic view is that we live in the midst of the *kali-yuga*, a world age characterized by spiritual and moral decline. This is bad news only in the short run. Taking a telescopic view of history, the traditional cosmologists of India did not succumb to pessimism. For, at the end of a dark age, they envisioned the birth of a new golden age. They saw this cyclic succession of world ages (*yuga*) as an integral aspect of time-bound existence in which humans and other beings are given the opportunity to ripen morally and spiritually in repeated incarnations.

The Sanskrit language has a number of words that denote "world," but none captures this endless recycling of human experience through the mechanism of time more strikingly than the term *samsāra*.[1] It means literally "that which flows together" (from the prefix *sam*, corresponding to the Greek *syn*, and the verbal root *sri*, "to flow"), signifying the perpetual flux of existence that brings subjects and objects together in fateful combinations. Sometimes the Sanskrit term is expanded into compounds like *samsāra-mandala* (round of cyclic existence), *samsāra-cakra* (wheel of cyclic existence), *samsāra-sāgara* (ocean of cyclic existence), or *samsāra-vriksha* (tree of cyclic existence). *Samsāra* is often somewhat flatly rendered as "conditioned existence" or "mundane existence." These two English equivalents fail to convey the rhythmic or cyclic nature of our individual worldly lives, which ride on the current of time, now submerging into the invisible, "subtle" realms, now reemerging into material visibility.

Samsāra is the round of birth, life, death, rebirth, renewed life, and then again death, ad infinitum. It is existence determined by fate (*daiva*), the intricate and inviolable web of karmic indebtedness that

exists between beings. *Samsāra* is *karma*. This means, as the contemporary Tantric adept Vimalananda pointed out, that it is mostly memory.[2] Cyclic or conditioned existence is governed by all kinds of laws
(which are the frozen memories of nature), the most important of
which is the law of cause and effect. Newton captured its physical
aspect in his formulation that every action has an equal but opposite
reaction. India's sages assure us that this law applies with equal force
in the realm of the mind to our thoughts and volitions. Because science looks only at the material realm, it fails to appreciate the comprehensive nature of causation and therefore also allows for
meaningless chance events. From a deeper, spiritual perspective, however, all events are governed by causation. Existence is an infinitely
complex network of conditions giving rise to other conditions. This
is what *karma* signifies.

Samsāra, as the British mathematician and philosopher Alfred
North Whitehead would say, is "process." And what is being pro-
cessed is the human psyche (*jīva*), which must undergo repeated
world experience in order to realize its true destiny beyond all manifestation, consisting in the realization of Being-Consciousness, or
Spirit. The world is a school, which is an idea given expression in
non-Indic spiritual traditions as well. If human life can be said to
have an overarching purpose at all, it is to graduate through the awakening of wisdom (*vidyā, jnāna*).

From yet another angle, *samsāra* is *māyā*. That is to say, it is a
finely woven mesh of illusions, rooted in our fundamental misappre-
hension of ourselves and the world. The misconception about ourselves consists in looking upon ourselves as ego-personalities rather
than the indivisible pure Being-Consciousness. The misconception
about the world consists in looking upon it as an external reality
rather than as being identical with our own nature. This root error
(*avidyā*), which is a matter of spiritual blindness, is what keeps the
karmic nexus going. It is at the bottom of our limited and limiting
experience of space and time and is the primary cause of our experience of suffering (*duhkha*) as seemingly individuated beings.

The Hindu texts describe in graphic terms the nature of cyclic existence. Thus the *Mahābhārata* (11.5), one of India's two great na-tional epics, contains a noteworthy passage that for easy comprehen-sion I will paraphrase rather than translate literally.

Once a brahmin went astray in a lush jungle abounding in dan-gerous animals and plants, which would have terrified even Yama, the Lord of Death. Little wonder that the poor brahmin was seized with panic. However much he tried to hew himself a path out of the thicket, he only succeeded in going deeper and deeper into it. Look-ing up, he realized that the jungle was covered with an impenetrable net, beyond which he glimpsed a giant female with outstretched arms. Five-headed serpent monsters loomed in the sky.

Then the terrified brahmin fell into a pit that had been con-cealed with brushwood. Hanging upside down with his legs entangled in the shrubbery, he saw a gigantic serpent at the bottom of the pit and a huge elephant with six heads and twelve legs near the opening. Enormous bees swarmed around him, and the honey that trickled from their honeycombs dripped into the brahmin's mouth, increasing his thirst by the minute.

Black-and-white rats were gnawing at the tree near the edge of the pit, and it was clear to him that before long it would topple and crush him under its weight. Almost out of his mind with fear, and without any hope of rescue, he nevertheless still desperately clung to life.

This nightmarish picture is a portrayal of the world in its whole absurdity and insidiousness. The jungle of course represents life, and the ferocious beasts are symbols of the diseases and misfortunes that can befall us. The giant female stands for the transiency of life. The pit is the human body. The serpent in the pit represents time. The brushwood in which the brahmin becomes entangled is our greed for existence. The elephant symbolizes the year, his six heads and twelve legs depicting the six Indic seasons and twelve months respectively. The rats gnawing at the tree of life are the days and nights, messengers of death. The bees are our desires, and the honey drops symbolize the transient pleasure that can be derived from their fulfillment.

The kind of thinking expressed in the above passage is not

unique to the *Mahābhārata* or its era. It also offers a key to understanding the *Tantras*, which were composed many hundreds of years
later. For instance, in the *Kula-Arnava-Tantra* (1.61–63), Shiva declares:

> *Samsāra* is the root of suffering. He who exists [in this world]
> is [subject to] suffering. But, O Beloved, he who practices re-
> nunciation (*tyāga*), and none other, is happy.

> O Beloved, one should abandon *samsāra*, which is the birth-
> place of all suffering, the ground of all adversity, and the abode
> of all evil.

> O Goddess, the mind that is attached to *samsāra* is bound
> without binds, cut without weapons, and exposed to a terrifying
> potent poison.

> Because suffering is thus everywhere at the beginning, the
> middle, and the end, one should abandon *samsāra*, abide in Real-
> ity, and thus become happy.

To be trapped in *samsāra* means to be doomed endlessly to repeat
oneself, that is, one's karmic patterns. Those sensitive to this fact have
always sought to escape *samsāra* by burning the karmic seeds of future
rebirths into the conditioned realms of existence. This is also the view
of the masters of Tantra. As I will show, however, their transcendence
of time does not take the form of mere escape from the round of
spatiotemporal existence but of actual mastery of space and time.
Propelled by the karmic forces set in motion by his or her own past
actions or volitions, the individual who is bound to the realm of cyclic
existence is called *samsārin*. The most common translation of this
Sanskrit term is "worldling"; another rendering is "migrator." By
contrast, the person who has succeeded in escaping *karma* and the
flux of time through the power of liberating awareness is known,
among other things, as a *mahā-siddha*, or "great adept" who has transcended or "cheated" time.[3] It is to such a one that *samsāra* reveals
its hidden, divine nature.

THE ARCHITECTURE OF THE WORLD

Similar to other traditional cosmologies, Hinduism conceives of *samsāra* as a vast, hierarchically organized field of experience, comprising many levels or mansions of existence, each containing countless beings of all kinds. The visible material world is thought to be only one of fourteen levels of manifestation extending above and below the earth. Both the realms above the earth and those stretching out below it, though invisible to the ordinary eye, can be seen by those gifted with clairvoyance (*dūra-darshana*, or "remote viewing"). As some Hindu texts insist, and as shamans around the world assert as well, it is even possible to visit these other realms in the subtle body. In fact, we can understand such paranormal abilities as the principal source of knowledge upon which traditional cosmologies are built.

Many Western interpreters, however, prefer to regard these cosmologies as mere products of the imagination. The many variations found in the traditional descriptions of the higher and lower realms are generally taken as proof of their origin in pure fantasy, yet we know that a description is only as good as a person's power of observation and linguistic facility. A dozen people witnessing the same event very likely will yield a dozen different descriptions of it, as in the well-known story of the blind men and the elephant.

When we examine the cosmologies of the various spiritual traditions, however, we find a remarkable overlap. We can either explain this as being due to a borrowing of ideas from one tradition by another, or, more reasonably, see this as evidence that actual observation-based knowledge was involved in their creation. This is not to say that creative imagination does not come into play in the traditional descriptions of the world, just as it is an ingredient of modern cosmology and indeed any branch of knowledge.

Why is it important to speak of cosmology in connection with Tantra? The Tantric goal, like the goal of all spiritual traditions, is to transcend the experienced world, which is both external and internal.

But to be able to transcend the world, we first need to know the territory.

The scriptures of Tantra by and large subscribe to the same cosmography that can also be found in the *Purānas*. The *Purānas*, as the name suggests, are "ancient" lore, combining myth with history (especially dynastic history), religion with folklore, and metaphysics with practical moral instruction. They are encyclopedic in style and purport to describe the unfolding of life from the beginning of time to the time of their own era. The *Purānas* belong to a stream of knowledge that runs parallel to the Vedic revelation. Originally, they gathered all the knowledge that was not deposited in the *Vedas*, the *Brāhmanas*, the *Āranyakas*, and the *Upanishads*, as well as the extensive exegetical literature based on these revealed scriptures. Later, as the Vedic revelation became more and more preempted by the brahmins, the spiritual authorities and creative minds outside the orthodox core produced their own literatures—the *Purānas*, *Āgamas*, *Samhitās*, and *Tantras*.[4] These alternative literatures, considered sacred by their respective communities, share many teachings, ideas, and linguistic expressions with the Vedic corpus while in many ways representing a distinct orientation and style. In traditional terms, they all belong to the *kali-yuga*. There are also numerous commonalities between these various literatures themselves, cosmography being one of them.

According to the Puranic-Tantric picture of the world, our earth is at the center of a vast multidimensional and multilayered universe, which is known as the "brahmic egg" (*brahma-anda*, written *brahmānda*).[5] Tradition speaks of countless such universe-islands floating in the infinite cosmic ocean. The observable material earth is merely the coarsest and least spectacular aspect of the universe. The universe reveals its true splendor only to trained meditative vision. As the *Purānas* and *Tantras* describe it, the earth is really part of a vast circular plane called *bhū-mandala* (earth round), with a diameter of 500 million *yojanas* (c. 4 billion miles).[6] This curiously corresponds with the size of our solar system if we consider Pluto's mean distance from the sun, which is approximately 3.6 billion miles.[7]

The *bhū-mandala* comprises seven concentric rings of land, or continents, which are separated from each other by equally concentric great oceans. The innermost island, or continent, is known as *jambū-dvīpa*, or "Jambū island," which has a diameter of 100,000 *yojanas* (c. 800,000 miles). It is named after the Jambū tree that grows on top of Mount Meru, or Sumeru, which is situated as the center of the continent and thus at the heart of the entire *bhū-mandala*. Mount Meru, the cosmic mountain made of solid gold, is said to be 84,000 *yojanas* (c. 672,000 miles) high. It is sometimes described as a cone that widens with increasing height. The Vedic seers and the visionaries of other traditions and cultures speak of this as the tree of life. The Jambū island is subdivided into nine regions (*varsha*), eight of which are semiheavenly realms, while the ninth is the heartland of *bhārata-varsha*. This term is generally applied to India, but originally may have referred to the entire earth. However, because scriptures like the *Bhāgavata-Purāna* give *bhārata-varsha's* north-south axis as being 9,000 *yojanas* (c. 72,000 miles), it is clear that the earth envisioned by the ancient authorities was considerably bigger than the earth that is perceptible by the five senses.

Below the enormous higher-dimensional earth plane are the seven successive planes of the underworld, each of which is inhabited by various kinds of beings. Starting at the bottom, they are respectively known as *pātāla*,[8] *rasatala*, *mahātala*, *talātala*, *sutala*, *vitala*, and *atala* (the word *tala* meaning simply "plane" or "level"). Sometimes various hells (*naraka*) are said to be situated between the earth plane and *pātāla*.

Above the earth plane (also called *bhūr-loka*) are the six higher planes, or "realms" (*loka*), each of which has its own species of beings—demigods and deities corresponding to the hierarchies of angels recognized in the Middle Eastern religions. In ascending order, these celestial realms are *bhuvar-loka*, *svarga-loka*, *mahar-loka, jana-loka, tapo-loka*, and *satya-loka*. The highest plane, inhabited by the Creator (be he called Brahma, Vishnu, or Shiva), is the only aspect of the brahmic egg that survives the periodic collapse (*pralaya*) of all the other planes, for the *satya-loka* serves as the seed for the next cosmic evolution. But even the Creator does not enjoy true immortality and forfeits his life after 42,200 *kalpas*, corresponding to 120 brahmic years. Since one *kalpa* (or brahmic daytime) is 4,320,000,000 human years long, Brahma's lifespan translates into a staggering 453,248,000,000,000 human years.[9] The present Brahma is said to be in his fifty-first year. His eventual death will coincide with the total destruction of the brahmic egg itself. This is the moment when our present universe will blink out of existence completely. For this reason, the spiritual traditions of India all consider the attainment of *satya-loka* as ultimately unattractive. In fact, the Indic teachings praise human life with its intensity of experience as a unique platform for escaping the cycle of birth, life, and death, which is found desirable even by the deities themselves.

Beyond the immensity of the brahmic egg lies the inconceivable dimension of the formless Divine, which, as the *Mundaka-Upanishad* (3.1.7) puts it, is "subtler than the subtlest." The Divine, equated in the *Tantras* with Shiva/Shakti, is outside the realm of causation or destiny and is the supreme object of the liberation teachings. This aspatial and atemporal Reality, which alone is immortal, simultaneously and paradoxically interpenetrates the cosmos in all its levels of manifestation and is therefore also the ultimate spiritual core of the human being. Without the immanence of the Divine, liberation would be impossible. Without its transcendence, liberation would be meaningless.

Because the various levels of the cosmos, apart from the visible aspect of our earth world, are accessible only through the pathway of meditation or inner vision, the three-dimensional cosmographic descriptions found in the *Tantras* and *Purānas* are little more than (perhaps even rather misleading) simplifications of what in fact is an enormously complex higher-dimensional reality. In any case, it is a reality that is an integral part of the experience of Tantric masters and that therefore should not be dismissed purely on the basis of our knowledge of the sensory world.

The higher and lower planes are quite like the layers of an onion, and they are to the macrocosm what the "sheaths" (*kosha*) are to the individual human being as a microcosm. This parallelism is fundamental to Tantric spiritual practice, and I will have occasion to discuss its symbolism in subsequent chapters in connection with the structures of the subtle body (such as the *cakras* and *nādīs*). To penetrate, in meditation, the subtle coverings of the physical body means to transcend the visible and the invisible realms and realize the divine Self, the ultimate Reality.

Escaping the Prison of the World

The goal of Tantra Yoga, as of any Yoga, is to crack the cosmic egg, to use Joseph Chilton Pearce's obliging metaphor. To do so implies the transcendence of the fabric of space-time. Since the world is not something that is merely external to us but is part of our consciousness, and vice versa, there is no question of any spatial trajectory out of the world. Liberation is an intrapsychic event. Hence Pearce was right when he offered a figurative, psychological interpretation of the cosmic egg:

> Our *cosmic egg* is the sum total of our notions of what the world is, notions which define what reality *can be* for us. The crack, then, is a mode of thinking through which imagination can escape the mundane shell and create a new cosmic egg.[10]

In our case, the crack is the path of Tantra Yoga. It creates the necessary opening in cyclic existence. Yet for the *yogin* it is not imagination that escapes, because imagination belongs to the realm of the mind and thus to the world. Imagination, however, has the capacity to grasp the nature of the reality in which we are caught up and show us a way out of it. When it has done so it must be jettisoned for liberation to occur. The mind, driven by imagination, does not itself escape. It is part of our worldly baggage. In fact, nothing really ever escapes the boundaries of the world. The crack in the cosmic egg is only a crack in our limited understanding, a fissure in our imagination through which genuine wisdom can manifest. In a certain sense, liberation is something of a nonevent, for there is neither loss nor gain in it. Rather, when wisdom fully manifests, the world becomes transparent, revealing our true nature, which is inherently free. The idea that we are bound is the first and the last illusion.

Nor is it the *yogin*'s ambition to create a new cosmic egg after abandoning the old one. On the contrary, practitioners of Tantra do their utmost to penetrate all veils of illusion, that is, all mental constructs of Reality. In this way they can be sure to be rid of all possible bondage to cosmic existence now and forever.

From a yogic perspective, the brahmic or cosmic egg is a prison. Many people, under the influence of *māyā* (fundamental illusion), are not in the least aware of their self-perpetuated state of incarceration. But those in whom wisdom has dawned can see that the world, or rather how they experience it, is confining. They also are sensitive to the fact that worldly existence is suffused with suffering (*duhkha*). At first, they may not see a way out of the cosmic prison, but as wisdom increases, there is a growing sense of a Reality that transcends the cosmos. Then they understand that the Divine, though transcending space and time, dwells within themselves in the form of the eternal Self (*ātman*) and that it is the hidden doorway to liberation. In other words, the prison gates were never locked. As Shankara, the great preceptor of Advaita Vedānta, puts it in his popular *Viveka-Cūdāmani* (571):

> Fools wrongly project bondage and liberation, which are attributes of the mind, upon Reality, just as the shade cast upon the eyes by a cloud [is projected upon] the Sun itself. For this immutable [Reality] is nondual, unattached Consciousness.

When we realize the imperishable Self, previously obscured by karmic habit patterns, we overcome the world, which means we overcome our particular restricted world experience. In that instant the world loses its hostile quality and instead reveals itself to us as the benign ever-present Reality itself. Until that moment of *metanoia*, however, we are entrapped by our own representations of Reality, our idiosyncratic (though largely shared) mirrorings of Truth. This is the meaning of bondage (*bandha*) in the Hindu liberation teachings, including Tantra.

What is so objectionable about cyclic existence is that it is shot through with suffering. And suffering is primarily caused by the experience of impermanence, manifesting as change and death. These, in turn, are a function of time (*kāla*), which is the subject of the next chapter.

Time, Bondage, and the Goddess Kālī

Because you devour time, [you are] Kālī,
the primal form of everything.
—*Mahānirvāna-Tantra* (4.32a)

TIME IMMANENT, TIME TRANSCENDENT

Samsāra signals both spatial and temporal confinement. Above all, however, *samsāra* is time. The *Maitrāyanī-Upanishad* (6.16) speaks of embodied time as the great ocean in which all creatures (including the time-pacing solar deity, Savitri, himself)[1] have their being and are "cooked," or ripened. Time means change, be it in the form of natural rhythms or abrupt transitions. Most of us Westerners are so used to dwelling in cities that we have become relatively oblivious to the natural rhythms of nature. The fast pace of life and the substitute reality created through both the extensive use of electricity for light and warmth and the use of drugs (especially pain killers) have alienated us from our own somatic cycles, or biorhythms. Our consciousness is dominated by a linear conception that understands the passage of time as an arrow pointing from the past to the future rather than as consisting of self-repeating cycles. Correspondingly, we are forever chasing time, either by aspiring after the future or by tracking down the memories of the past, while often forgetting to be mindful in the present. The traditional consciousness, by contrast, fears to be caught in the cycles of time, which ultimately bring little more than physical and mental suffering.

Time (*kāla*) has been a favorite theme of the Indic sages ever since the early Vedic era.[2] In the *Atharva-Veda*, two highly metaphoric hymns are dedicated to the mystery of time. One hymn (19.53) speaks of time as the first god among the deities, "throned in the loftiest realm," creator of all creatures and of energy (*tapas*) itself. The other hymn (19.54), in a similar vein, reads as follows:

> From Time the cosmic waters evolved.
> From Time came prayerful meditation (*brahman*),[3] energy
>   (*tapas*), and the spatial directions.
> Because of Time the Sun rises and in Time it sets again. (1)
>
> Because of Time the wind purifies [everything].
> Because of Time the Earth is great.
> Upon Time the great heaven is fixed. (2)
>
> Long ago, Son Time engendered the past and the future.
> Through Time the hymns of praise came into being.
> Through Time the sacrificial formulas came into being. (3)
>
> Time inaugurated the sacrifice providing the gods with oblation.
> In Time are the *gandharvas* and *apsarases*.[4]
> In Time the realms are established. (4)
>
> In Time are set these heavenly Angiras and Atharvan.
> For both this realm and the highest realm,
> the virtuous realms, and the virtuous interspaces
> —all realms conquered through prayerful meditation,
> this Time moves on as the highest god. (5)

I have quoted this Vedic hymn in full because it also captures the philosophy of time found in the *Tantras*, composed several millennia later. Because the *Atharva-Veda* foreshadows the Tantric heritage in many ways, some scholars and adherents of Tantra regard this Vedic hymnody, or the cultural environment in which it was created, as one of the historical roots of Tantra.

Time as the "highest god," however, must not be misconstrued as referring to mere conventional time. It is the supreme Reality itself in its life-giving, sustaining, and ordering aspect—what in Buddhist Tantra is known as *kāla-cakra*.[5] A similar notion is present in the *Devī-Māhātmya*, popularly known as the *Candī*, after the name of the goddess to whom it is addressed. This hymn is to pious Shāktas (worshipers of Shakti, the great goddess) what the *Bhagavad-Gītā* is to votaries of Vishnu in his earthly incarnation as the god-man Krishna. Both hymns consist of seven hundred verses and are chanted daily.

The *Candī* is a heartfelt eulogy to the goddess as the universal matrix, or divine mother. Although she is eternal, she manifests in countless ways (1.64–65), is the primordial cause of everything (1.78), supports the worlds (1.71), causes change by manifesting as time (*kāla*) in its various divisions (11.9), and has the power to destroy the universe (11.9); but she also leads to liberation (4.9). She is the repository of the Vedic hymns of praise and the sacrificial formulas (4.10), is adored even by the Lord of Gods himself (5.81), illuminates the spatial directions (5.92), owns all the treasures of the deities, *gandharvas*, and *nāgas* (5.111),[6] and abides as higher understanding (*buddhi*) in the hearts of all beings (11.8). But, as is clear from the core story of this hymn, the goddess also has her destructive side. She not only conquers all demonic forces but also annihilates the universe at the appropriate time. To her devotees, however, she shows her most benign maternal aspect, protecting and ultimately liberating them. After having been propitiated with praise, the goddess responds:

> Whosoever with concentration worships Me constantly with these [hymns], his every difficulty I will remove without a doubt. (12.2)

KĀLĪ, SHIVA, AND THE COSMIC DANCE

Even a short précis of the Tantric view of time, as attempted here, would be incomplete without introducing the Divine Female, or Shakti, in her most startling manifestation as the goddess Kālī. The name is the feminine form of *kāla*, meaning "time," "death," and "black." These three connotations are all fused in the symbolism of the goddess Kālī. Black results from the absorption of all colors, whereas white is their copresence. The saintly Ramakrishna, *guru* of Swami Vivekananda, offered a devotee's complementary explanation of the name Kālī when he remarked, "You see her as black because you are far away from her. Go near and you will find her devoid of all color."[7] In *The Gospel of Sri Ramakrishna*, which chronicles the life and teachings of this great nineteenth-century master, we find the following hymn:

> In dense darkness, O Mother, Thy formless beauty sparkles;
> Therefore the yogis meditate in a dark mountain cave.
> In the lap of boundless dark, on Mahanirvana's waves upborne,
> Peace flows serene and inexhaustible.[8]
> Taking the form of the Void, in the robe of darkness wrapped,
> Who art Thou, Mother, seated alone in the shrine of samadhi?[9]
> From the Lotus of Thy fear-scattering Feet flash Thy love's
>   lightnings;
> Thy Spirit-Face shines forth with laughter terrible and loud![10]

To absorb, devour, or destroy the universe is one of the terrifying functions of the black goddess. She brings death not just to the individual but to the cosmic egg itself in which individuals, high and low, live out their respective separative lives over and over again. In the *Mahānirvāna-Tantra* (4.29–31) the goddess is addressed as the supreme *yoginī* because at the end of time she devours the devourer of time himself, Shiva in his form as Mahākāla.

In many temples in Bengal and Nepal, Kālī is depicted as a black or dark blue block of stone. In her humanoid form, Hindu iconography pictures Kālī as a fierce-looking female whose naked, full-breasted

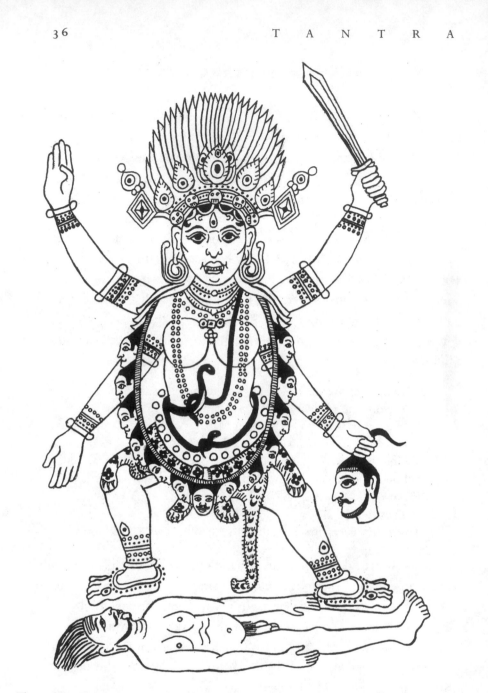

The goddess Kālī, representing the destructive aspect of the Divine. (Illustration by James Rhea)

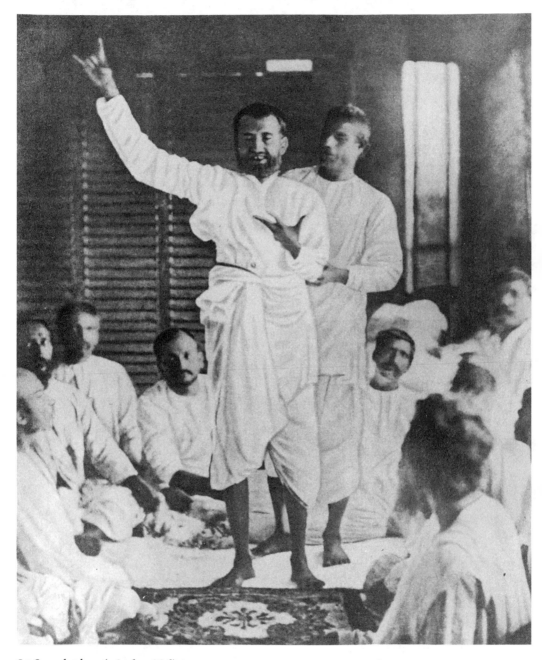

Sri Ramakrishna (1836–1886) in ecstasy. (PHOTOGRAPH COURTESY OF RAMAKRISHNA-VIVEKANANDA CENTER, NEW YORK)

body stands astride or straddles the prostrate nude body of her divine partner Shiva, with ashen skin and erect penis. Her eyes are wide open and her long red tongue protrudes from her teeth-baring mouth dripping with blood. Around her neck she wears a garland of fifty human skulls, around her waist a girdle of human hands. The skulls stand for the fundamental energies of the cosmos (also represented by the fifty letters of the Sanskrit alphabet); the hands symbolize action and its karmic fruition. In the middle of her forehead is a third eye, indicating her omniscience. She usually has four arms, but two-, six-, eight-, and ten-armed versions are also known. One left hand holds a severed human head by the hair, suggesting the death of the ego-personality that must precede liberation; the other left hand holds a bloody sword that cuts all bondage to the world. One right hand is in the fear-dispelling gesture, the other in the gesture of blessing. Encircling her ankles, wrists, and upper arms are serpents, which are symbols of both temporal cycles and the arcane knowledge that liberates the initiate from space and time but is dangerous to the uninitiated. The serpents are also associated with the mysterious *kundalinī-shakti*, the serpentine psychospiritual energy residing in the human body as the instrument of both bondage and liberation. Artistic imagination has created numerous variations of Kālī's dread-instilling image.

Kālī's devotees, however, experience her as a loving, nurturing, and protecting mother. With tear-filled eyes and a longing heart, they invoke her as Kālī Mā, asking her for health, wealth, and happiness, as well as liberation. Like a doting mother, she bestows all boons upon her human children. Sri Ramakrishna, who was a great devotee of the goddess, prayed to Kālī for the fruit of all Yogas and, as he confirmed, "She has shown me everything that is in the Vedas, the Vedanta, the Puranas, and the Tantra."[11] Toward her devotees, Kālī always presents her most benign aspect. Even her destructive side is modulated in a benevolent way, as a force that removes all inner and outer obstacles, especially spiritual blindness, and grants the highest realization beyond space and time. "Because You devour Time (*kāla*), You are called Kālī," declares the *Mahānirvāna-Tantra* (IV.32). At the end of time, the great Goddess also swallows up all the myriad forms filling space. Then she alone remains, in intimate union with her divine Beloved, Shiva—until the next Big Bang, when the cosmic egg newly arises from its own ashes.

The Feminine Divine and the Masculine Divine are never really separate. Consequently Kālī's destructive function is also often attributed to the supreme god Shiva. He is also called Mahākāla, meaning "Great Time." Thus the *Mahānirvāna-Tantra* (5.141) has this pertinent verse, spoken by a devotee of the goddess:

> I worship the primal Kālikā [i.e., Kālī] whose limbs are like a [dark] rain cloud, who has the moon in her crown, is triple-eyed, clothed in red, whose raised hands are [in the gestures of] blessing and dispelling fear, who is seated on an open red lotus with her beautiful smiling face turned toward Mahākāla [i.e., Shiva], who, drunk on sweet wine, is dancing before her.

Like Kālī's grisly image, Shiva's dance is one of the grand archetypes of Hinduism. The dancing Shiva is known as Natarāja, or "King of Dancers." His performance extends throughout the universe. His repertoire, or dance steps, include the creation, preservation, and destruction of the world, as well as concealment of the truth and grace by which the ultimate Reality is revealed in its true form. What is not often appreciated outside India is that Shiva's dance has several forms, each conveying a distinct but related message. Its best known form is that of the *tāndava*, which Shiva dances in wild abandon in the cemetery and cremation ground.

According to Hindu mythology, Shiva once visited a group of sages in their forest huts. Ignorant of his true identity, they began to curse him. When their curses had no effect, they set a ferocious tiger upon him. Shiva skinned the animal alive and put its hide around his waist. Still blinded by their own delusion, the sages next set a monstrous serpent upon him. Shiva simply seized it and draped it around his neck like a harmless necklace.[12] Finally, the forest hermits set a vicious black dwarf upon him, but with a single blow Shiva knocked him to the ground and then planted his right foot on the dwarf's back. The demonic dwarf, named Muyalaka, represents the karmic energies that must be subdued to achieve liberation.

Then Shiva started his cosmic dance, attracting even the deities from the highest realms to watch the spectacle. As he danced, he rhythmically beat his drum, which emanated a blinding light. Bit by bit the universe around him started to dissolve. In due course, however, his dance restored the world out of nothingness. The cardinal witness of Shiva's dance was Kālī, the great Goddess in her fierce form. According to one myth, she was even the cause of his destructive dance. She had hoped to defeat him but ended up worshiping him. After her submissive gesture, Shiva explained to her that he had performed the dance not because of her challenge to him but because he wanted to grant a vision of the dance to the sages of the forest.

Typically, Shiva Natarāja is depicted with four, six, or ten arms and cobralike strands of wildly flowing hair, the dwarf trapped under his right foot, the left foot raised in a dancing step, and surrounded by a ring of fire, representing the holocaust at the end of time. In his four-armed form, Nātarāja holds a drum (*damaru*) in his upper right hand and a flame in his upper left hand. The lower right hand is in the fear-dispelling gesture, while the lower left hand points to the raised leg that bestows liberation.

For the Shāktas, it is Kālī who performs the rhythmic dance that weaves and disentangles the gossamer threads of cosmic existence. According to one myth, the goddess Durgā once fought the demon Raktabīja (Blood Seed), but however much she severed his limbs with her sword, she was unable to kill him, for every drop of the demon's blood that fell on the ground promptly gave rise to a thousand new demons as powerful as Raktabīja. When Durgā's fury reached its peak, the dark goddess Kālī sprang from her forehead and mercilessly attacked the demons, whirling about in a blur of motion. Between the infallible strikes from her sword, she licked the blood that had spilled to the ground, preventing the generation of new demons. At last she destroyed Raktabīja himself.

In triumph, she started to dance, and the more she danced the more she lost all sense of self. Her frenzied dance caused the earth to quiver and soon threatened to annihilate the universe itself. At the behest of the terrified deities, the supreme god Shiva begged the goddess to stop dancing. When she ignored his request, Shiva lay prostrate before her. She promptly jumped on his body, placing one leg on his chest and the other on his extended legs, continuing her dance. After some time she realized that she was dancing on her husband's body, grew ashamed, and stopped. The destruction of the universe was halted, and deities, humans, and all other beings were able to resume their respective lives governed by the rhythm of time.

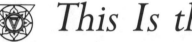 *This Is the Other World*

SAMSĀRA EQUALS NIRVĀNA

The Lord has the universe for a body.
—*Pratyabhijñā-Hridaya* (4) of Kshemarāja

THE TWO TRUTHS

Ever since the emergence of religious and cultural pluralism in the Western hemisphere, more and more people have been wondering, What is the truth about anything? Under the spell of Einstein's relativity theory, many have adopted the extremist view that truth itself is relative and completely dependent on the position of the observer. This viewpoint is not entirely without merit because it may lead one to practice humility and tolerance toward other perspectives. But it is not very satisfactory when one is looking for a higher purpose in life that can bring lasting happiness. In that case, one must go beyond the pedestrian level of understanding that takes truth to be variable. As the great spiritual traditions of the world affirm, truth is always one, though there are many pathways to it. Truth is Reality, which is singular. What is relative are our angles of perception and comprehension.

The masters of Tantra therefore distinguish between two levels of understanding, corresponding to two levels of reality. First there is the worldly (*laukika*) point of view, which believes in a solid material universe and which tends to be partial and often corrupted. And then there is the spiritual (*ādhyātmika*) point of view, which is informed by wisdom and leads one to *the* truth, that is, the ultimate Reality. The worldly understanding, shot through with desire and delusion, is hardly a reliable guide for those seeking lasting happiness. It is of course very useful in worldly matters, though it is ineffectual in spiritual matters. Similarly, wisdom does not enable us to repair a motorcycle, but it does enable us to live a harmonious life that is conducive to higher realizations. It contributes to our handling of material knowledge and skills by freeing us from negative emotions and attitudes. Thus even from a mundane perspective, wisdom can be said to make us more functional. That wisdom is senior to worldly knowledge is obvious from the fact that in the absence of guiding wisdom, worldly knowledge all too easily turns destructive. Many critics of our postmodern technological society have argued precisely this way.[1]

THE DIVINE NATURE OF CYCLIC EXISTENCE

To the ordinary, unenlightened mind, the world is a place of mixed experiences, affording both pleasure and pain. At times it even gives rise to the impression that it is the best of all possible worlds— until illness, loss, or death make their point again. This describes the naive, unexamined attitude to life.

To a more perceptive intelligence, however, the world is far from an ideal place, for it can give no abiding happiness. Everything is subject to impermanence, the bloody tooth of time. Human beings especially are quite short-lived and harvest numerous unpleasant experiences. As Gautama the Buddha put it in a nutshell, "Birth is suffering. Life is suffering. Death is suffering. Everything is suffering."

This famous declaration is echoed in many Tantric and other texts. Thus Patanjali, the author of the *Yoga-Sūtra*, declares in one of his aphorisms: "To the discerning person everything is suffering."[2] But beyond this recognition of the omnipresence of suffering in the sphere of finite reality, and far beyond the naive attitude of the thoughtless individual, there is a third, surprising possibility in understanding the nature of existence. This is the Tantric view, according to which, as one contemporary adept put it, our conditional universe (*samsāra*) *is* the "other" world.[3] In more traditional (Buddhist) terms, *samsāra* equals *nirvāna*.

What does this mean? It is clearly not the naive perspective that looks upon ordinary life as if it were paradise. No delusion or self-deception is involved here. Rather, the formula "*samsāra* equals *nirvāna*" implies a total cognitive shift by which the phenomenal world is rendered transparent through superior wisdom. No longer are things seen as being strictly separated from one another, as if they were insular realities in themselves, but everything is seen together, understood together, and lived together. Whatever distinctions there may be, these are variations or manifestations of and within the self-same Being. As Lama Anagarika Govinda explained:

> Thus, good and bad, the sacred and the profane, the sensual and the spiritual, the worldly and the transcendental, ignorance and Enlightenment, *samsāra* and *nirvāna*, etc., are not absolute opposites, or concepts of entirely different categories, but two sides of the same reality.[4]

Strictly speaking, the equation of *samsāra* with *nirvāna* belongs to the language and conceptual framework of Buddhism. Both the word *nirvāna* and the concept for which it stands are also found in Hinduism, however. Likewise, the idea that the world is none other than the ultimate Reality is as much at home in Hinduism as it is in Buddhism. As early as the *Chāndogya-Upanishad* (3.14.1), which is now thought by some scholars to have been composed in the second millennium BCE, we find a veteran sage declaring: "Verily, all this is the Absolute."[5] That is to say, this entire universe is nothing other than the singular Being, which contains within itself every conceivable thing.

This ancient notion reached its climax in the medieval Sahajiyā movement, straddling both Hinduism and Buddhism. *Sahaja* means literally "born (*ja*) together (*saha*)" and refers to the essential identity between the finite and the infinite, the phenomenal and the noumenal reality. The term has variously been translated as "the innate," "the natural," or "spontaneity"—all denoting the indivisible Reality. The Sahajiyā movement is thoroughly Tantric in orientation and crystallizes the highest metaphysical insight of Tantra. The Tantric adept Sarahapāda (800 CE?), one of the Buddhist *mahā-siddhas*, characterized *sahaja* thus:

> Though the house-lamps have been lit,
> The blind live on in the dark.
> Though spontaneity is all-encompassing and close,
> To the deluded it remains always far away.
>
> Bees that know in flowers
> Honey can be found.
> That Samsāra and Nirvāna are not two
> How will the deluded ever understand?
>
> There's nothing to be negated, nothing to be
> Affirmed or grasped; for It can never be conceived.
> By the fragmentations of the intellect are the deluded
> Fettered; undivided and pure remains spontaneity.[6]

According to the *Ratna-Sāra*, a text of the medieval Vaishnava Sahajiyā tradition, beings are born out of *sahaja*, live in *sahaja*, and again vanish into *sahaja*.[7] In the two extant versions of the *Akula-Vīra-Tantra*, a scripture of the important Kaula tradition, *sahaja* is described as a state of being characterized by omniscience, omnipresence, and goodness. When the spiritual practitioner attains it, all cognitions merge into it and the mind becomes utterly silenced. Then all duality is banished, all suffering is eliminated, and all karmic seeds are burned to ashes, so that the tree of unenlightened existence cannot sprout again.

The Tantric declaration that *samsāra* equals *nirvāna* can be read on at least two levels. First, it can be interpreted to mean that the finite world is really the infinite Reality and that, in other words, what we perceive to be the limited universe is fundamentally an illusion. Second, it can be understood to mean that the sage who made the declaration experiences the world to be none other than the perennial, unchanging Reality. Both readings are correct and go together. A third interpretation would be to take the statement to be a prescription, and this too is implied in the traditional formula. The prescription or admonition is this: because world and Reality are not truly distinct, therefore realize this to be so in your own case. This encapsulates the approach of Tantra, which is emphatically practical. As noted in the introduction, the *Tantras* are first and foremost *sādhana-shāstras*, or teachings designed to aid spiritual discipline. Our true nature, *sahaja*, is always with us. It is like honey in our mouth. Yet, out of ignorance, we continually look for it outside ourselves. Tantra teaches us to enjoy the sweet-tasting honey that is already on our tongue by enhancing our awareness.

VERTICALIST, HORIZONTALIST, AND INTEGRAL TEACHINGS

In another book, I have made a distinction between verticalist, horizontalist, and integral approaches to life.[8] The Sanskrit equivalents for the first two are *nivritti-mārga* (path of cessation) and *pravritti-mārga* (path of activity) respectively. The third orientation can be dubbed *pūrna-mārga* (path of wholeness).

The horizontalist approach characterizes the typical extroverted lifestyle of the worldling (*samsārin*), who is preoccupied with his or her job, family, belongings, status, and prospects. At a certain stage of spiritual development, these horizontalist concerns are appropriate enough, and the Hindu authorities have produced textbooks (*shāstra*) on a wide range of topics enabling worldly-minded people to live a better life. In the West perhaps the best known such work is the *Kāma-Sūtra*, which deals with the subtleties and technicalities of sexuality and was originally designed for the privileged class of Hindu society.

To the category of horizontalist teachings belongs also the vast legal literature of Hinduism, known as *dharma-shāstra*. Here the best known work is the encompassing *Mānava-Dharma-Shāstra* (or *Manu-Smriti*), which consists of 2,685 verses ascribed to the legendary Manu. All such Sanskrit scriptures seek to provide guidance on the first three goals or pursuits of human existence, namely, material welfare (*artha*), passionate self-expression (*kāma*), and moral virtue or lawfulness (*dharma*).

Manu, who is remembered as the progenitor of the present human race, divided the course of human life into four stages—those of a student, householder, renouncer, and liberated being. Each stage is thought to extend over a period of twenty-one years, yielding an ideal total of eighty-four years. In the first stage the foundations for a solid intellectual, moral, and spiritual life are laid. In the second stage, the Vedic training is applied in everyday life. Then when one's children are grown and have their own children, it is time to renounce the lifestyle of a householder and retire to the forest or a similar remote area. This is the beginning of the verticalist approach. The renouncer in the third stage of life intensifies his or her ritual practices, meditation, and prayer, increasingly focusing on the ultimate ideal of liberation. This ideal is traditionally recognized as the fourth and highest human pursuit (*purusha-artha*, written *purushārtha*). When one's renunciation has born fruit and one has realized the transcendental Reality, or innermost Self of oneself and all beings and things, it is appropriate to adopt the spontaneous lifestyle of a liberated being. The lifestyle of the fully illumined sage is inherently integrated but may tend toward verticalism or horizontalism without, however, being confined to either orientation.

In the West, which is driven by the philosophy of horizontalism, we have no equivalent to the last two stages of human life as envisioned in Hinduism. Our concept of retirement does not include the ideal of striving to realize our higher human potential. Rather, we commonly see it as an extension of the pursuit of pleasure that also governs much of our active life. Our materialist approach does not permit the notion of inner work, never mind the grand ideal of liberation. Exceedingly few people seize the opportunity of retirement to deepen their self-knowledge and dedicate themselves to exploring the spiritual dimension of existence. Our modern society is dominated by horizontalist concerns. It offers much knowledge but precious little wisdom. Attempts at verticalist teachings, as we find them for instance in the New Age movement, often remain on the level of mere intellectualization, popularization, psychologization, and quasireligious exhortation. All these are substitutes for genuine spiritual practice that aims not at knowledge, pleasure, personal growth, or moral goodness but at the transcendence of the self and the complete transformation of human nature.

Genuine liberation and the liberated life are the focus of the body of wisdom known as *moksha-shāstra,* which comprises scriptures belonging to both revelatory authority (*shruti*) and traditional authority (*smriti*). To the former belong the *Vedas, Upanishads, Brāhmanas, Āranyakas*, and—for adherents of Tantra at least—the *Tantras.* The category of traditional teachings is vast and diversified. It includes, among other things, such works as the *Mahābhārata* epic (of which the *Bhagavad-Gītā* is a part), the numerous *Purānas* (though some, like the *Bhāgavata-Purāna*, are counted as revealed literature by certain groups), and the *Sūtras* (notably the *Yoga-Sūtra*) and their many commentaries and subcommentaries.

A large proportion of India's liberation literature avows teachings that fall into the category of what I have called "verticalism." They show a pathway out of the karmic entanglements of the horizontal, worldly life. Their declared goal is some otherworldly state of freedom. They view liberation as being opposed to the condition of ordinary life, which is equated with one of bondage (*bandha*). All their recommended techniques are geared toward liberating the seeker from his or her self-imposed confinement in a human body and a finite world. The metaphor that best describes this orientation is that of a flight from the world straight up into a dimension beyond the conditional universe.

The verticalist approach to liberation has been enormously influential on Indian culture. Its beginnings can be witnessed in the early *Upanishads*, such as the *Brihad-Āranyaka* and the *Chāndogya*. It reached its peak in the teachings of Advaita Vedānta, as popularly expressed, for instance, in the *Viveka-Cūḍāmani*, ascribed to the great preceptor Shankara. Here the objective world is characterized as being more virulent than the poison of a cobra and the body as being worthy of little more than condemnation.[9] Since the body and the world as a whole are deemed insignificant, the spiritual seeker is further advised to focus exclusively on the Self, abandoning all conventional pursuits. That Self is said in verse 132 to be luminously present in the "cave of the mind" (*dhī-guha*), that is, within oneself, in the heart. The path to it is described in verse 367 as consisting in restraint of speech, nongrasping, nonhoping, nonwilling, and always cultivating solitude. These means comprise the foremost gateway of Yoga—clearly understood here as the vertical pursuit of enlightenment.

Had India produced only verticalist liberation teachings, its gift to modern seekers would perhaps not be as pertinent and valuable as it really is. But long ago the Indic sages also won through to an integral orientation that holds special significance for today. Integrative trends can be detected, for instance, in the above-mentioned two *Upanishads*, and the earlier-cited statement "Verily, all this is the Absolute" is a classic expression of these early trends. A fuller manifestation of integralism can be found in the *Bhagavad-Gītā*, which describes itself as a *yoga-shāstra* but has gained the status of a revealed scripture.

The flowering of the integral orientation occurred with the

emergence of Tantra. Although the Tantric scriptures are not free
from notions and practices belonging to the verticalist approach,
many of them clearly tend toward integralism. Above all, they view
the world as a manifestation of the ultimate Reality and the body as a
temple of the Divine. For this reason, they look askance at the kind
of extreme asceticism favored by verticalism and criticized already by
the Buddha around 500 BCE. Thus in the *Kula-Arnava-Tantra* Shiva
addresses the goddess in the following way:

> Fools deluded by your power of illusion (*māyā*) aspire to the
> Invisible (*paroksha*) by such means as asceticism of the body and
> abstention from food.

> How can there be liberation for the ignorant through the
> punishment of the body? What great serpent has ever died from
> striking an anthill?

> Are asses and the like *yogins* because they roam in the world
> naked without shame and for whom house and forest are the
> same?

> O Goddess, if people could become liberated by smearing
> themselves with mud and ashes, then villagers who live amid
> mud and ashes should all be liberated.

> O Goddess, are parrots and myna birds great scholars because
> they talk and repeat amusing things before people?[10]

Integral teachings emphasize the inner work, or inner sacrifice
(*antar-yāga*), rather than any outward ritual, though without dismiss-
ing external worship altogether. The *Kula-Arnava-Tantra* (5.70) puts it
this way:

> Just as a king favors those who move inside [the palace] over
> those who are outside it, so, O Goddess, you favor those who
> cultivate the inward sacrifice over others.

The discovery of the inner sacrifice was made long before the
appearance of Tantra. But it remained the province of a select few
because of the inveterate tendency in human beings to neglect the
inner world of consciousness and be overly active in the external

realm. Many Tantric teachers reacted against this tendency, which was strongly present in the mainstream priestly culture of Hinduism. They also reacted against the parallel tendency, fueled by the priestly philosophy of nondualism (*advaita*), that fled the Many to attain the One. Although in many respects Tantra continued the metaphysics and language of nondualism, it often sought to express new meanings through them. The Tantric One (*eka*), for instance, is not the life-negating Singularity of some brahmanical teachers but the all-encompassing Whole (*pūrna*), which is present as the body, the mind, and the world yet transcends all of these. At its best, Tantra is integralism. This is hinted at in the word *tantra* itself, which, among other things, means "continuum."

This continuum is what the enlightened adepts realize as *nirvāna* and what unenlightened worldlings experience as *samsāra*. These are not distinct, opposite realities. They are absolutely the same Being, the same essence (*samarasa*). That essence merely appears different to different people because of their karmic predispositions, which are like veils or mental filters obscuring the truth. To ordinary worldlings, the One remains utterly hidden. To spiritual seekers, it seems a distant goal, perhaps realizable after many lifetimes. To initiates, it is a reliable inner guide. To the Self-realized sages, it is the only One that exists, for they have *become* the Whole.

The Secret of Embodiment

As Above, So Below

> The psyche is composed of everything [that exists].
> —*Spanda-Kārikā* (2.3) of Kallata

The Preciousness of Human Life

One of the greatest contributions of Tantra to spirituality is its philosophy of the body. Unlike the vertical teachings preceding and surrounding it, Tantra has taken the human body seriously. A classic expression of the verticalist view of the body can be found, for instance, in the *Maitrāyanī-Upanishad* (1.3), a work probably belonging to the third century BCE:

> O Venerable one, what good is the enjoyment of desires in this ill-smelling, insubstantial body, a mere conglomerate of

bones, skin, sinews, muscles, marrow, flesh, semen, blood, mucus, tears, rheum, feces, urine, wind, bile, and phlegm? What good is the enjoyment of desires in this body, which is afflicted with desire, anger, greed, delusion, fear, despondency, envy, separation from the desirable, union with the undesirable, hunger, thirst, senility, disease, sorrow, death, and the like?

Philosophical verticalism views the body as a breeding ground for *karma* and an automatic hindrance to enlightenment. The common Sanskrit word for "body" is *deha*, which stems from the verbal root *dih* ("to smear" or "be soiled"). It hints at the defiled nature of the body. Yet the same verbal root can also signify "to anoint," which gives the noun *deha* the far more laudatory meaning of "that which is anointed." The older Sanskrit word for "body" is *sharīra*, derived from the verbal root *shri* ("to rest upon" or "to support"), which has a more positive connotation: the body serves as the prop, or framework, by means of which the Self can experience the world. This notion led to the still more positive interpretation of the body as a temple of the Divine—an idea intimated in the early *Upanishads* but not fully elaborated until the emergence of Tantra much later.

Tantra's body-positive approach is the direct outcome of its integrative metaphysics according to which this world is not mere illusion but a manifestation of the supreme Reality. If the world is real, the body must be real as well. If the world is in essence divine, so must be the body. If we must honor the world as a creation or an aspect of the divine Power (*shakti*), we must likewise honor the body. The body is a piece of the world and, as we shall see, the world is a piece of the body. Or, rather, when we truly understand the body, we discover that it is the world, which in essence is divine.

Because the human body has a complex nervous system allowing higher expressions of consciousness, it is especially valuable. Indeed, the Tantric scriptures often remind students of the preciousness of human life. Thus in the *Kula-Arnava-Tantra* (1.16–27) Lord Shiva declares:

> After obtaining a human body, which is difficult to obtain and which serves as a ladder to liberation, who is more sinful than he who does not cross over to the Self?

Therefore, upon obtaining the best possible life form, he who does not know his own good is merely killing himself.

How can one come to know the purpose of human life without a human body? Hence having obtained the gift of a human body one should perform meritorious deeds.

One should completely protect oneself by oneself. Oneself is the vessel for everything. One should make an effort in protecting oneself. Otherwise the Truth cannot be seen.

Village, house, land, money, even auspicious and inauspicious *karma* can be obtained over and over again, but not a human body.

People always make an effort to protect the body. They do not wish to abandon the body even when sick with leprosy and other diseases.

For the purpose of attaining knowledge, the virtuous person should preserve the body with effort. Knowledge aims at the Yoga of meditation. He will be liberated quickly.

If one does not guard oneself against that which is inauspicious, who, intent on the good, will ever cross over to the Self?

He who does not heal himself from hellish diseases while here on earth, what can he do about a disease when he goes to a place where no remedy exists?

What fool starts digging a well when his house is already on fire? So long as this body exists, one should cultivate the Truth.

Old age is like a tigress; life runs out like water in a broken pot; diseases strike like enemies. Therefore one should cultivate the highest good now.

One should cultivate the highest good while the senses are not yet frail, suffering is not yet firmly rooted, and adversities have not yet become overwhelming.

When we unpack the conceptual content of the above stanzas, we find that human life is so extraordinarily precious because it can serve as a platform or ladder for Self-realization. It endows us with sufficient self-awareness to reflect on our existence and thereby give us valuable options in life. One of the fundamental choices we have is in fact to go beyond the *karma*-producing automatisms, beyond the unconscious behavior patterns, by which life tends to perpetuate itself. We can choose to grow ever more conscious of the forces pushing and pulling us and thus also to become increasingly capable of shaping our destiny. Finally, we can opt to identify with the very principle of awareness, the Self (*ātman*), rather than the diverse displays of the body-mind. Concretely, we can choose to stop thinking of ourselves merely as an individual of a particular race, creed, gender, age, social setting, or educational and professional background.

Hindus, including almost all teachers of Tantra, believe that death is not the end but that we undergo numerous rebirths and repeated deaths. They also believe that this cycle can be interrupted only by intervening in the processes of the mind itself, by shifting our sense of identity from the body-mind to the Self. When this shift is complete and irreversible it is called liberation. Since our present life is the sum total of all our previous unenlightened volitions (*samkalpa*) and actions, it is impossible to say which seeds sown in previous lives have already borne fruit and which are still awaiting fruition. This also means that we cannot know with absolute certainty the particular quality of a future embodiment. As we all know, life is full of surprises, and many of these surprises stem from our activities in past lives both on the material plane and on more subtle planes of existence. According to some schools of Hinduism, we cannot even be sure that our next incarnation will necessarily be into human form. Hence it is traditionally considered most auspicious to have achieved a human birth. More fortunate still is a human life in which we encounter a spiritual teacher and teaching that potentially can free us from the entire cycle of repeated incarnations.

As precious as human life is, it is also extremely fragile and short. Therefore all liberation schools are agreed that we must seize every opportunity to develop the art of self-understanding, self-transformation, and self-transcendence—which is called spiritual discipline, *yoga*, or *tantra*. In the *Bhāgavata-Purāna* (7.6.1–9), the sage Prahlāda explains the significance of human life in these words:

> When still young, the wise person should cultivate the virtues dear to the Divine. A human birth is difficult to obtain here on earth, and even though human life is fleeting, it is full of significance.

> Thus one should approach the Lord's feet, for he is the good-hearted ruler of the self of all creatures and is dear to them.

> Sensory pleasures, like pain, are harvested effortlessly by embodied beings everywhere, simply on account of their destiny.

> One should make no effort to obtain pleasure, for that would be a waste of life and would not bring the supreme peace that springs alone from the Lord's lotus feet.

> Therefore, an intelligent person who is caught up in the world should struggle for peace while the human body is still flourishing rather than failing.

> The span of human life is a hundred years. Half of this is wasted by a person lacking self-control, because he sleeps stuporously in the dark of night.

> Twenty years go by in early childhood when one is bewildered and in youth when one is preoccupied with playing; another twenty years go by in old age when one is physically impaired and lacking in determination.

> The remaining years are wasted by that person who, out of great confusion and insatiable desire, is madly attached to family life.

> How can a person who is attached to family life, with his senses uncontrolled and bound by strong ties of affection, liberate himself?

Liberation presupposes the radical inner act of renunciation of all worldly objects and relations. It must be accompanied by an equally radical focus on the divine Reality. Prahlāda's "ultimate concern" was Vishnu, who, after many trials, granted him the highest realization.

Prahlāda's father, King Hiranyakashipu, likewise merged with Vishnu, because his mind was constantly fixed on the Divine. In Hiranyakashipu's case, however, it was not love but intense hatred of Vishnu that proved liberating. This is a Tantra-style teaching story, and only Tantra can offer a plausible explanation for this surprising feat: Whether the mind is focused by love or hatred, so long as its target is the Divine itself, the alchemical process of *solve et coagula* can occur. For the mind must point beyond itself to burst through its limitations by merging with a higher principle. As the *Shata-Patha-Brāhmana* (10.5.2.20) stated long ago, one becomes that which one contemplates.[1] Tantra explored and elaborated on the deeper implications of this arcane truth.

AGELESS BODY, TIMELESS MIND

If we aspire to lasting happiness, which coincides with our full awakening in enlightenment, we must pay attention to our bodily existence here and now. All too frequently spiritual seekers look for ultimate fulfillment apart from their corporeal existence. And all too frequently they end up not in genuine states of higher being and consciousness but in mental states conjured by the power of imagination, which of course are neither liberating nor ultimately satisfying. By contrast, Tantra takes the body seriously—not in the sense of granting it a finality that it does not have, but in understanding it as the ground for all higher realizations.

The Tantric approach is expressed well in the *Yoga-Vāsishtha* (4.23.18–24), a remarkable and huge Sanskrit work by a Kashmiri adept who probably lived in the eleventh century CE and was influenced by Tantra.[2] He put the following words into the mouth of the great sage Vasishtha:

> For the ignorant person, this body is the source of endless suffering, but to the wise person, this body is the source of infinite delight.

For the wise person, its loss is no loss at all, but while it persists it is completely a source of delight for the wise person.

For the wise person, the body serves as a vehicle that can transport him swiftly in this world, and it is known as a chariot for attaining liberation and unending enjoyment.

Since the body affords the wise person the experience of sound, sight, taste, touch, and smell as well as prosperity and friendship, it brings him gain.

Even though the body exposes one to a whole string of painful and joyous activities, the omniscient sage can patiently bear all experiences.

The wise person reigns, free from feverish unhappiness, over the city known as the body, even as Vāsava [the god Indra] dwells in his city free from distress.

It does not cast him into the pit of pride like a high-mettled horse, nor does it cause him to abandon his "daughter" of wisdom to evil greed and so forth.

The body, then, is the field in which we grow and harvest our experiences, which may be positive or negative, painful or pleasant. While negative, painful experiences do not bring us immediate joy, they do so in the long run because—if we are wise—we relate to them rightly by regarding them as useful lessons. No experience need be devoid of merit. People have had major spiritual breakthroughs as a result of deep suffering and debilitating illness. Even physical pain does not have to be a merely unpleasant experience. In fact, it can sometimes be a doorway to ecstasy. I once underwent a painful three-hour session at the dentist. The Novocaine injections were not working properly, and after writhing in the chair during a complicated procedure, I finally was brought to the point of simply surrendering to the situation. Suddenly, as my resistance to the pain was removed, I found myself in a state of ecstasy, which lasted for the remainder of the operation. I had discovered the attitude underlying much of the world's asceticism, known in India as *tapas*. Instead of shying away from the pain, I had allowed myself to pay full attention to it and thus pass beyond it. Women have reported making a similar discovery during childbirth.

In their widely read book *In the Zone*, Michael Murphy and Rhea A. White mention well-known football players and boxers who continued in a contest despite broken bones, entirely oblivious to the pain. But more than that, some athletes—especially distance runners—invite pain to convert it into ecstasy and surplus energy. As Gerald Heard, one of the early spokesmen for Vedānta in the West, pointed out in his thought-provoking book *Pain, Sex, and Time*, pain is far more than a mere warning signal; it is an indicator of the store of available evolutionary energy in us:

> Traditional and current opinion assumes that man's evolution is over. Any sensation he experiences, whether painful or pleasant, can only be for conservation and comfort, for restoring a disturbed stability, for keeping him where he is. Acute sensation cannot be intended to spur him to creativeness and to urge him to a new level of being. It must then be shown that there is unmistakable proof that we are developing actual capacities and faculties which so draw out and employ our vital energy that when this is done we are rendered painless. Strange as it may seem, enough evidence has already accumulated to make this highly probable. . . .
>
> The new principle is simple. It may be stated as a proposition: The more mentally active anyone is, the less is he capable of pain. . . . The half-awake suffer most; the most intensely attentive are least aware of pain.[3]

The principle stated in the last sentence has been amply demonstrated by *yogins* and fakirs, who seem immune to pain because of their intense mental concentration. Heard rightly believed that the energy, or vitality, that typically causes us to experience pain points to the possibility of our further evolution—not on the physical level but on the level of consciousness. This possibility is in fact a challenge to us, for in order to translate it into actuality we must respond to it consciously. And this is precisely the purpose of all Yoga and Tantra.

To be clear, Tantra does not recommend that initiates pursue pain. Its goal is that of all Indic liberation teachings: to move beyond all suffering and discover the indescribable bliss of Being. But Tantra understands that life on earth and in the other conditional realms brings us mixed experiences to which we must apply a measure of dispassionate, patient acceptance and self-discipline. Fearful avoidance of what we think are negative experiences merely reinforces the very attitude—namely, the exclusive identification with a limited body-mind—that breeds negative experiences. Likewise, blind attachment to what we consider positive experiences merely creates another kind of karmic bind by which we persist in our state of unenlightenment.

Significantly, Tantra asks us to go beyond the traditional stance of the cool, utterly detached observer of all our experiences. It recommends the more refined position of witnessing while at the same time understanding that observer and observed are not ultimately distinct. The Tantric approach is to see all life experiences as the play of the same One. Whether positive or negative, all experiences are embedded in absolute joy, the great delight (*mahā-sukha*) of Reality. When we have understood that what we dread the most—be it loss of health, property, relationships, or life itself—is not occurring *to* us but *within* our larger being, we begin to see the tremendous humor of embodiment. This insight is truly liberating.

The Tantric scriptures hammer on what may be the most important discovery of ancient spirituality, namely, that we *are* the world. The world is our true body. Therefore we are truly ageless, for according to Hindu cosmology the Big Bang that gives birth to the world is, after the demise of our present universe, followed by another Big Bang, ad infinitum. Cosmic existence unfolds and enfolds itself perpetually. Moreover, since body and mind are only conceptually separate and in actuality form aspects of the same world process, our mind is timeless as well. This profound finding is articulated in the archaic teaching of the identity of microcosm and macrocosm.

The Mystery of Microcosm and Macrocosm

The age-old isomorphic teaching that the microcosm is a reflection of the macrocosm is fundamental not only to all magic but also to arcane arts like astrology, as well as to the spiritual traditions, including Tantra. An oft-quoted statement of the *Vishva-Sāra-Tantra* puts it this way: "What is here is elsewhere; what is not here is nowhere."[4] Western students of esoterica are familiar with this principle from the famous saying of Hermes Trismegistus, "As above, so below." Moreover, without this hermetic insight, which has been rediscovered by modern science in the idea of the "holographic universe," we cannot adequately understand the *Vedas* and much of later Hindu sacred literature.[5] For instance, it is a master key to a deeper interpretation of the symbolism of many stories contained in the *Mahābhārata* and the *Purānas*, which have a spiritual significance. It is certainly fundamental to Tantric theory and practice.

It is within the microcosm (body-mind) that, according to the *Tantras*, we find the doorway to the outer cosmos. The entire architecture of the universe is faithfully mirrored in our own body-mind. As the *Shiva-Samhitā* (2.1–5), a seventeenth-century Hatha Yoga manual composed under the influence of Tantra, states:

> Within this body exist Mount Meru, the seven continents, lakes, oceans, mountains, plains, and the protectors of these plains.
>
> In it also dwell the seers, the sages, all the stars and planets, the sacred river crossings and pilgrimage centers, and the deities of these centers.
>
> In it whirl the sun and the moon, which are the causes of creation and annihilation. Likewise, it contains ether, air, fire, water, and earth.
>
> All beings embodied in the three worlds, which are connected to Mount Meru, exist in the body together with all their activities.
>
> He who knows all this is a *yogin*.[6] There is no doubt about this.

We can access the cosmos by going within ourselves because objective and subjective realities coevolve from and always subsist in the same Reality. In the transcendental dimension, they are absolutely

identical. In the subtle realms, they are barely distinct, and they manifest as seemingly separate lines of evolution only in the visible material
dimension. All this means nothing of course to materialists, who believe only in the existence of material elements and (reluctantly) in
consciousness as a by-product of matter (i.e., the brain). The Tantric
view is much more comprehensive and sophisticated because it pays
due attention to humankind's psychological and spiritual capacities.

According to one prominent school, Kashmir's Pratyabhijnā,
Tantra's ontology (model of existence) comprises thirty-six principles
or categories (tattva). These evolve out of the ultimate Reality, or
Parama-Shiva, who or which is called a metaprinciple (atattva).[7] In
descending order, these are as follows:

I. Universal Principles

1. *Shiva* (the Benevolent)—the masculine or consciousness aspect of the ultimate bipolar Reality

2. *Shakti* (Power)—the feminine or power aspect of the ultimate bipolar Reality, which polarizes Consciousness into
   "I" (*aham*) and "this" (*idam*), or subject and object, but
   without separating them dualistically

3. *Sadākhyā* (That which is named Being [*sat*]) or *Sadā-Shiva*
   (Ever-Benevolent)—the transcendental will (*icchā*) that recognizes and affirms "I am this," with the emphasis still on
   the subjective "I" rather than the objective "this" of the
   universal bipolar One

4. *Īshvara* (Lord)—the Creator, corresponding to the realization of "this I am," subtly emphasizing the objective side of
   the One and thereby setting the stage for cosmic evolution

5. *Sad-Vidyā* (Knowledge of Being) or *Shuddha-Vidyā* (Pure
   Knowledge)—the state of balance between the subjective
   and the objective, which are now clearly distinguishable
   within the One

II. Limiting Principles

6. *Māyā* (She who measures)—the power of delusion inherent
   in the ultimate Reality by which the One appears to be

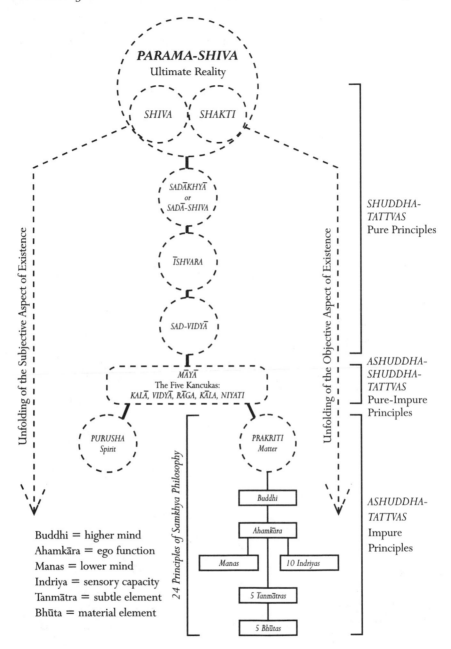

The thirty-six principles of existence according to Tantra.

limited and measurable through the separation of subject and object, which marks the beginning of the impure order of existence

The Five "Coverings" (Kancuka) Associated with Māyā:

7. *Kalā* (Part)—the principle by which the unlimited creatorship of Consciousness becomes limited, causing limited effectiveness

8. *Vidyā* (Knowledge)—the principle by which the omniscience of Consciousness is curtailed, causing finite knowledge

9. *Rāga* (Attachment)—the principle by which the wholeness (*pūrnatva*) of Consciousness is disrupted, giving rise to the desire for partial experiences

10. *Kāla* (Time)—the principle by which the eternity of Consciousness is reduced to temporal existence marked by past, present, and future

11. *Niyati* (Necessity)—the principle by which the independence and pervasiveness of Consciousness is curtailed, bringing about limitation relative to cause, space, and form

III. Principles of Individuation

12. *Purusha* (Man) or *Anu* (Atom)—the conscious subject, or Self, which experiences the objective reality

13. *Prakriti* (Creatrix)—the fully objectified reality, or nature, which is particular to each conscious subject

IV. Principles of the "Inner Instrument" (Antahkarana)

14. *Buddhi* (Understanding)—the mental faculty of intelligence, which is characterized by the capacity for making distinctions

15. *Ahamkāra* (I-maker)—the principle of individuation by which a person appropriates experiences ("I am such and such," or "I possess such and such")

16. *Manas* (Mind)—the mental faculty that synthesizes the incoming sensory impressions into whole concepts and images

V. Principles of Experience

The Five Powers of Cognition (Jnāna-Indriya, written Jnānendriya):

17. *Ghrāna* (Smell)—the olfactory sense

18. *Rasa* (Taste)—the gustatory sense

19. *Cakshus* (Eye, i.e., Sight)—the visual sense

20. *Sparsha* (Touch)—the tactile sense

21. *Shravana* (Hearing)—the auditory sense

The Five Powers of Conation (Karma-Indriya, written Karmendriya):

22. *Vāc* (Speech)—the faculty of communication

23. *Hasta* (Hand)—the faculty of manipulation

24. *Pāda* (Foot)—the faculty of locomotion

25. *Pāyu* (Anus)—the digestive faculty

26. *Upastha* (Genitals)—the procreative faculty

The Five Subtle Elements (Tanmātra):

27. *Shabda-Tanmātra* (Subtle Element of Sound)—the potential for auditory perception

28. *Sparsha-Tanmātra* (Subtle Element of Touch)—the potential for tactile perception

29. *Rūpa-Tanmātra* (Subtle Element of Sight)—the potential for visual perception

30. *Rasa-Tanmātra* (Subtle Element of Taste)—the potential for gustatory perception

31. *Gandha-Tanmātra* (Subtle Element of Smell)—the potential for olfactory perception

VI. *Principles of Materiality*

32. *Ākasha-Bhūta* (Element of Ether)—the principle of vacuity produced from the subtle element of sound

33. *Vāyu-Bhūta* (Element of Air)—the principle of motility produced from the subtle element of touch

34. *Agni-Bhūta* (Element of Fire)—the principle of formation produced from the subtle element of sight

35. *Āpo-Bhūta* (Element of Water)—the principle of liquidity produced from the subtle element of taste

36. *Prithivī-Bhūta* (Element of Earth)—the principle of solidity produced from the subtle element of smell

Tantric ontology seeks to answer the question of how the One can become Many, or how the ultimate Reality, which is singular, can give rise to the countless objects that we perceive through our senses. All liberation teachings provide some kind of an answer to the riddle of creation, because in order to be liberated we must trace our way from the Many back to the One. In Advaita Vedānta, as articulated by the eighth-century teacher Shankara, the world of multiplicity is simply the product of our spiritual ignorance (*avidyā*). The world is a phantom produced by the unenlightened mind. When the root ignorance is removed, the world reveals itself in its true nature, which is none other than the universal singular Being-Consciousness-Bliss (*sac-cid-ānanda*).[8] According to Shankara, the phenomenal world is not inexistent (because in the final analysis it is the eternal ultimate Reality); however, it is unreal (*asat*) because it appears as something other than what it truly is. To describe this curious condition the Vedantic sages often invoke the term *māyā*, which signifies illusion. What is implied by this concept is, among other things, the idea that the transition from the One to the Many is not a genuine emanation but only an apparent evolution (*vivarta*).

Like Advaita Vedānta, most schools of Tantra also maintain that the ultimate Reality is singular. However, they tend toward the view that the Many actually and not merely apparently evolves out of the

One (while still being contained within the One as the eternal back-drop of cosmic existence). They reject any metaphysics of illusionism. This emanationism is technically known as *sat-kārya-vāda*, which de-notes that the effect (*kārya*) is preexistent (*sat*) in the cause: the world could not come into existence if it did not already exist in potential form in the ultimate Being. Perhaps four thousand years ago—long before the rise of Tantra—the sage Āruna taught his twenty-four-year-old son Shvetaketu this metaphysical principle. He pointed out that a clay pot, a clay vase, or a clay statue all are made from clay, though they are given different names to indicate their respective functions. Then Āruna expressly challenged the metaphysical credo that something can come out of nothing (*creatio ex nihilo*):

> Dear one, in the beginning [all] this was being only, singular, without a second. Some say that [all] this was nonbeing only, singular, without a second and that out of nonbeing being was produced.

> He said: But how indeed, dear one, could this be? How could being be produced from nonbeing? To be sure, dear one, in the beginning [all] this was being only, singular, without a second.[9]

More than a millennium later, the *Bhagavad-Gītā* (2.16a) fol-lowed up on this idea, expanding it as follows:

> Nonbeing (*asat*) does not come into being (*bhāva*); being does not disappear (*abhāva*).

In any case, the importance of the Tantric emanationism lies not in the sphere of philosophy but in the realm of spiritual practice. For the existential categories serve the *yogins* or *tāntrikas* as a map by which they are able to find their way out of the maze of multiplicity back to the simplicity of the nondual Reality.

The basic categories of Tantric ontology were worked out long ago by the Sāmkhya school of thought, the rudiments of which can be found already in the *Rig-Veda*. In its classical form, as delineated in the *Sāmkhya-Kārikā* of Īshvara Krishna, Sāmkhya recognizes twenty-four ontological principles, the twenty-fifth being the principle or

category of the supremely conscious Self (*purusha*). The twenty-four
principles belong to the province of nature (*prakriti*), and they are
essentially the same as those given by the Tantric philosophers (and
summarized above). However, they added twelve more principles
based on a careful analysis of their experiences in the most subtle
states of meditation and ecstasy.

The ultimate principle is pure Consciousness, the irreducible
Identity of all beings and things. The Pratyabhijñā school calls it
Parama-Shiva, or "He who is supremely benign."[10] In contrast to Advaita Vedānta, however, the Pratyabhijñā system contends that the
ultimate Reality, though singular, includes the principle of transcendental Power (called *shakti*). The two are inseparable. As the *Tantras*
state, Shiva without Shakti is powerless, and Shakti without Shiva is
equally impotent.

This is a quintessentially Tantric doctrine. As the Shaiva *tāntrikas*
are fond of pointing out, their understanding of the nature of reality
has a distinct advantage over the metaphysics of Advaita Vedānta. For
they do not have to conjure up a separate agency—namely, *māyā*—to
explain the existence of the world, nor do they have to deny the
reality of the world. As they see it, their nondualism is more self-
consistent than that of Advaita Vedānta. For the Shaiva metaphysi-
cians, both *māyā* and world are integral to the One, and the world is
not a shadow to be abandoned but a glorious manifestation of Shiva.
However, Advaita Vedānta in their eyes is not truly nondualistic because in addition to the existence of the One it also affirms the begin-
ningless effectivity of *māyā*, which is separate from the One and is the
cause of the Many. Shankara anticipated this criticism when he explained *māyā* as being neither a reality in itself nor a phantom (which
would be ineffective) but as inherently indeterminable (*anirvacanīya*).

Working with the power or energy aspect of Reality is the spe-
cialty and unsurpassed strength of the Tantric adepts. Hence Tantra is
sometimes wrongly identified with Shaktism. Both are really distinct
historical streams of spirituality, though they have greatly influenced
each other over the centuries. I will discuss the doctrine of Shiva-
Shakti in the next chapter. Suffice it to say here that the ultimate

Reality, which has two aspects (Consciousness and Energy), manifests as the universe. It is for this reason that we, who are that Reality, can awaken to our true nature even while we are in the embodied state.

We *are* the world, as modern ecological-minded philosophers have rediscovered, and we also are that which transcends, creates, and sustains the world and again withdraws it into its infinite and timeless expanse.

The Divine Play of Shiva and Shakti

> Yoga is undoubtedly the union (*samāyoga*) of
> Shiva and Shakti.
> —*Tantra-Sāra* (702)

GODS, GODDESSES, AND THE ULTIMATE REALITY

The Tantric worldview affirms the existence of deities—long-lived higher beings on subtle planes who are endowed with extraordinary powers. The *tāntrikas* seek out their help through invocation, prayer, ritual, meditative visualization, and not least *mantra* recitation. At the same time, however, they understand that these deities, despite their elevated status, are not yet fully mature spiritual beings like the perfected masters (*siddha*). The gods and goddesses are powerful but not liberated. According to a widely held view in Hinduism, they can attain liberation only by first incarnating as a human being. The Tantric pantheon includes a large number of deities, some of which can also be found in Vajrayāna Buddhism. They are typically invoked for protection against interferences and karmic obstacles. The Western mind tends to hastily dismiss this aspect of Tantra as mere superstition or, at best, as a projection of archetypal imagery resident in the human psyche. For the Tantric practitioners the deities are very real, however, each corresponding to a particular energetic presence that can be palpably felt in meditation and even at other times. The *tāntrikas* tap into those energetic presences to accomplish their goal of self-transformation, to block or dispel negative forces impinging upon them, and also to help others in their spiritual life or material struggles.

The Tantric *sādhakas* are thoroughly at home in the subtle dimension of existence, and the adepts are masters of the energetic forces present in the invisible realms. From their vantage point, ordinary people are purblind, ignorant of the many forces that infiltrate and manipulate the flatland universe in which they live. As the *Bhagavad-Gītā* (2.69) puts it:

> That which is night for all beings, therein is the self-controlled practitioner (*samyamin*) awake. That in which beings are awake is night [i.e., irrelevant] for the seeing sage.

Terms like "primitive polytheism" that have been applied to Tantra and Hinduism in general are ready-made labels that fail to do justice to the actual situation. The masculine and feminine deities worshiped in the Tantric rituals are personifications of specific intelligent energies present in the subtle dimension. Beyond this, the Tantric practitioners also understand that the gods and goddesses are ciphers, symbols that point beyond their immediate forms of manifestation to the absolute Godhead, the singular Being. In the scriptures, and in ritual worship, the boundaries between intelligent energy, personified symbol, and the divine background are often blurred. Thus the Tantric adepts also regard the deities as so many distinct but related aspects of the same Reality. When they invoke a particular deity, they mentally bridge the gulf between the personal and the impersonal, the concrete and the abstract, as well as the psychological and the ontological. They are cognizant of the singular Being looming large behind or shining through a specific deity. It is in fact the radiant omnipresence of Being that imbues a deity with sacredness and special significance. Yet the *tāntrikas* are well aware that a deity is a limited being and not the ultimate Reality itself. Gods and goddesses can, however, become portals to that Reality.

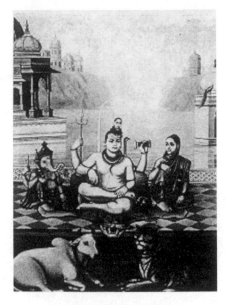

Lord Shiva and his consort Pārvatī.

In the *Tantras,* which comprise the two broad categories of *Āgamas* and *Nigamas,* various deities lend their name to the singular eternal Being. For instance, in the *Āgamas*, it is most often Shiva—but also Bhairava, Ganesha (Ganapati), and Vishnu—who is celebrated and worshiped as the Ultimate. In the *Nigamas*, the pure Being-Consciousness is characteristically remembered in its feminine guise as the Mother Goddess, or Power (*shakti*), under a diversity of names—Devī, Kalī, Durgā, Umā, Lakshmī, Kubjikā, and others. Together with the name, a deity's diverse attributes often are also bestowed on the Absolute, though always with the understanding that in its essence the Godhead is beyond all possible descriptive labels and categories. Such personifications of the Divine are in the service of devotion (*bhakti*), which Tantric practitioners cultivate to varying degrees. Especially most Shaiva schools of South India—the Siddhānta tradition—emphasize a devotional approach and insist that there is a subtle but definite divide between the ultimate Lord and the supraconscious Spirits. Yet even the practitioners of more strictly nondualist Tantra are steeped in the age-old mythology associated, for instance, with Shiva. They may draw on it for their devotional life, while at the same time being intellectually convinced of the featureless singularity of the ultimate Reality.

In this vein, many *Tantras* are presented as direct communications from Lord Shiva. They describe him as being seated on top of the paradisiacal Mount Kailāsa, the world mountain, in the company of his beloved spouse, recipient of his teachings. The *Mahānirvāna-Tantra* (1.1–2, 5–10), which is a relatively recent text, begins with these evocative words:

> At the beautiful summit of the foremost mountain, resplendent with various gems, covered with various trees and creepers, resounding with the songs of various birds,
>
> redolent with the fragrance of flowers from all the seasons, most delightful, fanned by plentiful cool, aromatic, slow breezes, . . .
>
> peopled by hosts of adepts, bards, celestial nymphs, and followers of Ganapati, there was the silent God, world teacher of moving and immobile things,
>
> who is ever benevolent, ever blissful, an ocean of ambrosial compassion, white like camphor or jasmine, consisting of pure *sattva*, all-pervasive,
>
> space-clothed [i.e., naked], lord of the destitute, master of *yogins,* beloved of *yogins*, upon whose topknot the Ganges splashes, who is adorned with locks of hair,
>
> besmeared with ashes, peaceful, wearing a garland of snakes and skulls, with three eyes, who is lord of the three realms, holding a trident,
>
> who is easily appeased, full of wisdom, bestower of the fruit of liberation (*kaivalya*),[1] formless, fearless, undifferentiated, untainted,
>
> the hale doer of good to all, God of gods. Seeing Shiva with his serene face, Goddess Pārvatī bowed respectfully and for the benefit of the entire world asked him [to teach her].

Then follow Shiva's teachings and further questions from his divine spouse, with yet more answers. This pleasant literary device is meant to convey to the reader that the contents of this *Tantra* is authentic, revelatory, and sacred. As Shiva declares at the conclusion of his teachings:

> In reply to your questions I have completely revealed in this *Tantra* what was the most secret discipline (*sādhanā*) and the most excellent knowledge. (14.200)

Then Shiva makes this promise:

> By listening to this great *Tantra*, he who is as it were blinded by ignorance, who is dull, or who is duped by action is released from the bonds of karma. (14.205)

The *Mahānirvāna-Tantra* is not unique in making such a claim. The study of the Tantric literature is thought to awaken the will to liberation, which in turn motivates the initiates to apply themselves diligently to the various Tantric practices. In due course their efforts will bear fruit, and then Shiva's promise will have been fulfilled.

All *Tantras* share this quality of optimism. They also uniformly assert that their revealed teachings are to be kept secret, as they must not fall into the hands of unprepared individuals who would neither appreciate nor benefit from them and for whom they could possibly even prove harmful. This admonition should be borne in mind by Westerners who attempt to practice Tantra without proper initiation and the lifelong commitment and responsibility this entails.

PARAMA-SHIVA: *the Ultimate Reality*

When the *Tantras* mention Shiva, they most often intend the Godhead, the ultimate Reality, or Parama-Shiva.[2] They characterize it as *sac-cid-ānanda*,[3] or Being (*sat*), Consciousness (*cit*), and Bliss (*ānanda*). What is meant by this? Being is the totality of existence, the Whole (*pūrna*). As we can readily appreciate, we experience only a minuscule slice of what there is. Our perception is confined to a fairly narrow range of frequency. We do not hear the full range of the pulsed shrieks of bats or the ultrasound echolocation of dolphins, nor the low-frequency calls of elephants. We do not have the visual acuity of an eagle, nor can we see into the infrared or the ultraviolet spectrum. Our taste buds are not as efficient as those of fish, which have taste buds over their entire skin surface, and compared to a dog, our sense of smell is exceedingly poor. Understandably, we tend to regard the sliver of existence we experience through our senses as if it were the entire cosmos. If we fail to check this naive attitude, however, we end up with an impoverished materialist philosophy that stunts our spiritual growth and keeps us entrapped in *samsāra*. To avoid this pitfall, we must resort to reason and intuition.

Accomplished *tāntrikas* generally enjoy greatly enhanced sensory and mental capacities, and therefore their testimony about the hidden or subtle aspects of existence carries weight. They all agree not only that the material world is a fraction of what there actually is but also that it constitutes the lowest vibratory level of cosmic existence. For them Parama-Shiva, the all-encompassing Being, is both utterly transcendental (*vishva-uttīrna*, written *vishvottīrna*) and immanent or "world shaped" (*vishva-maya*). The ultimate Reality is unfathomable creative vibration (*spanda*), the basis for all distinct vibrations composing the countless objects of the subtle and the material realms. David Bohm, one of the finest minds in modern physics, described reality as movement that occurs as "a series of interpenetrating and intermingling elements in different degrees of enfoldment *all present together.*"[4] This comes very close to the Tantric notion of Reality, which is omnipresent vibrancy. What is missing from Bohm's definition, though, is that this dynamic Being is supremely conscious.

The Tantric adepts speak of the ultimate Reality as *cit* ("conscious" or "consciousness"), *caitanya* (that which is conscious), or *parā-samvid* (supreme knowing), or *hridaya* (heart). The last designation is particularly interesting, as it connects with an age-old spiritual tradition that regards the human heart as the seat of consciousness. Thus the heart is the gateway to the Heart. To a spiritual practitioner, the term "heart" conveys "that which I truly am," which is not the body and not the mind, but pure Being-Consciousness-Bliss.

The transcendental Consciousness or Awareness is of course

quite distinct from what we mean by these terms in ordinary contexts, for in the ultimate Being there is no differentiation into subject and object. Our day-to-day experience of self-awareness is the closest approximation that we have to the self-illuminating nature of Being. *Cit* is eternal, pure, luminous Intelligence, which continuously illumines the myriad forms that make up its infinitude and are not different from it.

Parama-Shiva is described as being constituted of *prakāsha* and *vimarsha*. The former term means "luminosity," while the latter term stands for "examination." *Prakāsha* is the Light of lights, which has no source but is the source of everything. *Vimarsha* (from the verbal root *mrish*, "to touch") is the divine "mirror" in which the eternal Light is reflected. Without it, the supreme Light would never shine into any worlds or human hearts. It would be impotent. *Vimarsha*, the self-reflecting nature of Being, is responsible for creating the multidimensional cosmos in which the supreme Light manifests as lesser lights, or objects. To use another metaphor, it is a crystal splitting the singular Light into its inherent spectrum of colorful light that makes up the universe in all its many layers. Our own self-awareness replicates this mirroring capacity within Being itself. This allows us to stand back from our activities, examine them, and, ultimately, trace our way back to the Source Light.

Parama-Shiva is infinitely potent, the possessor of all powers (*shaktimat*). The five most important powers (*shakti*) intrinsic to the ultimate Reality are self-revealing Consciousness (*cit*), absolute Bliss (*ānanda*), unlimited Will (*icchā*), total Knowledge (*jnāna*), and universal Dynamism (*kriyā*). The notion of the inherently blissful nature of Reality is particularly attractive to those of us who are enmeshed in the conditional realms, which are full of suffering. This bliss, to be sure, has no object. When we are happy we are, by and large, happy *about* something. Our happiness is dependent on an outside agency and therefore is rather limited and short-lived. Only when we have developed a measure of contentment do we become independent of outside emotional nourishment. Our search winds down, and we begin to discover the joy within ourselves, which is an intimation of the unsurpassable bliss of Being.

Parama-Shiva's unlimited Will stands for omnipotence, while total knowledge stands for omniscience. By universal Dynamism is meant Parama-Shiva's capacity to assume any form whatsoever. Together the five powers (*shakti*) inherent in the ultimate Reality are the foundation for both self-concealment and self-revelation, the two aspects of Being by which it becomes immanent while yet remaining transcendental and whole.

SHIVA: *The Principle of Consciousness*

Shiva, as opposed to Parama-Shiva, is that aspect of the ultimate Reality which is Consciousness. It is pure subject, pure "I," without the slightest notion of "I *am*," or "I am *this*," or "I am *here*." Hence the philosophers of Kashmiri Shaivism also call this aspect *ahamtā*, or "I-ness." The great Tantric adept and scholar Abhinava Gupta assigns to Shiva, stationed at the heart, the mantric sound value *aham* (meaning "I"). From the perspective of evolution, the Shiva principle (*shiva-tattva*) is the first emergent within the ultimate Reality. It contains potentially all other subsequent principles or categories of existence, but manifests only the aspect of Consciousness without an object. This very first ontological principle must be carefully distinguished from the "I-maker" (*ahamkāra*), which comes much later in the evolutionary process from the One to the Many. In a certain sense, the ego is a stepped-down version of the transcendental "I." Shiva is the result of a preeminence of the fundamental power of consciousness (*cit-shakti*) inherent in Parama-Shiva. Admittedly, the word "preeminence" is somewhat misleading, because it evokes spatial imagery, whereas Shiva exists prior to space and time. But when talking about these metaphysical realities, we must resign ourselves to the limitations of language and be willing to resort to paradox and not entirely fitting metaphor.

In his *Tantra-Āloka* (3.201), Abhinava Gupta speaks of Shiva as the "Mother and Father" of the cosmos and as the universal agent. It is Shiva who (or which) is the seed of the multidimensional universe, giving rise to all other ontological categories. But there is no duality in Shiva, because he is still completely immersed in blissful union with Shakti.

SHAKTI: *The Principle of Energy*

Shakti, the second aspect or principle within the ultimate Reality, is the principle of creativity. Although it is typically listed after the Shiva principle, Shakti coexists with Shiva and cocreates the universe. It would therefore be incorrect to consider it as an emergent principle, or evolute. Therefore, in some schools Shakti is not listed as a separate principle but is described together with the Shiva principle.

If counted separately, Shakti is understood to be a manifestation of the Bliss aspect of the ultimate Reality. On that supreme level, it is the mirror in which Consciousness, the Shiva principle, is reflected. As such it also is the seed for the subsequent division into subject and object, experiencer and experience. It is also known as *spanda-shakti* or ultimate vibratory energy. As Shakti triggers the process of evolution or progressive manifestation, she obscures Consciousness. This bears the technical term *nimesha*, or "closing," as opposed to *unmesha*, or "opening," which describes the process involved in revealing the true nature of Shiva accompanying the dissolution of the cosmos either macrocosmically (at the end of a world cycle) or microcosmically (in meditation).

Concealment and revelation, or closing and opening, are relative terms that are primarily meaningful to the Tantric practitioners in reorienting their life. Philosophically, we need to appreciate that the evolution or emanation of the *tattvas* occurs within the ultimate Reality. As Jaideva Singh, one of the finest contemporary interpreters of Kashmiri Shaivism, explains in his commentary on the *Spanda-Kārikā* (1.2):

The world is not contained in Him as a walnut in a bag where the walnut has its own independent existence and the bag for the time being contains it. The world has no separate existence from Śiva as the walnut has from the bag. So also when we say that the world has come out from Him, it is not meant that the world has come out from Him as a walnut comes out from a bag where both the walnut and the bag are separate from each other. The world and Śiva are not two separate entities. Śiva is the world from the point of view of appearance, and the world is Śiva from the point of view of Reality.[5]

Another point that needs to be fully appreciated is that the veiling effect of Shakti does not block Shiva from our view entirely, or else spiritual life would be impossible. As a species, we can glimpse enough of our true nature—as Being-Consciousness-Bliss—that we can dedicate ourselves to its full recovery. We are free to rediscover our essential being, just as we are free to deny it and live the inauthentic life of the ordinary worldling, who follows the dictate of self-delusion (*moha*), greed (*lobha*), and aggression (*krodha*), as well as all the other *karma*-engendering negative emotions and attitudes. We are free to be free, just as we are free to be in bondage to our karmic conditioning. Tantra is a path to authenticity, integrity, and transparency beyond all mental limitation or emotional blockage. It is a means to realizing our innate freedom and splendor as Shiva-Shakti.

THE DIVINE LOVE PLAY AND CREATION

Hindu iconographers have made various attempts to depict in three-dimensional form the zero-dimensional relationship between Shiva and Shakti. One popular image is that of Ardhanārīshvara (lit. "Half-Woman-Lord"),[6] which is sometimes wrongly described as hermaphroditic. The left half of this figure is depicted as a female with one ample breast, while the right half is depicted as a male, often holding Shiva's trident. Obviously, this image is only a very imperfect depiction of the "union" between Shiva and Shakti, which is a seamless continuity of Consciousness and Power within one and the same

Reality. Even the term "polarity" does not describe this transcendental situation accurately. A somewhat more fitting analogy would be that of a hologram that yields one image when viewed from a certain angle and another image when viewed differently.

The same limitation inherent in the Ardhanārīshvara image also applies to Tantric paintings or statues depicting Shiva and Shakti in intimate embrace. Usually voluptuous Shakti sits astride her beloved's lap, wrapping herself around him like a creeper in what the Tibetans call the *yab-yum* (mother-father) position, face turned blissfully upward. This graphic motif suggests sexual love, which makes sense, since for many people sexual union affords the only experience of unity. When they lose themselves in the arms of their lover, they experience at least a semblance of the ego-transcending consciousness of the Tantric adept. It is therefore not surprising that so many Neo-Tantrics in the West look upon Tantra as a sexual discipline promising pleasure beyond all expectation, mostly in the form of prolonged or multiple orgasms. Neo-Tantrics seek to emulate the divine couple but typically forget that the union between Shiva and Shakti is transcendental and therefore also asexual. The fruit of their union—and hence also the goal of Tantra Yoga—is not bodily orgasm, however overwhelming, but perpetual bliss far beyond anything the human nervous system is capable of producing.

A third motif often exploited in paintings and sculptures is that of the reclining Shiva, with Shakti (mostly in the form of the fear-instilling goddess Kālī) towering above him, with weapons in her hands, a garland of skulls around her neck, protruding tongue dripping with the blood of her victims. This image gives us the most penetrating glimpse into the Shiva-Shakti symbolism. Here Shiva is depicted with a massive erection, yet with a body besmeared from toe to crown with ashes, clearly suggesting that he is indifferent to his sexual arousal and the world at large. The pale, almost translucent white color of his skin suggests the luminosity of the Divine. It is no accident that he resembles a corpse, lying in what is called the corpse posture (*shava-āsana*), for the image strongly points to a practice at the very heart of Tantra that many Western observers have found

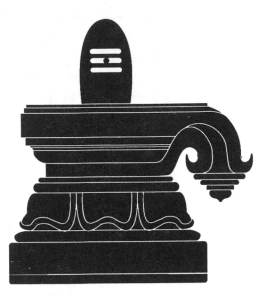

The *yoni-linga*, symbolizing the divine intercourse
between Shiva and Shakti. (ILLUSTRATION COURTESY
OF *HINDUISM TODAY*)

rather disquieting. This is the old custom of left-hand *tāntrikas* to
receive initiation from a female adept in the graveyard. The Tantric
male practitioner emulates Shiva, who is dead to all passion and pure
Consciousness. Even his blood is turned to ashes—a symbol of utter
dispassion.

A vastly simplified form of the divine intercourse between Shiva
and Shakti is the *yoni-linga* symbol, which can be drawn, painted, or
carved. It consists of a round or oval shape in whose center an upright
linga is placed. These represent the male and female generative organs
and their corresponding creative energies. The *yoni* (vulva) stands for
Shakti, energy, immanence; the *linga* ("mark" or "phallus") represents Shiva, consciousness, transcendence. Their juxtaposition symbolizes the creative union as a result of which multiplicity can arise
within the simplicity of Parama-Shiva. This particular imagery has also
been incorporated into the description of the psychoenergetic center
at the base of the spine, the *mūlādhāra-cakra*. This is the seat of the

serpent power, the localized presence of the nonlocal Shakti. The serpent power is depicted as being coiled three and a half times around a *shiva-linga*.[7] The spiral coils again suggest the inherent dynamism of Shakti.

Another strong image that is widely used in Tantra to depict the complementary relationship between Shiva and Shakti is the *shrī-yantra*, described in more detail in chapter 1 3. Here the five upward-pointing triangles represent Shiva, the four downward-pointing triangles Shakti. Their interweaving, giving rise to a total of forty-nine triangles, stands for cosmic existence as a whole.

What is significant for the present discussion is that in Hindu Tantra Shakti plays the active role, whereas Shiva, although aroused by Shakti's love play, remains passive and cool.[8] He manifests the absolute stillness of Consciousness; she expresses the unlimited potency of Power or Energy. Together they symbolize the play of life and death, creation and annihilation, emptiness and form, dynamism and stasis. This interplay is found on all levels of cosmic existence because, as we have seen, it preexists in the ultimate Reality itself. As we move down the ladder of cosmic existence—from the transcendental to the subtle to the coarse levels of manifestation—the transcendental "polarity" increasingly becomes one of stark oppositions. The Sanskrit texts refer to the *dvandvas* (two-twos), which are pairs such as light and dark, hot and cold, moist and dry, but also praise and blame, fame and obscurity, and so on. Tantric practitioners must learn to master these by raising their consciousness from the material plane to the transcendental dimension of existence, which is characterized as *nirdvandva,* or beyond all opposites. In this connection Carl Gustav Jung, archetypally voicing the Western approach to life, made these relevant comments:

> The Indian's goal is not moral perfection, but the condition of *nirdvandva.* He wishes to free himself from nature; in keeping with this aim, he seeks in meditation the condition of imagelessness and emptiness. I, on the other hand, wish to persist in the state of lively contemplation of nature and of the psychic images. I want to be freed neither from human beings, nor from myself,

nor from nature; for all these appear to me the greatest of miracles.[9]

Jung's observations suggest an orientation that approximates the ideal of what the Hindu scriptures call *prakriti-laya,* the state of absorption in the ground of nature. This term is also applied to those adepts who, by virtue of their single-pointed contemplation of nature, have merged with the transcendental core of nature rather than with Being-Consciousness-Bliss itself. Jung favored manifestation and diversity over the unqualified simplicity of the ultimate Reality. His critique of the Indian point of view, however, fails to appreciate that Hinduism includes not merely verticalist paths but also integral traditions such as Tantra.

The Tantric tradition, as we have seen, offers a positive evaluation of the manifest realms, which all arise within and as the Divine. True, the Tantric practitioners, like the adherents of what I have called verticalist traditions, endeavor to free themselves from the constraints of the world of opposites. However, they do not seek merely to escape the manifest realms but to master them from the vantage point of Self-realization, or liberation. Hence the great adepts of Tantra are all masters of the subtle dimension of existence. They "possess" not only the ultimate power (*siddhi*) of liberation but also the whole range of paranormal powers (also called *siddhi*) by which they master the conditions of the various subtle planes. From a Tantric point of view, Jung's chosen path remains on the level of intellectual fascination, which in the final analysis is a karmic state of mind. As such it is subject to the blinding power of *māyā.*

To return to the main discussion: Ontologically speaking, the "polarization" of the ultimate Reality into Shiva and Shakti is the matrix for the opposites experienced at the level of conditional reality. All polarities and dualities—notably male and female—that we can possibly encounter in the world are precontained in the Shiva-Shakti dimension. Psychologically speaking, the unitive relationship of Shiva and Shakti can be understood as a symbol for intrapsychic unity or, in Jung's terms, the integration of *animus* and *anima.* We could say that because Shiva and Shakti are ultimately in perfect union, we are capable of achieving a similar union within our psyche. Conversely, because the ultimate Reality has these two aspects, our psyche also exhibits a feminine and a masculine side. As above, so below. As without, so within. Tantric metaphysics is also a metapsychology with far-reaching practical implications.

The Guru Principle

SHIVA INCARNATE

The *guru* is Brahma; the *guru* is Vishnu;
the *guru* is God Maheshvara [i.e., Shiva].
He is the ferry [leading across]
the ocean of existence.
Only the *guru*, [who is ever] tranquil,
is the supreme Condition.
 —*Shrī-Tattva-Cintāmani* (2.36) of Pūrnānanda

THE GURU AS DIVINE AGENCY

Tantra is strictly an initiatory tradition, which means that its sacred and secret teachings are passed on in the age-old fashion of oral transmission from teacher to disciple. In this respect, Tantra is markedly different from Neo-Tantrism, which is all too often practiced and promulgated by enthusiasts who have not been properly initiated but have acquired their knowledge largely from books. But as the *Mahābhārata* (12.293.25) stated long ago, books are a burden so long as we do not know the reality behind their words. No amount of intellectual learning is liberating. The *Yoga-Shikhā-Upanishad* (1.4) even speaks of the "snare of textbooks" (*shāstra-jāla*). In the *Yoga-Bīja* (9) we can read:

> Those who through [their study of] endless logic, and grammar, and so on, have fallen into the snare of the textbooks become mentally confused.

The *Vīnā-Shika-Tantra* (137) points out that books are easy to come by, but the rules for actual practice are difficult to obtain. Without knowledge of the correct execution of the Tantric practices, however, especially *mantra* recitation, there can be little hope of success. It is, however, also true that the Tantric tradition has produced a large number of texts. Obviously the *sādhakas* and *siddhas* who composed them must have felt that the written word might be helpful to other practitioners.

In any case, the Tantric authorities are insistent that only that instruction which has been received directly from the teacher's mouth is potentiated and can bring genuine inner growth. "Initiation," declares Shiva himself in the *Mantra-Yoga-Samhitā* (5), "is the root of all victory." He goes on:

> O Goddess! He who is bereft of initiation can have no success and no fortunate destiny. Therefore one should endeavor to seek initiation from a [qualified] teacher.

The Tantric adepts consider initiation (*dīkshā*) crucial to one's progress on the spiritual path. And for initiation to be truly empowering, it must be granted by a qualified Tantric master. Such a master is known as a *guru*. This Sanskrit word is used both as a noun and as an adjective. Etymologically, it is derived from the verbal root *gur*, meaning "to be heavy." Thus the *guru* is someone whose wisdom or counsel is, by virtue of his or her personal attainment, weighty or of decisive importance to the spiritual process as it unfolds in the disci-

ple. Put more colloquially, the *guru* is a spiritual heavyweight. Esoterically, the word *guru* is explained in the *Kankāla-Mālinī-Tantra*
(1.17–18) as follows:

> The sound *gu* denotes "darkness." The sound *ra* [i.e., *ru*]
> denotes "causing the restriction of that [darkness]." Because he
> removes darkness, he is called a *guru*.

> The letter *ga* is said to denote "bestowing success (*siddhi*)."
> The letter *ra* denotes "removal of sin." The letter u denotes
> Vishnu, the triple Self, the teacher himself.

Here sin stands for the karmic tendency to perpetuate egoic
existence, as opposed to being present as the Self. The *guru* is the
agent who dispels spiritual blindness and through his or her transmission and teaching safely conducts the disciple to perfection (*siddhi*).
Little wonder that the Tantric scriptures pay considerable attention
to the figure and role of the *guru*.

Another esoteric etymology is given in the *Guru-Gītā* (46):

> The syllable *gu* [means] "transcending the qualities (*guna*)";
> the syllable *ru* [means] "devoid of form." He who grants the
> essence of transcending the qualities [of Nature] is known as a
> *guru*.

Nature is composed of three fundamental qualities (*guna*), representing the principles of luminosity, dynamism, and inertia respectively. Their interplay is responsible for all manifest existence,
including our chronically overactive mind. Self-realization, or liberation, presupposes transcendence of these basic forces. The teacher's
great gift to the disciple is the gift of pure witnessing prior to the
play of the *gunas*. In the *Shiva-Sūtra-Vārttika* (3.27) of Bhāskara, the
accomplished adept is said to wear the qualities like the sacred thread
worn by brahmins.

One way of explaining the function of the *guru* is to say that he
or she plants the seed of enlightenment in the disciple, which then
can be made to sprout and ripen through the tender care of the
disciple's daily spiritual discipline (*sādhana*). This function is what the

Tantras and Yoga scriptures call the grace of the teacher (*guru-kripā* or *guru-prasāda*). The *Shiva-Samhitā* (3.11 14) contains these stanzas:

[Only] knowledge imparted from the *guru's* mouth is productive [of liberation]; otherwise it is fruitless, weak, and the cause of much affliction.

He who makes an effort to please the *guru* [through his dedication to self-discipline and service] receives the [secret] knowledge. In due course he will also obtain the fruit of that knowledge.

The *guru* undoubtedly is father, the *guru* is mother, the *guru* is deity (*deva*). Therefore one should follow him in all one's actions, thoughts, and speech.

By the *guru's* grace one obtains everything auspicious. Hence one should always follow one's *guru*, or else there will be no benefit.

To practice Tantra Yoga without the initiatory grace of an adept amounts to a Sisyphean task; uninitiated seekers are engaged in pushing the massive boulder of their own *karma* uphill, and what awaits them in the end is either discouragement or self-delusion. Only the graceful intervention of an adept both lessens the weight of the karmic boulder and infuses the practitioner's muscles with the necessary strength to reach the top of the mountain of inner growth. Because spiritual initiation is not a concept in our modern Western culture, however, few people can appreciate the unique opportunity this represents. Instead they worry about issues of power and exploitation. Their concerns have been fueled in recent years by exposés in the news media about the irresponsible and even abusive behavior of several well-known spiritual teachers. But these frailties say nothing about the tradition of initiation itself, which is as potent and relevant as ever.

Whatever liabilities exists in the *guru* tradition, these pertain to individuals and not to the initiatory system as such. To illustrate this point, consider mathematics. It is a perfectly valid symbol system. But there are good and not-so-good math teachers, who either succeed or fail (sometimes completely) to communicate that system and its intrinsic intellectual beauty to their pupils. Once the principles of mathematics are grasped, however, the knowledge can be thought to have been successfully communicated, and henceforth any student of a certain aptitude can master higher levels of the mathematics game.

During initiation, whether formal (in a ritual context) or informal (e.g., by a mere glance), the *guru* transmits something of his or her own essential nature—as Being-Consciousness-Bliss—to the disciple. Another, perhaps more appropriate way of putting it is to say that the *guru* creates an opening within the pupil through which he or she can more clearly intuit, or become sensitive to, the ultimate Reality. The initiatory process is an initial purification of the disciple's mind, which must then be maintained and indeed augmented through steady application to spiritual practice. The entire path to liberation can be couched in terms of a progressive catharsis of the pupil's ordinary being to the point where it is like a clear crystal that faithfully reflects the light of Consciousness. The metaphor of purification is pervasive in the liberation literature of India, as are the purificatory practices themselves.

As with the mathematics example, the spiritual seeker must bring to initiation a certain aptitude. Some people are spiritually gifted; others are less so, depending on the work they have done in previous lives. Thus some initiates experience a major breakthrough at the first moment of initiation, while in others the process unfolds underground as it were. But in each case it inevitably melts down the walls of the ego and creates an increasing resonance with one's true nature, providing the disciple seriously follows the course of disciplines laid out by the *guru*. Swami Muktananda remarked:

> The initiation performed by the Guru takes place easily and simply. The Siddhas [adepts] state that when the Guru sows the seed of Shakti, the seed develops very naturally into a tree with flowers and fruit.[1]

Whether initiation will bear the ultimate fruit of liberation in this life depends on many circumstances, chiefly the spiritual maturity of the disciple and his or her application to the given *sādhanā*.

Guru-yoga

Westerners, who are educated to be individualists, have difficulty
in grasping the concept that the *guru* is not so much a person as a
function. Of course, the *guru* function depends for its performance
on a human being, and therefore it always occurs in the context of a
particular personality. This is what is the most confusing to Western
students, who tend to get caught up in externals. Their difficulty is
greatly exacerbated by the fact that most Eastern teachers also have a
personality type shaped by their own culture, which can clash quite
severely with the Western psyche. These psychological differences
prompted Carl Jung to completely dismiss any suggestion that yogic
and Tantric practices could be useful for Westerners.[2]

The *guru*, as stated in the above quote from the *Shiva-Samhitā*, is
to be thought of as father, mother, and deity. What does this mean?
Within traditional Hindu society, *gurus* unquestionably are imbued
with parental authority, and male teachers are widely addressed as
bāba ("grandfather" in Hindi), whereas female teachers are called
mātā (nominative of *mātri*, Sanskrit and Hindi) or *mā* (Hindi), both
meaning "mother." This formality is estranging and sometimes even
offensive to independent-minded Westerner seekers. Hindu teachers
working in the West have had to make adjustments, and those who
have not been able to do so have inevitably encountered problems
with their students.

While spiritual parentalism has its intrinsic difficulties when
transplanted into a Western context, the equation of the *guru* with
God is still more problematic. Western students, who are conversant
with psychology but may not have an in-depth knowledge of Eastern
spiritual traditions, are apt to dismiss this traditional equation as ego-
inflation and as an open invitation to spiritual tyranny and exploitation. Addressing this issue, His Holiness the Dalai Lama wisely recommended that *guru-yoga,* which revolves around seeing one's teacher
as the ultimate Reality, should not be engaged by beginners.[3] Of
course, as a Tantric adept, he fully endorses this traditional practice
at more advanced levels.

The *guru* is God not in the sense of having expanded (inflated) his or her human personality to divine proportions. Rather the *guru*, having transcended (not obliterated) the personality, is capable of assuming a liberating function in regard to the disciple. In other words, the *guru*—if he or she is a *sad-guru*, or "true teacher"[4]—is fully capable of suspending personal considerations when it comes to assisting the spiritual awakening of others. It naturally helps the disciple to know that the *guru* is himself or herself liberated, or enlightened. But even if that is not the case, the disciple is traditionally encouraged to look upon the *guru* as if he or she were enlightened anyway. Thus the disciple's faith (*shraddhā*) plays a large role in the success of his or her discipleship.

Of course, it makes sense to choose one's teacher carefully. If one cannot find a fully awakened *guru*, then one must at least make certain that one's teacher possesses absolute integrity and is completely committed to assist one's own awakening. The reason for treating even an unenlightened teacher as if he or she were enlightened is straightforward: Without this assumption one would constantly question the teacher's motives, which in turn would only handicap one's spiritual practice. Moreover, if one can learn to trust the *guru*'s guidance, even when it greatly challenges one's personal preferences and perceptions, then one can learn to trust life itself, develop patience, humility, and many other virtues.

For most Western students, *guru-yoga* is the great stumbling block in their discipleship. Having been brought up to "think for themselves" and "be their own person," they confuse obedience to the *guru* with childish dependency. But the *sad-guru* is not interested in playing a parental role. The *sad-guru*'s fatherhood or motherhood toward the disciple is merely one of absolute care for the disciple's spiritual growth. The teacher in whom the "*guru* function" is alive has no other interest in the disciple than, as one contemporary adept put it, to dissolve the phenomenon called "disciple."[5]

Unfortunately, not every teacher is a *sad-guru,* and therefore it is prudent to use one's intelligence and judgment before approaching a teacher for initiation and discipleship. This has manifestly been an issue for a very long time. For instance, in the *Kula-Arnava-Tantra* (13.104–5, 107–10), composed almost a thousand years ago, the following words are uttered by Shiva himself:

> *Gurus* are as numerous as lamps in every house. But, O Goddess, difficult to find is a *guru* who lights up everything like the sun.

> *Gurus* who are proficient in the *Vedas*, textbooks, and so on, are numerous. But, O Goddess, difficult to find is a *guru* who is proficient in the supreme Truth.

> *Gurus* who know petty *mantras* and herbal concoctions are numerous. But difficult to find here on earth is one who knows the *mantras* described in the *Nigamas, Āgamas,* and textbooks.

> *Gurus* who rob their disciples of their wealth are numerous. But, O Goddess, difficult to find is a *guru* who removes the disciples' suffering.

> Numerous here on earth are those who are intent on social class, stage of life, and family. But he who is devoid of all concerns is a *guru* difficult to find.

> An intelligent man should choose a *guru* by whose contact the supreme Bliss is attained, and only such a *guru* and none other.

The *Tantras* list additional qualities to be looked for in a true teacher. To cite the *Kula-Arnava-Tantra* (13.70, 86, 88–89) again:

> O Beloved, he whose vision is stable without object, whose mind is [equally firm] without support, and whose breath is stable without effort is a *guru*.

> He who really knows the classification of the principles of existence (*tattva*) from Shiva down to the earth element is deemed a supreme *guru*.

> O Beloved, he who really knows the identity of the body (*pinda*) and macrocosm (*brahma-anda*), [the secret about] the head, and the number of bones and hairs is a *guru,* and none other.

He who is skilled in the eighty-four distinct postures such as the lotus posture and who knows the eightfold Yoga is deemed a supreme *guru*.

The "*guru* function" primarily consists in constantly and faithfully mirroring the disciples back to themselves, while at the same time strengthening their intuition of the ultimate Reality, the transcendental Self. Because of this dual aspect, the *guru*'s work with disciples is both a demolition job and a rebuilding. From the disciples' perspective this is difficult but also rewarding. In his book *Secret of the Siddhas*, Swami Muktananda mentions how when he finally received the initiatory *mantra* from his teacher, the great Bhagavan Nityananda, it produced in him both "inner heat and the coolness of joy."[6]

The ego-personality, fortified by multiply reinforced habit patterns, is singularly resistant to change, especially the kind of radical change envisioned in Tantra. Therefore, in addition to strong faith in the teacher, in the process, and in themselves, disciples also must embrace self-transformation through diligent discipline. The *guru* can lead his or her disciples to the eternal fountain, but cannot make them drink the elixir. Both grace and self-effort are needed to attain liberation.

Faith in one's teacher deepens into love (*bhakti*). Whenever Swami Muktananda, who was himself a great adept, spoke of his beloved *guru* he would inevitably break into grateful praise and poetry:

> Only when I lost myself in the ecstasy of Nityananda did I realize who he was. He is the nectar of love which arises when everything, sentient and insentient, becomes one. He is the beauty of the world. He pervades all forms, conscious and inert. He is the luminous sun, the moon, and the stars in the heavens. He frolics and sways with love in the blowing of the wind. His consciousness glimmers in men and women. There is only Nityananda, nothing but Nityananda. He is the bliss of the Absolute, the bliss of the Self, the bliss of freedom, and the bliss of love. There is only love, love, nothing but love.[7]

To arrive at such a realization, Swami Muktananda had to release the grip of the conventional ego-personality. Only when one is willing to drop all egoic barriers can the "*guru* function" do its transformative work. Then the *guru*, as Being-Consciousness-Bliss, increasingly manifests in oneself. This is why Kshemarāja in his *Shiva-Sūtra-Vimarshinī* (2.6) speaks of the "teacher as the means" (*guru-upāya*, written *gurū-pāya*). This reminds one of the famous words of the founder of Christianity who, according to the Gospel of John (14.6), declared: "I am the way, the truth, and the life."

The goal is not being swallowed by the teacher's personality but merging with his or her true nature, which is the singular Reality that also is one's own true nature. In other words, when the *guru* has succeeded in dispelling one's inner darkness, the distinction between teacher and disciple, path and goal, and even liberation and bondage fades. There is only the all-encompassing blissful Reality. As the *Mahā-nirvāna-Tantra* (14.116, 135) affirms:

> One enjoys liberation when one knows that the Self is the Witness, the Truth, the Whole (*pūrna*), all pervasive, nondual, supreme, and though abiding in the body, is not body-bound.

> Knowledge of the Self (*ātma-jnāna*), O Goddess, is the only means to final liberation. He who knows it is truly liberated in this world. There is no doubt about that.

Initiation

BRINGING DOWN THE LIGHT

The *guru*'s consciousness is activated in the disciple's
consciousness . . . thus initiation that bestows
liberation is given.
  —*Parā-Trīshikhā-Vivarana* (p. 9) of Abhinava Gupta

APPROACHING THE TEACHER

When one has found a teacher who inspires faith and hope, one
should humbly and formally approach him or her requesting initiation. According to an old Vedic tradition, the aspirant should bring
"fuel sticks" as a sign of his (or, at that time extremely rarely, her)
inner readiness to have the ego burned to ashes. But since this is the
single most important step for a spiritual seeker to take, some of
the *Tantras* recommend that one should first carefully scrutinize one's
prospective teacher, taking, if necessary, up to twelve years to do so.

The Tantric authorities do not sanction irrationalism in matters of spiritual life, because so much is at stake. Discipleship involves a lifelong commitment, or at least until one has attained liberation oneself. The *Tantras* are quite outspoken about the qualities that one should look for in a *guru*. Thus the *Shārada-Tilaka-Tantra* (2.141−44) declares:

> A good disciple intent on the highest human purpose [i.e., liberation], who has a pure disposition, purified relative to mother and father and with his senses controlled, should resort to a *guru*.

> [The teacher should] understand the essence of all the *Āgamas*, know the reality behind all the textbooks, and be dedicated to serving others, as well as be absorbed in recitation, worship, and so on.

> [The teacher should be] someone whose words are not in vain, peaceful, devoted to the *Vedas* and the import of the *Vedas*, cultivating the Yoga path, and touching the heart of the deities.

> One who is endowed with such qualities is deemed by the *Āgamas* to be a *guru*.

According to the sixteenth-century *Shrī-Tattva-Cintāmani* (2.20−21), the *guru* should not only know *mantras* and *yantras* but, more importantly, have realized the innermost Self (*adhyātman*) and hence have a tranquil mind and be a fully accomplished (*siddha*). As the *Kula-Arnava-Tantra* (13.121−24) emphasizes:

> A knower of Truth (*tattva-vid*), even though he may be lacking all identifying characteristics, is known as a *guru*. Hence a knower of Truth alone is liberated and a liberator.

> He who knows the Truth, O Great Goddess, can illumine even a "beast" (*pashu*).[1] But how can someone lacking the Truth grasp the truth about the innermost Self?

> Those who are taught by knowers of Truth undoubtedly become knowers of Truth. But those, O Goddess, who are taught by "beasts" are known as "beasts."

> Only he who has been pierced [by the Truth] can pierce others, O Goddess.[2] But he who has not been pierced cannot be a piercer. Only he who is liberated can liberate one who is bound. How can he who is not liberated be a liberator?

The Tantric authorities stress the importance of acquiring a *guru* who is part of an established teaching lineage. "The deities," states the *Kula-Arnava-Tantra* (14.5), provide protection only to those teachers who preserve a lineage (*parampara*). The Sanskrit word *parampara* means literally "one after the other," referring to the unbroken succession of teachers, all linked by the empowered teachings passed down the line from teacher to student. The same *Tantra* (14.8) advises seekers to look for a teacher who belongs to an unbroken transmission (*avichinna-sampradaya*) originating with the supreme Being—Parama-Shiva—itself.

A lineage is like an uninterrupted electric current that does not diminish in power, at least not unless there is a weak link. Sometimes when the transmission has become interrupted, a great master incarnates to revive the teachings and the teaching lineage. A well-known example is that of the Buddhist master Asanga, who, receiving teachings directly from Buddha Maitreya, succeeded in reviving the teachings of Mahāyāna. Incidentally, Asanga's sibling Vasubandhu was most doubtful of his elder brother's claim to have been taught by Buddha Maitreya himself. Yet the wisdom pouring forth from Asanga soon changed Vasubandhu's mind and attitude. Another example, within Hindu Tantra, is that of Matsyendra Nātha, the founder of the Yoginī branch of the Kaula tradition.

According to legend, as told in the *Kaula-Jnāna-Nirnaya* (16.27–37), Lord Shiva himself imparted the Kaula secrets to his son Vatuka Kārttikeya (the god Skanda), who out of ignorance threw the occult text into the ocean.[3] Then Shiva rescued the holy book by killing the fish that had swallowed it. He hid it in a secret place, but it was stolen by Kruddha (Skanda), assuming the shape of a mouse. Again it was cast into the ocean, and this time it was swallowed by a fish of gargantuan size. Shiva, assuming the form of the fisherman Matsyendra Nātha, made a net woven by Shakti, caught the monster fish, and once more recovered the teachings of the *kula-āgama* (tradition of the *kula*).⁴

The traditional emphasis on the importance of lineage is especially relevant in our modern Western context. As I have said before, Neo-Tantrism is by and large a homespun movement whose teachers have not received the teachings and the accompanying spiritual transmission within a recognized lineage. There is a great advantage in belonging to a well-established lineage, because it contains certain safeguards against corruption. A lineage is a chain of authentic teachers who pass on their wisdom and empowerment to qualified disciples (who become teachers in turn). The close bond between *guru* and disciple, which traditionally continues beyond the grave, remains intact only so long as the disciple (even if he or she has become a spiritual authority in his or her own right) preserves the integrity of the transmission, both in regard to the oral teachings and the spiritual transmission received. To affirm this continuity, the *tāntrikas* include in their daily practice the formal veneration not only of their immediate *guru* but also the *parama-guru* (teacher's teacher), the *parāpara-guru* (teacher's teacher's teacher), other lineage teachers, and not least the root *guru*, or founder of the lineage.

Whenever a *guru* gives a disciple permission to teach, this means that he or she has been judged competent to teach and pass on the teachings to others. Each *guru* has a responsibility toward the lineage as a whole and is therefore eager to preserve its integrity, which is why permission to teach is never given lightly. The fate of those who break this rule is said to be not liberation but many years in the hell realms.⁵

Just as an aspirant should be prudent in his or her search for a *guru*, so the teacher should examine the petitioning seeker with equal care, because the esoteric teachings must not be imparted to an unqualified aspirant. To give initiation to an unsuitable individual is not only useless to the disciple but also extremely dangerous to both disciple and teacher. As the *Kula-Arnava-Tantra* (14.17–18) states:

> Knowledge imparted to untrue disciples lacking devotion becomes impure like cow's milk mixed with dog's fat.

If one initiates—out of fear, greed, or for monetary considerations—someone who is unfit, one invites the curse of deities
and the act is futile.

The *Kula-Arnava-Tantra* (14.19) recommends testing a seeker for
a period of three months to a year. The *guru,* this scripture goes on
to say, should during this probationary period reverse everything in
matters concerning life, money, prostration, orders, and so on. In
other words, he or she should trick the seeker, who, on the other
hand, must understand the teacher's crazy behavior as grace. The
aspirant should never lose sight of the true reason for the teacher's
disturbing actions, even when the *guru* appears to be cruel, indifferent, and biased. The text includes being pulled about and beaten by
the teacher.

The anonymous composer of the *Kaula-Avalī-Nirnaya* (p. 2, line
2off.) makes the somber statement that fools who study its teachings
without having obtained them from a *guru* will die, and all their actions will take them straight to hell. However, initiation given properly to a well-prepared disciple, according to the *Shrī-Tattva-Cintāmani*
(2.5), is capable of removing the sins accumulated in myriad lives.
The text further states (2.7–8) that initiation will enable a brahmin
to attain *brahma-loka* (brahmic realm), a member of the warrior estate
to attain the realm of Indra, a member of the merchant estate to
attain the realm of Prajāpati, and a member of the servile estate to
attain the celestial realm of spirits. Other *Tantras* do not divide the
fruit of initiation along these social lines but affirm that anyone, regardless of his or her social status, can reach the highest goal of
liberation if duly initiated. In fact, the Tantric tradition in many ways
opposed and undermined the rigid social structure of Hinduism, and
most early teachers of Tantra came from lower castes.

According to the *Mahānirvāna-Tantra* (1.130–31), the formal request for initiation may take the following form:

O compassionate one! Lord of the wretched! To you I have
come for refuge. O you who are rich in fame, cast the shadow
of your lotus feet upon my head!

Having thus prayed and venerated the *guru* according to his best ability, the disciple should remain before him in silence with folded hands.

This kind of supplication implies that the aspirant has undergone much heart searching and is now ready to submit to a rigorous discipline and the teacher's guidance. He or she may have had several contacts with the prospective *guru* and may even have been tested in various ways. But sometimes a teacher may decide to test a seeker's commitment further by repeatedly refusing to initiate him or her. Students of Tantric Buddhism are familiar with the well-known story of Milarepa, who sought instruction from Marpa but first had to accomplish one Herculean task after another. Marpa's teacher Nāropa was likewise severely tested by his *guru,* Tilopa. But these individuals had great spiritual competence (*adhikāra*) and were thus able to endure all the many tests, which in a way were already part of their training. In most cases, however, a *guru* will be far more lenient and, assuming the supplicant meets the basic qualifications, will not withhold initiation unduly. After all, genuine teachers are never tightfisted but are ever moved by a desire to promote the ultimate welfare of others.

THE INITIATION RITUAL

The Sanskrit word for "initiation" is *dīkshā.* In his *Parā-Trīshikā-Laghu-Vritti* (25), Abhinava Gupta etymologically associates this term with the words *dāna* (giving) and *kshapana* (destroying). Initiation destroys the bonds that keep the disciple in ignorance and gives him or her self-knowledge (*sva-pratīti*) leading to liberation. The *Kula-Arnava-Tantra* (17.51) explains *dīkshā* as that which gives the divine condition (*divya-bhāva*) and wipes away character stains, the worst of which is spiritual ignorance.[6] Sometimes the word *abhisheka* (consecration) is used synonymously with *dīkshā*, but in some contexts it denotes a separate ceremony, which is held either before or after initiation.

Progress on the spiritual path is thought to be slow or even impossible without initiation. As Shiva is made to say in the *Mantra-Yoga-Samhitā* (5):

> O Goddess! There can be no success or a good destiny for one who lacks initiation. Therefore one should make every effort to receive initiation from a *guru*.

When an aspirant has been accepted for initiation, the teacher may spontaneously initiate him or her on the spot. After all, as the *Mantra-Yoga-Samhitā* (10) reminds us, the *guru* is authoritative (*svādhīna*) and endowed with all powers. It is more common, though, for a teacher to fix a place and time for a formal initiatory ritual. Most often initiation takes place at the teacher's residence, but sometimes the *guru* prefers a special holy site, such as a temple, shrine, cave, or on the banks of a sacred river. The banks of the Ganges are thought to be especially auspicious.

Ever since the time of the Buddha, the cemetery (*shmashāna*) has been another favored place, particularly of the followers of the left-hand path and certain Kaula schools of Tantra.[7] As Mircea Eliade commented:

> The role that the cemetery (*śmaśāna*), together with meditations performed while sitting on a corpse, plays in a number of Indian ascetic schools is well known. The symbolism is frequently emphasized in the texts: the cemetery represents the totality of psychomental life, fed by consciousness of the "I"; the corpses symbolize the various sensory and mental activities. Seated at the center of his profane experience, the yogin "burns" the activities that feed them, just as corpses are burned in the cemetery. By meditating in a *śmaśāna* he more directly achieves the combustion of egotistic experiences; at the same time, he frees himself from fear, he evokes the terrible demons and obtains mastery over them.[8]

The adepts of the Aghorī sect, an extremist left-hand school of Tantra, are famous in India for frequenting cemeteries, stealing skulls, and even consuming bits of corpses. Their lifestyle is a stark demonstration of the reversal of values advocated in Tantra and seeks to drive home the point that Reality transcends conventional morality.

The *aghorins,* as the practitioners of this antinomian tradition are called, are celibates and generally live a life of radical renunciation.[9] Their forerunners, the Kāpālikas, likewise indulged in unconventional practices involving the cemetery, but they were orgiastic rather than ascetic. The name *kāpālika* means "skull bearer" and refers to the custom of these initiates to carry a skull that functions as a food bowl.

In his autobiography *The World of Tantra,* Brajamadhava Bhattacharya recollects an incident that happened in 1934.[10] While immersing his newly deceased sister's body in the Ganges for a final ablution at the end of the day, he noticed a skeletal figure of a man gnawing at the charred remains of a corpse he had fished out of the water. Bhattacharya was both shocked and disgusted. Tired from the day's events, he took a nap near the cemetery gates. Startled by something, he drowsily opened his eyes and found the same man, an *aghorin,* seated in front of him. Bhattacharya, who had been initiated into Tantra at an early age, reached deep within himself to subdue the rising terror. Then the *aghorin* challenged him to overcome his judgmental mind. Suddenly, he pushed Bhattacharya over, seated himself on his chest, and started to chant *mantras.* After spitting on and all around Bhattacharya's body, he disappeared into the night as quickly as he had come. Bhattacharya never found an explanation for that extraordinary incident, but undoubtedly some form of initiation or blessing had been given.

It is possible that initiations in the cemetery were quite common in the early days of Tantra. This should not surprise us, since Tantra originated in circles outside the brahmanic orthodoxy, at the margins of society, where different notions of purity prevailed. It is also likely that the earliest teachers of Tantra were often women, especially those who earned their livelihood as washerwomen (*dombī*).

Bhattacharya's first *guru* and initiator was a woman, the "Lady in Saffron," who was a coconut vendor and apparently a Tantric adept of no small accomplishment. His reminiscences read like an adventure novel. She lived on her own, refrained from socializing, but curiously cultivated an intimate relationship with the young brahmin boy who many years later would write the aforementioned book and many others, including a two-volume history of Shaivism.[11]

Wherever the *guru* may choose to grant the initiation, including the cemetery, that place should be regarded as hallowed, appropriate, and fortunate. As the *Mantra-Yoga-Samhitā* (19) affirms, there is nothing superior to the *guru*, whose word is comparable to revelation.

In choosing the right time, a *guru* may resort to astrology, which is a very ancient craft in India. The *Mantra-Yoga-Samhitā* (11–18) gives detailed instructions about the auspicious and inauspicious astrological signs and annual seasons. Overall the best month is deemed to be Caitra (March), and solar and lunar eclipses are considered to be particularly auspicious. The time must match the specific deity and its *mantra,* which will be imparted during initiation. The *Vīnā-Shikha-Tantra* (15) favors the fourth, fifth, ninth, and especially the eleventh days of the month.

At least one day prior to initiation, the disciple must abstain from sexual activity, and he or she may also be required to observe certain preparatory rituals, such as fasting and pondering the teacher's lotus feet. According to the *Mantra-Yoga-Samhitā* (10), on the day preceding initiation, the teacher should tie the student's topknot (*shikhā*) while reciting a *mantra* for dreaming (*svāpa-mantra*), which the disciple must repeat thrice before going to sleep. The *mantra* runs as follows:

> Obeisance, victory to the Three-Eyed One, to Pingalā, the Great Self. Obeisance to the universal Rāma, Lord of Dreams. Tell me in my dreams completely the truth about what is to be done. By my grace I, Maheshvara [i.e., Shiva], bestow on you the power of action.

On the morning of the day of initiation, the disciple tells the *guru* his dreams. The following dream images are thought to be favorable: a girl, umbrella, chariot, lamp, palace, lotus, river, elephant, bull, garland, ocean, tree with fruit, mountain, horse, sacrificial meat, wine, and liquor. The last three play an important role in left-hand Tantra and also on the Kaula path. As dream images, they are bound to have a somewhat different significance in a Western context, where these

TABLE 1. THE *KULA-AKULA-CAKRA*.

WIND	FIRE	EARTH	WATER	ETHER
a, ā	i, ī	u, ū	ṛ, ṝ	ḷ, ḹ
e	ai	o	au	aṃ
ka	kha	ga	gha	ṅa
ca	cha	ja	jha	na
ṭa	ṭha	ḍa	ḍha	ṇa
ta	tha	da	dha	na
pa	pha	ba	bha	ma
ya	ra	la	va	śa
ṣa	kṣa*	laḷ†	sa	ha

For a more accurate representation of the Sanskrit alphabet, this table employs the commonly accepted scholarly transliteration of Sanskrit instead of the simplified version used in the rest of this book.

*This is strictly speaking not a letter of the Sanskrit alphabet. It serves as a substitute for the omitted *anusvara* sound (transliterated as ṃ).

†This odd duplication was presumably made to fill the gap left by the omission of the *visarga* (transliterated as ḥ), the fiftieth letter of the Sanskrit alphabet.

substances are widely used in a secular way. The teacher, too, will prepare for the initiation. He or she may, as the *Vīnā-Shikha-Tantra* (23) stipulates, stay up all night continuously reciting a *mantra* for protection.

In determining the right *mantra* for a prospective disciple, the teacher resorts to his or her intuitive knowledge of the disciple's character and spiritual destiny, but may also make use of various traditional charts (called *cakra*). Since the *mantra* is the very essence of the deity that henceforth forms the pivot of the disciple's spiritual practice, it is most important to impart the correct *mantra*. The *Mantra-Yoga-Samhitā* (21) describes in some detail the *kula-akula-cakra*,[12] which arranges the fifty letters of the Sanskrit alphabet according to the five material elements (see Table 1).

This table allows the teacher to impart the proper *mantra* corresponding to the disciple's character. For instance, if the *guru* has determined that the neophyte's essential character belongs to the ether element, then it would be appropriate to initiate him or her into the mystery of Shiva and consequently impart one of Shiva's *mantras,* such as *om namah shivāya.* The earth and water elements are deemed compatible, as are the fire and wind elements, while the ether element is thought compatible with all others. Thus it is possible to give a *mantra* that is not drawn directly from the letters found in the column showing the disciple's characteristic element but from any of the letters listed in the column of the compatible element.

Since certain days and even hours of the day are associated with specific deities, the *guru* may postpone initiation until that time. In every case, however, the vitally important ingredient of initiation is the teacher's actual empowerment of the disciple. *Mantras* that are not empowered are considered almost, if not completely, useless.

The *Vīnā-Shikha-Tantra* (25ff.) describes how the teacher designs a beautiful *mandala* with colored powder, having four gates at the cardinal directions. He or she then makes various offerings and visualizes the main deity and other deities, as well as protectors. When the sacred space has been created and the aspirant has been duly purified, the *guru* invites the aspirant into the *mandala.* Characteristically, the teacher faces east or south, with the initiate opposite, though the *Mahānirvāna-Tantra* (3.133) has the teacher facing east or north, with the disciple on the left.

Further visualization and rital worship take place, and finally the teacher instructs the neophyte in the preliminary modes of worship, the essential teachings of the school, and in some cases also in the art of breath control and meditation. After admonishing the initiate to keep the *mantra* absolutely secret, the *guru* finally imparts the *mantra* he or she has selected for the neophyte. Usually, the *mantra* is whispered into the right ear and is repeated three times. The *Mahānirvāna-Tantra* (3.132), however, prescribes that the *mantra* should be whispered seven times into the right ear of a brahmin disciple and into the left ear of disciples of all other estates or castes. This is an indication of the variation in theory and practice existing between the various schools.

The ceremony often ends with the new disciple doing a full-body prostration before the teacher who, according to the *Mahānir-vāna-Tantra* (3.137), should utter:

> Rise, dear one, you are liberated! Be devoted to the knowledge of the Absolute (*brahma*)! May you always be self-controlled, truthful, strong, and healthy!

The same *Tantra* (139) makes it clear that as soon as the disciple has received the *mantra*, his or her entire being is suffused with the deity. Henceforth, obedient to the *guru*, the disciple roams the world "like a deity." This means that the seed for the creation of the "divine body" (*divya-deha*) has been planted.

After making an offering to the *guru* of fruit, money, or his or her own being, the disciple sometimes circumambulates the *guru* three times clockwise. Then he or she will receive some of the food that was offered to the deities during the ceremony, and at last the disciple is expected to go to the temple to worship in gratitude.

THE DESCENT OF DIVINE POWER

Initiation has many forms, depending on its purpose and the particular tradition or school. According to Swami Agehananda Bharati, the contemporary Nātha order distinguishes three types of initiation: *Yoga-dīkshā* is initiation into certain yogic practices in which no *mantra* is given. *Upayoga-dīkshā* is initiation into *mantra* practice for purposes other than Self-realization. *Jnāna-dīkshā* is initiation into wisdom with the help of a *mantra*, leading to one's personal realization of the ultimate Reality.[13]

Another distinction made in the *Tantras* is between the *sāmayī-dīkshā* (conventional initiation) and the *putraka-dīkshā* (initiation of a son). The former aims at the purification of the disciple and consists of a variety of rituals, of which the *Tantra-Sāra* (13, p. 148) describes no fewer than forty-eight. The latter initiation lifts the disciple, or spiritual "son" (*putraka*), at once into a higher level of consciousness, simply by the *guru*'s grace. It is generally granted only after the conditions of the other type of initiation have been fulfilled.

The *Shrī-Tattva-Cintāmani* (2.6ff.) classifies initiation into *shāmbhavī-, shākteyī-,* and *māntrī-dīkshā*. The first is initiation that occurs spontaneously simply because of the teacher's grace and by virtue of his or her attainment of Shivahood (*shivatā*); it becomes effective through the *guru*'s mere glance, touch, or spoken word. A well-known example is that of Swami Vivekananda, who entered the state of trans-conceptual ecstasy (*nirvikalpa-samādhi*) when his *guru*, the great Ramakrishna, planted his foot on the unsuspecting disciple's chest. The second form of *dīkshā* uses the adept's inner power (*shakti*). The third and lowest form is initiation by means of a *mantra*.

The *Shārada-Tilaka-Tantra* (4.3ff.) speaks of four kinds of initiation:

1. *Kriyā-vatī-dīkshā*—initiation by means of ritual activities for all ordinary disciples; this by and large coincides with above-mentioned *māntrī-dīkshā*.

2. *Varna-mayī-dīkshā*—initiation consisting in the teacher's placing the letters of the Sanskrit alphabet into the disciple's body and thereby awakening the power of sound in him or her, leading to the awakening of the power of Consciousness.

3. *Kalā-ātma-dīkshā*—initiation consisting in the teacher's placing the *kalās* (subtle forms of energy) into the disciple's body and thereby awakening their power.

4. *Vedha-mayī-dīkshā*—initiation by "piercing," in which the *guru* focuses his or her mind on the disciple's serpent power (*kundalinī-shakti*), awakens it in the psychoenergetic center at the base of the spine, and conducts it safely to the center at the crown of the head, thereby bestowing on the disciple the gift of liberation. According to the *Kula-Arnava-Tantra* (4.64), "piercing" (*vedha*) may cause the disciple to experience intense bliss, bodily tremor, a sensation of reeling, a sense of being reborn, sudden deep sleep, or fainting.

The last three modalities are possible only in the case of extraor-dinary spiritual practitioners, who have had much preparation in this life or previous lives. Rāghava Bhatta, in his commentary on the *Shar-adā-Tilaka-Tantra* (5.121), mentions that the famous adept Utpaladeva was initiated in the fourth fashion by the great ninth-century master Somānanda.

The Kashmiri schools of Shaivism have their own fourfold classi-fication scheme, while the *Kula-Arnava-Tantra* (14.39) lists seven kinds of initiation. Other classifications are also known, but these are all very similar.[14] What they have in common is the graceful transforma-tive agency of the divine Shakti. Whether the initiate will realize the ultimate Reality at once or only gradually depends on his or her prep-aration and capacity.

The initiatory process is typically described as involving what is called *shakti-pāta*, meaning literally "descent of the power." This expression is somewhat misleading, because the divine Shakti is omni-present and does not need to go anywhere. However, from the view-point of the unliberated individual there appears to be a descent of grace, followed in due course by the ascent of the *kundalinī-shakti,* which also is a form of the divine Power. As the *Kula-Arnava-Tantra* (4.86) puts it, through the play of Shakti the "beast" (*pashu*) is trans-formed into Shiva. The same text (14.89–80, 95–96) also states:

> O Beloved! Just as iron turns into gold when penetrated by mercury, so the self attains Shivahood when its is penetrated by initiation.

> When *karmas* are burned by the fire of initiation, the fetters of *māyā* are severed. One who is without [karmic] seed and has attained the supreme condition of wisdom becomes Shiva.

> The initiate does not need to accomplish anything through asceticism, rules, or vows, nor by going to sacred places or by controlling the body.

> But, O Beloved, the recitation, worship, and other rituals of those who are uninitiated bear no fruit and are like seed sown on rock.

Because of the superlative importance of initiation, the *Tantras* unanimously advise spiritual seekers to find a teacher who will initiate them. As we have seen, the *guru* is Shiva, and as Shiva he or she comes fully equipped with Shakti. According to the *Sadyojyoti* commentary on the *Svāyambhūva-Sūtra-Samgraha* (1.2.), the ultimate Reality (Shiva) manifests as wisdom (*jnāna*) and initiation (*dīkshā*), and both are of the nature of Shakti. Like the teacher, the disciple is of course also Shiva-Shakti but is not in touch with this truth. During initiation, thanks to the mysterious alchemy of Consciousness and Energy, the disciple is reconnected with that deeper level of his or her being. From then on, the Goddess inexorably grinds away at the many layers of impurity obscuring the initiate's inner vision. Contingent on the disciple's conscious collaboration by means of steady discipline, this cathartic process will sooner or later lead to enlightenment, or liberation. The *Svāyambhūva-Sūtra-Samgraha* (2.24) declares:

> Initiation alone releases one from the extensive bondage obstructing the supreme Abode and leads upward to the Abode of Shiva (*shaiva-dhāman*).[15]

But "upward" means also "downward" and "diagonally," since the ultimate Reality is everywhere at the same time, or nowhere at any time. As the *Svāyambhūva-Sūtra-Samgraha* (3.7) itself acknowledges:

> A path is a road to be traveled. Yet there is no such road to the Lord, and there also is no feasible motion for the Spirit (*pums* = *purusha*), because both are omnipresent.

Liberation is always the case, and through the process triggered by initiation this truth will dawn on us when the mind has grown tired of constructing an alternative reality. Until then we will either remain completely caught in the web of the great limiting power of *māyā* or struggle to extricate ourselves gradually through voluntary spiritual discipline.

Discipleship

THE ORDEAL OF SELF-TRANSFORMATION

> The teacher is the first letter [of the alphabet].
> The student is the last letter. Knowledge is the
> meeting place. Instruction is the link.
> —*Taittirīya-Upanishad* (3.1.1)

THE QUALIFICATIONS OF A DISCIPLE

The *Tantras*, as we have seen, have firm ideas about the credentials of a genuine teacher. They are equally specific about the qualifications or competence (*adhikāra*) of a good disciple (*shishya*). The *Shārada-Tilaka-Tantra* (2.145–52), for instance, lists the following characteristics:

> The disciple should be noble,[1] of pure self, intent on the [highest] human purpose, well read in the *Vedas*, skillful, focused on being liberated in due course;

he should be ever benevolent toward [all] living beings, orthodox,[2] free from unorthodox views, adhering to his own duty (*sva-dharma*), lovingly striving to be good to his father and mother;

he should be fond of listening to the teacher in matters of body, speech, and mind, free from conceit about teachers, status, knowledge, wealth, and so on;

and he should be prepared to yield his life in order to obey the *guru*'s orders, giving up his own plans and always delighting in working for the teacher.

The last stanza in particular makes stipulations that modern secular readers will find troubling. Taken out of its sacred context or followed by emotionally immature disciples it indeed ought to alarm us. Within a traditional framework, however, such complete obedience to the *guru* is meant to serve as a vehicle for the alchemical process between teacher and disciple. The more *shishyas* drop their egocentric motivations, emotions, and activities, the more they are able to duplicate the *guru*'s inner state for themselves. And this is not any loss but instead an inestimable gain. The *shishyas* do not become weak-willed, mindless zombies who merely copy the teacher. Rather, they are called to realize their true nature through a process of self-understanding, self-transcendence, and self-transformation that is necessarily unique for each individual.[3]

The *Kaula-Jnāna-Nirnaya* (14.4–14) complements the above-cited description by telling us who is undeserving of the initiatic wisdom imparted by the *guru*:

O Goddess, my Beloved, this supreme *kaula* [teaching] must not be told to those who lack devotion to the *kula* and are without devotion to the teacher,[4]

nor should the essential *kaulika* [Kaula teaching] be given to pupils who are found to be slow-witted, nor to the deceitful, the doleful, the foolish, the deficient, or those scorning the truth.

One should not bestow this grace upon those who hate deities, fire, or ascetics. Those teachers who give this [secret teaching] to such pupils will fall short of perfection.[5]

But, continues the *Kaula-Jnāna-Nirnaya* (14.9), those teachers who impart the liberating wisdom upon duly qualified disciples will be long lived. This statement alludes to the extremely close connection between *guru* and *shishya*. Once initiation has been granted, teacher and disciple are, in the words of a contemporary master, "joined at the hip." The *guru* in a way feeds the disciple with his or her own life substance, and if it is squandered on an unworthy pupil, the teacher's life is thought to be shortened. Reluctant or otherwise undeserving disciples are a drain on the *guru*'s energies. If the teacher is fully enlightened, he or she will always have an inexhaustible store of spiritual energy (*shakti*) to draw from, but this energy is not necessarily freely available for the maintenance of the teacher's physical body. In fact, the negative energy of an unworthy disciple acts as an obstruction for the teacher. If the blockage is severe enough, the teacher may even abandon the body to continue his or her spiritual work elsewhere, giving the disciples on the physical plane the opportunity to ripen through the hard knocks of life.

PRECONDITIONS FOR THE TANTRIC PATH

As a consequence of initiation by a qualified teacher, the spiritual seeker becomes transformed into a disciple. This is a profound change, which requires the disciple to choose awareness over unconsciousness, responsibility over negligence, and reality over self-delusion. An integral part of this new life is the adoption of the spiritual discipline recommended by the *guru*. This is the yogic path or what the *Tantras* call *sādhanā*. As I have explained in the introduction, this Sanskrit term is derived from the verbal root *sidh* ("to be accomplished"), which also forms the words *siddhi* ("accomplishment," "attainment," or "perfection") and *siddha* ("he who is accomplished/perfected").

Etymologically, the word *shishya*, generally translated as "pupil" or "disciple," means someone who is being taught or instructed. The *Kula-Arnava-Tantra* (17.30) explains it as someone who dedicates body, wealth, and life energies to the *guru* and learns (*shikshate*) from the teacher. The word stems from the verbal root *shās*, which also forms the words *sāsha* ("command"), *shāsana* ("instruction"), *shāstra* ("instruction" or "textbook"), and *shāstrin* ("scholar"). Interestingly, the same verbal root also connotes "to chastise." This conveys the close association of education with training and corrective punishment (*danda*), which is also present in the English word "discipline."

Most teachers, I would suspect, have dealt with recalcitrant disciples simply by ignoring them or asking them to leave the hermitage (*āshrama*) or monastery (*matha*). But tradition also knows of teachers who did not hesitate to administer physical punishment to wayward or lazy students. For contemporary Westerners, who operate with strong bodily boundaries, the idea of physical chastisement is abhorrent. Therefore this punitive method is also very unlikely to be effective. Yet when studying traditional accounts we must appreciate their different cultural context. More importantly, we must bear in mind that all genuine *gurus* have always been acutely aware of the supremacy of the moral virtue of nonharming (*ahimsā*). If, in bygone times, they resorted to physical punishment at all, it was with the long-range vision of wisdom.

This is perfectly illustrated in the case of the Buddhist Tantric master Marpa, who is known to have been liberal with blows for his disciples. However, it was precisely his fierce nature that brought out the best in his pupils. His rough treatment of Milarepa even provoked Marpa's wife to protest, yet it proved beneficial to this star pupil, who is fondly remembered as one of Tibet's greatest masters. Even after Milarepa had firmly attained enlightenment, he still continued to praise his guru with profound gratitude. In one of his songs, he addresses Marpa thus:

> Pray, always remember me, this ignorant disciple!
> Pray embrace me ever with your great compassion![6]

According to the *Shāradā-Tilaka-Tantra* (25.4), the foremost obligation of the disciple is to conquer the "six enemies," namely, desire, anger, greed, delusion, pride, and envy. These are the same qualifications that the *Tantras* specify for a suitable aspirant. No paradox is involved here, because the *guru* is fully aware that if an individual were to possess all these virtues, he or she would already be enlightened and no longer in need of initiation and instruction. What the teacher, therefore, is really looking for in the disciple is the relative absence of negative emotions and attitudes and the presence of at least a modicum of understanding and a healthy will to change and grow spiritually. A disciple lacking in these virtues will, as the *Mantra-Yoga-Samhitā* (8) puts it, merely bring sorrow (*duhkha*) to the teacher.

Without at least the desire for liberation, the pupil is not only unlikely to undertake the difficult task of self-transformation but is bound to experience much frustration and pointless hardship. The desire for liberation is known as *mumukshutva*, which is contrasted with *bubhukshutva*, or the desire for worldly experience exclusively. In Tantra, of course, both these impulses are not ultimately irreconcilable. The Tantric adept who has realized the ultimate identity of the world of change and the transcendental Reality—*samsāra* and *nirvāna*—is both liberated and capable of deep enjoyment of the world. But for the beginner, the challenge is to overcome worldliness and find greater delight in spiritual actualities.

To this end, the Tantric masters prescribe for their students a more or less rigorous course of disciplines, called *sādhanā*. This varies from school to school, or lineage to lineage, but it typically involves a whole range of practices, notably *mantra* recitation, prayer, ritual worship, and visualization. These various elements of the Tantric path will be discussed in more details in the following chapters. Here I am mainly concerned with the question of how they relate to discipleship in general.

All aspects of *sādhanā* are designed to chip away at the disciple's conventional ideas and subconscious tendencies. Consequently this process is of the nature of a sacred ordeal that must be endured. It is difficult for us contemporary Westerners, who tend to be afraid of pain just as we are fearful of disease and death, to grasp the underlying rationale of the initiatory process. We are inclined to look at the extremely austere life of *yogins* and *yoginīs* partly with dismissive amusement and partly with apprehension. Why, we ask ourselves, would they want to go to such length to punish themselves?

But what we regard as mere self-mortification is, for the initiates, a necessary discipline of self-limitation by which they mobilize a great deal of inner energy directed toward the radical transmutation of the personality. The *Tantras* occasionally use the ancient term *tapas* (singular case) to describe this sacred ordeal. The word means "glow" or "heat" and is widely used in the sense of "asceticism" or "austerity." In Vedic cosmogony, *tapas* is the process whereby the original Singularity (*eka*) multiplied itself, giving birth to the many-layered universe with its myriad forms. Thus the ultimate Reality itself is thought to have voluntarily undergone the ordeal of self-sacrifice in order to create the cosmos. All creation involves an element of such self-sacrifice, and therefore it is also present in discipleship, which can be understood as a comprehensive re-creation of oneself, or the creation of a new identity. Strictly speaking, the new identity that the disciple sets out to create or discover is really not new at all, but is the original and eternal Identity of all beings and things, called *ātman*, or "Self." Only for the unenlightened onlooker caught in the relativity of space-time is there the appearance of change. For the enlightened being, enlightenment is the realization that there has always been and will always be only the one self-same Reality, or Self-Identity.

Discipleship, then, is the process whereby an individual who deems himself or herself unenlightened, or bound, realizes that liberation is always the case. This awakening is dependent on self-purification, that is, on polishing the mirror of the mind. The entire game of liberation or bondage is enacted on the stage of the mind. Unenlightenment is a matter of being ignorant of what is always true of us. Discipleship is a matter of unlearning the way we think about ourselves and reality at large.

Another way of speaking about this fundamental ignorance (*avidyā*) is to say that we are typically caught in the web of our ideas about everything. Those ideas in turn shape our attitudes, which tend to crystallize into habits or tendencies. It can be rather difficult to change an idea, but to rid oneself of a habit can at times pose a seemingly insurmountable problem. Often we are even quite unaware of our habitual way of thinking and our behavioral tendencies.

Spiritual discipleship is designed to bring both into our awareness, and the *guru*—spontaneously or otherwise—seeks to undermine all the habit patterns that bind the disciple to the illusion of being a separate entity isolated from all others by the skin draped around flesh and bones. The teacher is not primarily interested in whether the disciple likes spicy food or ice-cold drinks, so long as these preferences are not habitual obstructions to his or her awakening. In principle, though, the *guru* expects the disciple to completely remodel his or her life, because then all the habit patterns are thrown into stark relief for ready self-inspection. Not being able to eat spicy food or savor ice-cold drinks can provoke a crisis and lead to significant insights into one's character (or habit patterns).

The *guru* prods the disciple wherever attachment (*sanga*) creates a block to self-understanding and self-transcendence. Attachment is the big stumbling block, at least attachment to worldly things. Tantra does not consider worldly things baneful in themselves, as they too are Shiva. The problem with attachment to them is simply that we experience them as external to ourselves, and thus they continuously reinforce our false self-identity (as the limited ego-personality rather than the universal Self). The *tāntrikas* do not seek to dissipate the energy present in attachment as such, but they redirect it to the ultimate Reality. When attachment to Shiva (or Shakti) outshines all other attachments, liberation is close at hand.

Tantric practitioners endeavor to gather all their energies into a laser beam focused on the Divine. All the many techniques and approaches of Tantra serve this purpose. They fall into two broad categories, as has been clearly enunciated in the *Yoga-Bhāshya* (1.12), which describes dispassion (*vairāgya*) and spiritual practice (*abhyāsa*) as the bipolar means for attaining liberation. All forms of Tantric discipline (*sādhanā*) contain both these aspects of the sacred work leading to inner purity (*shuddhi*). "In the purified mind," states the *Mahānirvāna-Tantra* (7.94), "knowledge of the Absolute is engendered." The Absolute (*brahman*) is Shiva, who is eternal Being-Consciousness-Bliss. Dispassion is nonattachment. In the words of the *Kula-Arnava-Tantra* (1.55):

> Nonattachment (*nihsanga*) alone is [the means] of liberation. All defects spring from attachment. Therefore one becomes happy by abandoning attachment and relying on Reality.

Practice is essentially self-purification. Until the moment when gnosis dawns, the practitioner must be completely willing to endure this cathartic process, which is enacted entirely in the disciple's mind. It consists in voiding one's mind of all impure notions (*ashuddha-vikalpa*). In the average disciple, initiation may bring an immediate, if only momentary, intuition of the glory of the ultimate Being, but will not remove impure notions permanently. Rather, the experience of duality, which marks the unenlightened state, will promptly return. This, in turn, gives rise to all the other factors by which we maintain ourselves in the state of unenlightenment.

Yet the *guru*'s grace—spiritual transmission—imparted during initiation will have opened the doorway to enlightenment, providing the disciple faithfully adopts the purificatory disciplines. The *guru*'s grace also is available to the disciple in the form of direct instruction. On this point the *Mantra-Shiro-Bhairava* (as quoted in the *Shiva-Sūtra-Vimarshinī* [2.6]) states: "The *guru*'s power resident in the *guru*'s mouth is greater than the guru himself." In other words, the *guru* is a vehicle of grace—a blessing power that exceeds his individual knowledge and talents. The *Tantras* universally acknowledge continuity of practice as one of the most important elements of a successful *sādhanā*. As the *Yoga-Sūtra* (1.14) emphasizes, practice must be cultivated uninterruptedly and over a long period of time. Only a seasoned teacher can tell how quickly, or slowly, a disciple might be successful on the path. It is, however, considered prudent not to overestimate one's capacities and to be fully prepared to practice for any length of time.

Tantra often presents itself as the quick path, and the scriptures promise success after a certain number of years, in any case at least during this lifetime. But this always presupposes that the practitioner has the necessary karmic preconditions and is capable of Herculean exertion. Therefore "quick" means "as quickly as possible for a certain individual." Similarly, the *tāntrikas* sometimes speak of their path as "easy," yet this too is a relative term. It is easy only insofar as other paths are deemed unsuitable for the dark age (*kali-yuga*) and therefore require more of their practitioners. Tantra, as I have explained in the introduction, was from the outset specifically designed for the needs of spiritual seekers in the present dark age. Because of the overall spiritual and moral degeneracy of the *kali-yuga,* those born into it are already at a disadvantage; hence, as the *Tantras* urge, they should resort to the most potent teachings: the Tantric heritage.

In appraising the fitness (*yogayatā*) of their disciples, the Tantric adepts distinguish the following three dispositional types, or temperaments (*bhāva*):

1. The *pashu-bhāva* (beastly character) is the result of the strong interplay of *rajas* and *tamas* (the dynamic and inertial qualities of nature), with almost a complete absence of *sattva* (lucidity factor). This fateful combination produces such undesirable traits as delusion (*bhrānti*), enervation (*tandrā*), and indolence (*ālasya*). Yet not every individual of this type will necessarily manifest these tendencies. According to the *Kula-Arnava-Tantra* (13.90), the *pashu* is bound by eight bonds (*pāsha*), namely, contempt, doubt, fear, self-consciousness (*lajjā*), disgust, family, custom, and caste. It would not be difficult to apply all of these to a contemporary Western context.

The psychological immaturity responsible for these traits disqualifies practitioners of the "beastly" temperament from certain rituals and practices. They are expected to adopt a more conventional approach to spiritual life and are particularly excluded from the ritual of the "five substances" (*panca-tattva*), which are explained in chapter 14. According to the *Kaula-Avalī-Nirnaya* (p. 11), they should not even mentally participate in this ritual. Instead they should make every effort to serve the *guru* in order to purify their inauspicious traits. The "beastly" temperament is not uniformly explained in the *Tantras*, presumably because many, if not most, practitioners fall into this category. Often the term *pashu* denotes practitioners who practice Tantra in a more conventional way, that is, treating the "five substances"—meat, fish, wine, grain, and sexual intercourse—literally rather than figuratively. Notably, in place of actual sacred intercourse with women initiates, male practitioners make an offering of two kinds of flowers representing the male and female sexual organ respectively.

2. The *vīra-bhāva* (heroic character) is the product of the interplay of predominantly *rajas* and *sattva*, with minimal interference from *tamas*. According to the *Mahānirvāna-Tantra* (1.54), practitioners of this temperament alone are suitable for the practice of Tantra. This scripture even denies the existence of the other two temperaments in the dark age, but this makes little sense, since the characteristics of the "beastly" temperament appear widespread.

3. The *divya-bhāva* (divine character) is also the product of the interplay of *rajas* and *sattva*, but with the latter quality predominating. Practitioners who have this godlike character are very rare, especially in the *kali-yuga*. The difference of this character from the heroic temperament seems to be one of degree, with the latter being more dynamic, which suits the Tantric approach well.

Tantra is the path of the spiritual hero (*vīra*), who is defined as follows:

> Because he is free from passion, pride, affliction, anger, envy, and delusion, and because he is far removed from *rajas* and *tamas* [i.e., the qualities of agitation and inertia], he is called a "hero."[7]

According to the *Kaula-Avalī-Nirnaya* (p. 11), the heroic practitioner has gone beyond the play of opposites in the mind. This is an important requirement, considering that Tantra often employs unconventional means that might otherwise entrap the practitioner in feelings of guilt or awkwardness. The Tantric hero must be immune to social disapproval or ostracism and firmly stay on the path regardless of any opposition or adversity. In the dark age, declares the *Mahānirvāna-Tantra* (4.19), only the heroic discipline (*vīra-sādhanā*) bears visible fruit. For this scripture, the heroic discipline is that of the prominent Kaula school, which I will introduce in the next chapter.

The Tantric Path

RITUAL AND SPONTANEITY

> Take the wisdom that grows on Shiva's
> soil, possesses special desirable qualities,
> is medicine for oneself, and leads to joy.
> —*Shata-Ratna-Samgraha* (5) of Umāpati Shivācārya

FIRST STEPS ON THE PATH

The Tantric path unfolds as a play between fluid responsiveness to the everyday challenges of *sādhanā,* or spiritual discipline, and adherence to the traditional forms of one's particular school or lineage. The situation is comparable to playing a virtuoso piece of classical music, where creative self-expression occurs within the overall structure of the musical score. Most schools of Tantra are highly ritualistic, but it is understood that this must not kill the disciple's spontaneity, without which inner growth could not take place. The numerous observances and formalities that are integral to the Tantric path are intended to stabilize the practitioner's mind and fortify his or her will.

In the previous chapter I have described the qualifications of a disciple, which are considerable. Not only must the Tantric initiate possess great strength of will and character, but he or she must also excel in faith (*shraddhā*). Once initiation has been granted, one should not doubt the efficacy of *guru* and teaching, nor the reality of liberation and one's own spiritual potential. Faith, which is no mere blind belief, is a deep-level, high-energy state of mind. The *Bhagavad-Gītā* (4.39) states that faith is in accordance with the very essence of a person. "Whatever his faith is," this scripture declares, "that verily is he." The *Yoga-Bhāshya* (1.20) likens faith to a caring mother, since it protects the *yogin and yoginī*. Vācaspati Mishra, author of the *Tattva-Vaishāradī* (1.20), speaks of faith as "the root of Yoga." The *Shiva-Samhitā* (3.16, 18–19) observes:

> Success comes to a person of faith and self-confidence, but there is no success for others. Hence practice hard.
>
> The first sign of success is confidence that [one's efforts] will bear fruit. The second is being firm in that faith; the third is worship of the *guru*;
>
> The fourth is equanimity (*samatā-bhāva*); the fifth control over the senses; the sixth is moderate eating; there is no seventh.

After faith, devotion to the teacher (*guru-bhakti*) is the single most important practice and virtue. The reason for this requirement should have become obvious by now. Without such devotion, the teacher is unlikely to transfer consciousness energy to the disciple in the Tantric initiation ritual or, afterward, transmit the necessary teachings and monitor the disciple's progress both on the physical and the subtle levels. The relationship between *guru* and disciple is of course not a business arrangement but a heart-to-heart connection. Just as the teacher is completely dedicated to awakening the student, the disciple must be willing to engage this process by cultivating loving regard for the teacher. It is through the pipeline of love and devotion that spiritual transmission flows. This must not be confused with affection or romantic attraction. Devotion to the *guru*, above all, consists of deep respect and gratitude.

The third aspect of *sādhanā* is earnest application to all the disciplines given by the teacher, however difficult, arbitrary, or incongruous they may seem. The teacher has no reason to burden the disciple with an unnecessary program of self-purification. Very likely the *guru* will recommend a course of action that has borne fruit in his or her own case, and he or she also will take the disciple's needs and abilities carefully into account. Milarepa was given the apparently senseless chore of building a tower only to have it torn down again and again. This was Marpa's way of helping his disciple to rid himself of the inauspicious karma he had acquired as a former black magician.

Underlying faith, devotion to the teacher, and application to the path comprise the fundamental understanding that the Divine is omnipresent and that one therefore must be mindful of the Truth in all circumstances. It is knowledge, whether generated through self-effort or grace or both, that is liberating. Rituals, *mantras,* and all the other practices are auxiliary means. They are designed to remove those factors from the lens of the mind that distort Reality. "In the purified heart," declares the *Mahānirvāna-Tantra* (7.94), "knowledge of the Absolute grows." While the Tantric means are numerous, knowledge or wisdom is singular, just like the Reality that it reveals.

If knowledge or wisdom is the actual liberating agent, then why should one want to pay attention to any other practices? Tantra itself includes a "noninstrumental" (*anupāya*) approach, a pathless path. Here the descent of grace automatically and promptly removes the veil of ignorance. Western students are naturally drawn to this effortless path, but they must realize that this works only for those very few who have the necessary preconditions. All others have traditionally been advised to purify themselves duly by means of whatever conventional practices may be prescribed by the teacher. In themselves those auxiliary disciplines are not liberating. According to the tenth-century Tantric master Abhinava Gupta, the limbs of Yoga can at best lead to the ecstatic state in which the contemplator achieves identification with the idealized object of contemplation (e.g., the visualized deity), though not with the object itself.[1] In other words, they are not finally liberating, because they fail to awaken pure ideation (*shuddha-vikalpa*), which springs directly from one's essential nature.

Without a teacher, who has great insight into the disciple's strengths and liabilities, there is the ever-present danger of overestimating one's spiritual capacity. Western students, who tend to be impatient, easily fall prey to self-delusion. They may practice the pathless path or "direct approach" for years, perhaps after reading a book or attending a talk or workshop, and become convinced they have attained a high state of realization. In reality, their attainment is almost entirely mental. Discipleship would quickly dispel their erroneous self-perception. As one writer observes, "even after long years of effort, relatively few people using the direct approach manage to get beyond the elementary stage of stilling the mind for a little while."[2]

Even when one has received *shakti-pāta*—and there are nowadays a number of teachers offering initiation to one and all—there still remains a great deal of work to be done in most cases. Some think that now that they have been granted initiation they can continue on their own, unencumbered by the expectations and demands of a *guru*. This in itself shows a lack of readiness and the need for instruction and discipleship. During *shakti-pāta* everything may indeed be given, but whether a seeker is able to use this awakening wisely or at all is another matter.

Knowledge of the Truth itself is the way but, as the *Kula-Arnava-Tantra* (1.107) affirms, this way must be revealed by a qualified teacher. This scripture (2.31–33) also states:

> The wisdom of *kula* shines forth, O Goddess, in a person whose impurities have dwindled through past austerities, charity, sacrifices, pilgrimages, recitation, and vows.
>
> The wisdom of *kula* shines forth, O beautiful Goddess, in one who pleases both you and me because of his devotion to deity and teacher.

The wisdom of *kula* shines forth in one who is pure minded, tranquil, engaged, dedicated to the teacher, very devotional, and hidden [i.e., capable of practicing without drawing attention to himself or herself].

THE TANTRIC PATH IN OUTLINE

The Tantric path varies from school to school. Over the centuries the Tantric masters have developed numerous *sādhanās*, all of which have led practitioners to higher realizations and possibly even liberation. For instance, the Buddhist *Sādhanā-Mālā* describes 3 1 2 distinct *sādhanās*, or programs of worship, complete with visualizations, *mantras*, and rituals. It has been estimated that about 80 percent of the subject matter in the *Tantras* deals with ritual, and this gives one a good sense of the typical Tantric approach.[3] The rituals comprise both external rituals and what is called the "inner sacrifice" (*antar-yāga*), which is the self-transcending attitude to be maintained in all respects. Together these two types form a comprehensive Yoga of self-transformation. Some *Tantras* avail themselves of the well-known model formulated in the *Yoga-Sūtra* of Patanjali, who delineated in succinct aphorisms the following eight "limbs" (*anga*):

1. *Yama*—moral restraint consisting of nonharming, truthfulness, nonstealing, chastity, and greedlessness, which are said to be valid on all levels, at all times, and everywhere

2. *Niyama*—self-restraint through purity, contentment, austerity, study, and devotion to the Lord

3. *Āsana*—posture, which makes the practitioner immune against the onslaught from the pairs of opposites (*dvandva*), such as heat and cold or dry and moist

4. *Prānāyāma*—lit. "extension of the life energy" by means of breath control

5. *Pratyāhāra*—sensory inhibition

6. *Dhāranā*—concentration, or fixing one's attention upon a selected object, be it a *mantra* or the graphic representation of a deity

7. *Dhyāna*—meditation, which is a deepening of concentration marked by a progressive unification of consciousness

8. *Samādhi*—lit. "putting together," or ecstasy, which consists in one's complete merging with the object of meditation

The *Shārada-Tilaka-Tantra* (25.5ff.), a hitherto untranslated Sanskrit text, gives an expanded interpretation of the eight limbs that differs from the definitions proffered by Patanjali in significant respects. For instance, it includes in the category of moral restraint five additional virtuous practices, namely, compassion, rectitude, patience, stability, and moderate eating, and instead of greedlessness names cleanliness (*shauca*). Rāghava, the fifteenth-century commentator on this *Tantra*, has interesting quotations that show how these virtues are applied. Thus desire is mastered by means of nonharming and chastity; anger by means of compassion and patience; greed by means of nonstealing, truthfulness, and rectitude; delusion by means of moderate eating and cleanliness; pride by means of patience and rectitude; jealousy (or envy) by means of nonharming, compassion, rectitude, and patience.

The category of self-restraint, again, is expanded to include belief in the sacred tradition, charity, worship of the deities, listening to the teachings, modesty, discernment, recitation of *mantras*, and ritual offerings.

Furthermore, while Patanjali prescribes no particular posture, the *Shārada-Tilaka-Tantra* singles out the following five to illustrate the category of *āsana*: lotus posture, *svastika* posture, thunderbolt posture, auspicious posture, and hero's posture.[4]

Prānāyāma and *pratyāhāra* are explained along more conventional lines. The former is defined as inhalation through the left channel (*idā*) for sixteen units, retention for sixty-four units while guiding the life force into the central channel (*sushumnā*), and exhalation through the right channel (*pingalā*) for thirty-two units. Breath control can be with seed (*sagarbha*) or without seed (*vigarbha*), that is, with or without accompanying mantric recitation.

Withdrawal of the senses, again, is explained as the forceful pulling back of the roaming senses from their respective objects.

This *Tantra,* moreover, explains *dhāranā* as one's holding the vital air (*prāna-marut*) in various locations of the body, such as the toes, ankles, knees, thighs, perineum (*sīvanī,* lit. "suture"), penis, navel, heart, neck, throat, uvula, nose, between the eyebrows, forehead, top of the head, and the mystical place twelve digits above the head. This technique removes obstructions in the subtle channels (*nādī*) and enhances the flow of the vital force, which in turn focuses the mind and thus permits a deepening identification with one's meditational deity.

Dhyāna, again, is defined as contemplation of one's chosen deity as the very Self. In Tantra, this practice generally stands for meditative visualization in which one's deity assumes a lifelike vividness.

In stark contrast to Patanjali, the *Shāradā-Tilaka-Tantra* explains the term *samādhi* as signifying the constant contemplation of the sameness between the individual psyche (*jīva*) and the ultimate Self. This definition illustrates the nondualistic metaphysics of this *Tantra* and is an important point of difference with Patanjali's Yoga, which is traditionally held to be plainly dualistic.

By no means do all *Tantras* subscribe to the kind of strict nondualism that, for instance, marks the *Mahānirvāna-Tantra.* In fact, the more uncompromising nondualistic metaphysics is a fairly late development within Tantra. For example, the *Āgamas* of South India favor a somewhat more dualistic metaphysics, making a clear distinction between the Lord and his creation. Early Tantra appears to have inclined toward the kind of qualified nondualism that also characterizes the teachings of many *Upanishads*. In the *Kula-Arnava-Tantra* (1.19) Shiva himself reminds us that ultimately such distinctions belong to the finite realm and are a matter of opinion:

> Some choose nondualism, others choose dualism. But they know my Reality as transcending dualism and nondualism.

On the level of practice, these philosophical distinctions are mostly quite irrelevant. While the aspirant is engaged in the process of becoming enlightened, there always is a more or less pronounced sense of duality or polarity, with the practitioner looking at the Divine, or the Self, as the object of worship and aspiration. Prior to enlightenment, the human heart seems to require an alter ego for its outpourings of love and an objective foundation for its hope and yearning. Even advanced practitioners, who intellectually understand and also have a strong intuition of the Divine as their own essential nature, may still choose to practice dualistic worship. Even such a radical nondualist and abstract philosopher as Shankara, who is also remembered as a consummate Tantric adept, composed beautiful hymns to the Divine in the form of God and Goddess, though some scholars have contested his authorship of these works.

While Patanjali's eightfold path commends itself as an overall schema, it does not account for a number of uniquely Tantric features. As far as I know, these have never been presented in a structured fashion in the *Tantras*, and so it seems useful to provide a rough framework here. The following practices, which are not necessarily found in all schools, are to be understood as complementing the eight limbs of Yoga:

1. Preparatory purification: (a) purification of oneself chiefly by means of the purification of the elements (*bhūta-shuddhi*); (b) purification of the place of ritual or spiritual practice by cleansing until it is like a spotless mirror and by decorating it with flowers, garlands, incense, camphor, and lights; (c) purification of the principal *mantra* by linking the *mantra* to the letters of the alphabet both in forward and reverse order; (d) purification of the ritual substances by sprinkling water on them while reciting a purificatory *mantra* and making appropriate symbolic hand gestures (notably the *dhenu-mudrā*); (e) purification of the image of the deity by sprinkling water and reciting the principal *mantra* (which is the essence of the deity). More is said about *bhūta-shuddhi* in chapter 11.

2. Preliminary practice (*purashcarana*) is undertaken in order to qualify for full consecration (*pūrna-abhisheka*) and consists in extensive repetition of *mantras* to remove obstructions and build up energy for visualization (*dhyāna*) and ritual. In the *Kula-Arnava-Tantra* (15.8), however, this practice is de-

scribed as follows: "The worship at the three times [i.e., dawn, noon, dusk], daily recitation, water offering (*tarpana*), sacrifice, and feeding of brahmins are called preparation."[3] This scripture (15.7) also calls preliminary practice the five-limbed worship (*panca-anga-upāsana*), which can be done in pure locations, on riverbanks, caves, mountain peaks, pilgrimage centers, confluences of rivers, sacred groves, deserted gardens, the foot of bilva trees, mountain slopes, temples, the seashore, and one's own home (15.22–23). *Purashcarana* can also be practiced to avert danger or combat ill health. In every case, the *mantra* is recited a thousand times or more. An instance of this in Buddhist Tantra is the recitation of the *mantra* of Vajrasattva, which neophytes are asked to perform 100,000 times. The *Mahānirvāna-Tantra* (3.113) sanctions 32,000 repetitions of a *mantra*. The *Kankāla-Mālinī-Tantra* recommends the preliminary mantric practice on certain auspicious days, when it should be done from dawn to dusk. Alternatively, it suggests that one should pick any day and repeat the *mantra* a total of 12,000 times. The *Vīnā-Shikha-Tantra* (367) recommends 1,008 repetitions to render a *mantra* "supreme," that is, to strengthen it. This type of mantric practice, which potentiates the *mantra* and prepares the mind for the rigors of full discipleship, overlaps with the category of preparatory purification.

3. *Mantra* recitation is the universal means of Tantra and is described in detail in chapter 12.

4. Construction of a *mandala* (or *yantra*) serving as the deity's seat is a major aspect of the Tantric ritual. The construction creates sacred space that is properly protected against unwelcome entities and negative energies. Details about this are given in chapter 13.

5. *Nyāsa* is the ritual infusion of life force into an object, including one's own body, by which it is divinized. This is explained in chapter 13.

6. *Mudrā* also is an important aspect of *sādhanā* in many schools. It refers to hand gestures used during rituals as described in chapter 13.

7. *Devatā-pujā* is the worship of one's chosen deity. This involves the following means: preparing a seat (*āsana*) for the

deity; welcoming him or her; washing the feet; offering un-
boiled rice, water, milk, honey, flowers, sandal paste, *dūrvā*
grass (a kind of millet grass), cloth, jewels, scented items,
incense sticks, food, and other substances; presenting water
for bathing; waving lights; and prayer. Worship also includes
the fire sacrifice (*homa*), which goes back to Vedic times.
Substances are offered into the fire, which then carries
them to the deity in purified form.

8. *Guru-pūjā* is the ritual worship of the teacher, who is treated
as an embodiment of the Divine. This not only honors the
teacher but also strengthens the spiritual link between *guru*
and disciple. In the absence of the teacher, his or her san-
dals (*pādukā*) are used as a substitute during this ritual.

9. *Dakshina* is the ceremonial gift for the teacher. The gift is
symbolic of the reciprocity without which spiritual transmission cannot occur. It is a sign of the disciple's voluntary
submission to the spiritual process as initiated and maintained by the *guru*.

10. *Yātrā* refers to pilgrimage to sacred places or power spots
where the practitioner can further his or her *sādhanā*. For
Tantric practitioners the most important holy sites are those
that were sanctified by a body part of the Goddess. According to Tantric mythology, as told in the *Kālikā-Purāna* (chapter 18), Shiva's wife, Satī (i.e., Devī), immolated herself
after being insulted by her father, Daksha. Shiva was so
disconsolate at her death that he wandered aimless around
the earth carrying her dead body on his shoulders. The deities entered the body and disposed of it piece by piece.
Wherever a body part would fall, the ground became hallowed. These sites are called "seats" (*pītha*), and the texts
mention from 4 to 108 such sacred places. The most es-
teemed are generally accepted to be Oddiyāna in northwest-
ern India, Jālandhara in the Punjab, and Kāmarūpa (or
Kāmākhya) in Assam. The last-mentioned is thought to be
especially powerful because it is the resting place of Devī's
genitals (*yoni*). However, since the body mirrors the macrocosm, all pilgrimage centers can be found within it as well,
and hence some *Tantras* recommend the inner pilgrimage
along the sacred river Sarasvatī (i.e., the central channel) to

the sacred confluence of the two rivers Ganges (Gangā) and Yamunā (i.e., *idā* and *pingalā*) at the place of the *ājnā-cakra*.

11. *Vrata* means "vow" and consists in various observances, notably the *durgā-pūjā*, or daily worship of the goddess Durgā, which is known as the "great vow" (*mahā-vrata*). In addition, the practitioner may make certain pledges (*samaya*), such as fasting or staying awake for a certain period of time in order to intensify his or her *sādhanā*.

12. *Latā-sādhanā*, or "discipline of the creeper," is a special aspect of left-hand Tantra and the Kaula tradition and is described in chapter 14.

13. Protective amulets or spells (both of which are called *kavaca*, "armor") play an important role in some schools of Tantra. Sometimes these are associated with the planets, which are understood to be distinct forms of energy in close relationship to specific deities. The *Kirana-Tantra* contains instructions for sacrifices to the nine planets (*nava-graha*). Each deity is petitioned to protect a particular part of the body, a practice mentioned in the *Varāda-Tantra*. The *Sādhu-Sam-kalinī-Tantra* (cited in the *Prāna-Toshanī*, 127) mentions *kava-cas* for each day of the week. These amulets are connected with their own planets and deities and are to be fastened on the neck or the right arm (for men) or left arm (for women).

14. Alphabetic diagrams (*cakra*) are used to determine which *mantra* is suitable for a practitioner. The *Kula-Arnava-Tantra* (2.78ff.) mentions six such diagrams: *akathaha-cakra, aka-dama-cakra, nakshatra-cakra, rāshi-cakra, rini-dhana-cakra,* and *kula-akula-cakra*. The last-mentioned is shown in chapter 7.

15. The acquisition and exercise of paranormal powers (*siddhi*) for white and black magic is almost universal in Tantra. This aspect is discussed in chapter 15.

The initiate's daily schedule typically entails the following practices: purification of the elements; infusion of the life force (*nyāsa*), by which the body is transformed into a divine body; mental and physical worship of one's chosen deity, complete with a fire sacrifice (*homa*); and *mantra* recitation. Whatever external rituals may be performed, the mental component (through intense visualization) is never absent and is the crucial factor. Ritual calls for a high degree of concentration and extraordinary punctiliousness, and hence the laity of some schools regard a *sādhaka* with almost the same awe as an enlightened master.

Ritual worship (*pūjā*) is generally divided into four types. The lowest type is held to be that which consists in external acts involving either a statue or picture of a deity or its abstract representation in the form of a *yantra* or *mandala*. Somewhat higher is worship involving mantric recitation and the singing of hymns of praise (*stava*). The next higher category is yogic contemplation of one's chosen deity, and the highest form is identification with the Divine in which there is no otherness. A famous *stava* is the *Mahimnā-Stava,* whose authorship is attributed to Pushpadanta (Flower-Toothed), the leader of the musical spirits (*gandharva*).[6] It is a poetic tribute to the greatness (*mahimnā*) of Shiva, who is invoked as the giver of lasting happiness and the *guru* of all deities. Another popular Tantric hymn, ascribed to Shankara, is the *Ānanda-Laharī,* a tribute to the Goddess whose waves of bliss wash over the devout practitioner, removing every trace of sin.[7] Integrally connected with this work and also attributed to Shankara is the *Saundarya-Laharī,* which is the most revered text of the Shrī-Vidyā tradition.[8] Of particular appeal also is the Kashmiri hymn *Panca-Stavī* (c. 900 CE), addressed to the Goddess in the form of Tripurā, who is praised as the "mother of the universe."[9]

One final facet of ritual worship needs to be mentioned. When a practitioner commits a ritual faux pas, he or she must promptly correct the error by an appropriate expiation rite known as *prāyash-citta.* Depending on the gravity of the mistake, this type of remedial action can consist in the recitation of a *mantra* or a very complex ritual.

As can be seen, Tantra endorses a highly ritualized lifestyle. Its purpose is to focus the practitioner's attention as exclusively as possible on his or her *sādhanā,* leaving little or no room for diversion. But, as I noted at the beginning of this chapter, all this structure must not squelch the spontaneous unfolding of the spiritual process, which is unique to each individual. The practitioner must learn when to push harder and when to ease off and also when to adhere strictly to the traditional rules and when to follow the promptings of the inner wisdom. Once enlightenment is attained, all conventional ideas and rules are transcended and life is lived spontaneously out of the fullness of Being.

The Rule of Secrecy

Secrecy is an important aspect of Tantra and many other spiritual traditions. The *Kaula-Avalī-Nirnaya* (p. 1), for instance, demands that the teachings are kept as carefully concealed as a mother would sexual intercourse. The esoteric reason for this requirement is that by talking about the initiatory process or one's spiritual experiences one dissipates energy. Apart from this, by divulging Tantric secrets to the uninitiated one is likely to invite disapproval and ill will, particularly in regard to the left-hand practices. In addition, the Tantric knowledge will merely bring disaster upon those who are not ready for it. Some *Tantras* guarantee severe karmic consequences for initiates who divulge the secrets of their tradition to unworthy recipients.

This rule of secrecy seems to stand in contrast to a surprising statement found twice in the *Mahānirvāna-Tantra* (4.79–80, 8.190), which explicitly declares that when the *kali-yuga* has grown strong, the Tantric path should be practiced openly, without concealment. This presumes, however, a favorable environment for the practice of Tantra (see 1.147). In its declared liberal spirit, the *Mahānirvāna-Tantra* does indeed disclose many previously secret rituals, which can now readily be studied by anyone. Yet it would be naive to think that the text that today is widely available in translation contains all the secrets of *sādhanā*. Besides, without initiation none of the rituals are effective. This affords some protection to those seekers who want to learn Tantra from books.

Apart from the difficulty of comprehending the meaning of the

Tantric texts without access to the living tradition, there is an added obstacle for noninitiates delving into the *Tantras*. This is the "twilight language" (*sandhyā-bhāshā*). A mysterious time of day, twilight is especially charged with power—both for good and for evil—and therefore initiates have since ancient times performed special rituals at dawn and dusk (as well as the transition point at noon). The twilight language is thus a language of potency that simultaneously illumines and obscures. Its metaphors create a rich context while at the same time concealing to the outsider the real meaning. As Lama Anagarika Govinda, an initiate of Buddhist Tantra, wrote:

> This symbolic language is not only a protection against the profanation of the sacred through intellectual curiosity and misuse of yogic methods and psychic forces by the ignorant or un-initiated, but has its origin mainly in the fact that everyday language is incapable of expressing the highest experiences of the spirit. The indescribable that can only be understood by the initiate or the experiencer can only be hinted at through similes and paradoxes.[10]

Examples of *sandhyā-bhāshā* are:[11]

vajra (lit. "thunderbolt") = *linga* (lit. "mark," phallus) = *shūnya* (void)

sūrya (sun) = *rajas* (menstrual blood) = *pingalā* (right channel) = right nostril

avadhūtī (female renouncer) = *sushumnā* (central channel) = *prajnā* (wisdom)

samarasa (lit. "same taste," unitive state) = coitus = breath retention = mental focusing = arrest of semen

The phrase *sandhā-bhāshā*, found in some Tantric texts, has caused some confusion and a lively debate in scholarly circles. Some authorities understand it as a shortened form of *sandhāya-bhāshā*, meaning "intentional language." Since the scriptures use both *sandhā-* and *sandhyā-bhāshā*, we may assume that if their meaning is not identical, it is at least not mutually exclusive either. In any case, both terms refer to the same thing, which, in Mircea Eliade's words, is "a secret, dark, ambiguous language in which a state of consciousness is expressed by an erotic term and the vocabulary of mythology or cosmology is charged with Hatha-yogic or sexual meanings."[12]

RIGHT, LEFT, AND BEYOND

Because Tantra is such a complex tradition, its teachers have early on looked for ways to categorize it in order to make it more easily comprehensible. Thus they invented the idea of lineage traditions (*āmnāya*), seats (*pītha*), and currents (*srota*).[13] The best known division of the Tantric heritage is into the three categories of right-hand path, left-hand path, and Kaula path. These roughly correspond to a particular mode or style in which Tantra is practiced.

The right-hand path (*dakshina-mārga*) is what can be called conventional (*samaya*) Tantra. In particular, this approach understands the Tantric core ritual of the "five substances" (*panca-tattva*) in a symbolic rather than literal manner. The word *dakshina* means both "right" and "south." This dual meaning is readily explained by the fact that when facing east (the cardinal ritual direction), south is on one's right. According to one tradition, all teachings issued from the five faces of Shiva, and some classical authorities undertook to assign certain *Tantras* to each face.[14] All these schemas, however, are woefully inadequate when we look at the tangled historical reality of Tantra.

The so-called left-hand path (*vāma-mārga*), connected with the north, is frequently characterized as revolving around the acquisition of *siddhi* in the dual sense of "perfection" (i.e., liberation) and "power" (i.e., paranormal ability). There is a particularly strong magical current running through the schools of the left-hand path. Almost all the *Tantras* of this branch have been lost, and we know some of them only by name. The left-hand schools are those that are farthest removed from mainstream (Vedic) Hinduism, occupying the margins of Hindu culture and society.

The right-hand path (*dakshina-mārga*), symbolically associated with the south, has in many ways stayed close to the Hindu orthodoxy. It avoids extremist practices and seeks to uphold the Vedic social order. It is also known as *dakshina-ācāra* or "right-hand conduct." According to the *Prāna-Toshanī* (7.4), everyone belongs to this path by birth and can enter the left-hand path only through proper initiation, but this idea is not universally accepted. For instance, the *Kula-Arnava-Tantra* distinguishes seven types of "conduct":

1. *veda-ācāra*— the Vedic way of life (orthodox Brahmanism)

2. *vaishnava-ācāra*—the way of life of the Vishnu worshipers

3. *shaiva-ācāra*—the way of life of the Shiva worshipers

4. *dakshina-ācāra*—the right-hand approach

5. *vāma-ācāra*—the left-hand approach, which especially involves sacred intercourse with a consecrated woman (*vāma*)

6. *siddhānta-ācāra*—the Siddhānta way of life, which is defined as a higher form of the left-hand path, emphasizing inner worship

7. *kaula-ācāra*—the Kaula approach, which is introduced as the highest form of spiritual practice and as a synthesis of the left-hand and right-hand schools of Tantra

These seven types form a ladder of spiritual competence, with the Kula or Kaula approach at the apex. "There is nothing superior to *kaula*," declares the *Kula-Arnava-Tantra* (2.8). The text continues (2.9):

> O Goddess! The *kula* is the most secret of secrets, the essence of essence, the highest of high, given directly by Shiva, and transmitted from ear to ear [i.e., orally].

The Kaula branch of Tantra originated perhaps in the fifth century CE and achieved great prominence three or four centuries later.[15] It represents a synthesis of the *dakshina-* and *vāma-mārga* and produced a significant number of adepts and numerous scriptures, many of which, however, have been lost.[16] This lineage of transmission (*santati*) is made up of many schools and subschools, which are still inadequately understood.

An important early Kaula school, that revolving around the worship of the goddess Kubjikā, has produced many *Tantras*, of which over eighty are known by name. The name comes from the Sanskrit word *kubja*, meaning "crooked," a reference to the coiled energy of the *kundalinī* in its potential state, prior to awakening.

Kaula, or Kaulism, as this Tantric stream is sometimes called, quickly became almost synonymous with Tantra in the north of the subcontinent. By the thirteenth century, the greatly influential Kaula tradition had also penetrated many schools of South India's Siddhānta tradition.

What marks the Kaula branch of Tantra is a strong presence of the *shakti* element in both theory and practice. One manifestation of this is the teachings about the serpent power (*kundalinī-shakti*); another is the fact that women have always played a significant role in Kaula circles both as Tantric consorts and, more significantly, as initiators. According to one classification, the Kaula tradition is divided into Yoginī Kaula and Siddha Kaula schools; the former is transmitted by female adepts (*yoginī*) and the latter by male adepts (*siddha*). Kaula features can also be found in many other Tantric traditions, notably the Shrī-Vidyā tradition of South India and the Krama tradition of Kashmir.

An important Tantric cult is that of the sixty-four Yoginīs, to whom several circular temples are dedicated. The best-known temple is the one located at Khajuraho, where it is the oldest structure, dating back to 600—800 CE. Khajuraho is a popular tourist attraction because of the explicit sexual stone carvings on the walls of a number of buildings of this complex in Madhya Pradesh. Of the many explanations offered for what some have dubbed "lascivious iconography," Michael Rabe's is the most convincing.[17] He sees in these graphic depictions portrayals of the paradisaic pleasures awaiting the kings who ordered and sponsored the construction of such temples. The temples themselves are earthly models of paradise (*svarga*).

The Yoginīs, worshiped as deities, were originally probably female adepts and initiators into the secrets of Tantra. Their number is as highly symbolic as the sixty-four *Tantras* said to exist according to some texts. The sculptures of the Yoginīs are arranged in a circle around the central image of Shiva (either as an anthropomorphic statue or in the abstract form of a *linga*).

Some scriptures also mention sixty-four Bhairavas (forms of Shiva) and sixty-four Kalās (aspects of the supreme Goddess). Thus the number 64 is as meaningful and sacred to Tantra as the number 108 is to other Hindu traditions.

One of the great masters of Kaula Tantra was Matsyendra Nātha, who is credited with founding the Yoginī Kaula branch. He also is traditionally held to be the teacher of Goraksha Nātha, the creator of original Hatha Yoga. However, the two masters appear to have been separated in time by several centuries. Unless we assume the existence of another adept by the name of Matsyendra who lived in Goraksha's era, we are left with the yogic feat of mind-to-mind transmission as the only other explanation.

The term *kula* has twenty or so distinct lexicographical meanings, the primary ones being "group," "family," or "multitude." Technically, *kula* refers to the ultimate Reality, which is beyond the transcendental principles of Shiva and Shakti. But many schools and texts employ the term *kula* to denote the "cosmic family," that is the manifest universe and the power inherent in it, namely, Shakti. As the *Mahānirvāna-Tantra* (7.97–98) states:

> The individual psyche (*jīva*), the principle of nature, space, time, ether, earth, water, fire, and air are called *kula*.

> O Primordial one! *Kula-ācāra* is practicing formlessness (*nirvikalpa*) by recognizing the Absolute (*brahman*) in them, which produces virtue, wealth, pleasure, and liberation.

Similarly, *akula*, meaning "that which is not the *kula*," is sometimes used to refer to the Shiva principle, as opposed to the supreme Being as such.

The word *kula* can also stand for the state of union between

Shiva and Shakti and, by logical extension, to the bliss arising from this union. Finally, the esoteric group in which the Kaula teachings are practiced also bears the name *kula*.

Those who aspire to the realization of the ultimate *kula* are called *kaulas* or *kaulikas*. Hence the name of this Tantric branch is either Kula or Kaula. The latter word is explained esoterically in the *Kula-Arnava-Tantra* (17.45) thus:

> It is called *kaula* because it restricts youth (*kaumāra*), and so on, because it dispels birth, death (*laya*), and so forth, and because it is connected with the whole *kula*.[18]

According to Abhinava Gupta's *Tantra-Āloka* (29.29), the founder of Kaula Tantra was the adept Macchanda (alias Mīna). He may have been an Assamese ruler associated with the Tryambaka branch of early Tantra and is sometimes identified with Matsyendra.

The Subtle Body and Its Environment

Worshiping the *linga* of the body, one gains liberation
and enjoyment. Goddess, this is the *linga* of perfection
stationed in the body and granting proof.
  —*Kaula-Jnāna-Nirnaya* (3.27)

OUR LARGER ENVIRONMENT

Wedged between our familiar material universe and the ultimate
Reality are the multiple layers of subtle (*sūkshma*) existence. In their
endeavor to reach the One, the Tantric practitioners inevitably must
traverse those intermediate realms, which are invisible to ordinary
sight but nonetheless as real (or unreal) as the material world. The
idea of a subtle dimension of existence can be found already in the

ancient *Vedas* and is shared by many, if not most, other spiritual and religious traditions. These subtle realms are considered the home of deities, ancestral spirits, and other entities, including various kinds of earthbound demonic beings (called *bhūtas*, or "elementals").

We continuously participate in the subtle dimension of existence, though we generally remain unaware of it. Many adepts, in India and elsewhere, have emphasized that our visible universe is greatly influenced by the forces present in the subtle worlds. So long as we are not conscious of these forces, we are at their mercy. Therefore Tantric practitioners are urged to protect themselves against undesirable interference at all times, and especially during the performance of rituals. One way of accomplishing this is by cultivating the friendship and help of beings in the subtle realms, who then assume the role of protector. This is done through supplication in the form of regular ritual offerings and, at a more advanced level of practice, through mind-to-mind communication. An aspect of this protection against unwanted influence from the spirit world is the creation—both mentally and graphically—of a fiery surround encircling the sacred space, or *mandala*, in which the Tantric rituals are performed.

Great Tantric adepts (*mahā-siddha*) typically have a whole retinue of protectors, who belong to various levels of the subtle dimension. Since protectors can be effective only in their own subtle environment, each has a specific role and function. Protection is particularly necessary at the lowest levels of subtle existence, to which protectors of higher subtle realms generally do not have access, though they may have their own hierarchy of subprotectors for tasks to be done on those levels. But this subject is seldom discussed openly and requires initiation.

The Subtle Vehicle

How do we participate in the subtle dimension of existence? The answer is simple: through our own subtle energy field and the mind. These are often treated as separate "bodies" (*deha, sharīra*) or "sheaths/containers" (*kosha*), but some schools regard them as constituting a single structure named *ātivāhika-deha* (superconductive body),[1] *antah-kārana* (inner instrument), or *puryashtaka* (eightfold city).

The idea of simultaneously existing multiple bodies belonging to a single individual goes back to the *Taittirīya-Upanishad* (2.7), which was composed three thousand years ago. This scripture distinguishes five "sheaths," or envelopes, covering and progressively concealing the ultimate Reality:

1. *Anna-maya-kosha*, or "sheath composed of food," is our familiar physical body, by which we navigate in the material world.

2. *Prāna-maya-kosha*, or "sheath composed of life force," is the energy field associated with and sustaining the physical body. It is the connecting link between the physical body and the mind.

3. *Mano-maya-kosha*, or "sheath composed of the mind," refers to the mind in its lower function as a processor of sensory input. *Manas* is driven by doubt and volition (or desire) and vacillates between externalizing our consciousness and withdrawing it into the realm of imagination. This aspect of the mind is governed mainly by the factors of inertia (*tamas*) and dynamism (*rajas*).

4. *Vijnāna-maya-kosha*, or "sheath composed of intelligence," refers to the mind in its higher function as an organ of discernment between what is real and unreal, that is, as the seat of wisdom. Where the lower mind causes doubt and uncertainty, the higher mind (often called *buddhi*) also brings certainty and faith, as well as a sense of stillness, because the lucidity factor (*sattva-guna*) is predominant in it.

5. *Ānanda-maya-kosha*, or "sheath composed of bliss," is equated in the *Taittirīya-Upanishad* with the transcendental Self (*ātman*) itself, though subsequent Vedānta schools consider it to be the final veil surrounding the ultimate Reality, or Self. In any case, *ānanda* (bliss) must not be mistaken for an emotional

state, which is hierarchically higher than intellection or intelligence (*vijnāna*). Emotions belong to the *anna-maya-* and
prāna-maya-koshas.

While this archaic quintuple model is not typical of Tantra, Tantric initiates fully adopt its functional distinctions of body, mind, life
force, higher intelligence (*vijnāna* or *buddhi*), and bliss.

The philosophically well-developed Trika school of Tantra distinguishes between the physical body, the subtle body, and the causal
body. The subtle body, typically designated as *puryashtaka*, corresponds
to what we would call the psyche or mind. It is attached to an individual throughout his or her embodiments in the physical realm.

The causal body (*kārana-sharīra*), as the name suggests, contains
the karmic seeds that give rise to the other vehicles through which we
experience the world and create new *karma*, thus keeping cyclic existence going endlessly. It is the substratum for the subtle body. The
causal vehicle is also known as the "higher body" (*para-sharīra*) and,
according to the Trika philosophers, is composed of the ontic principle of *māyā* together with its five "coverings" (*kancuka*), as described
in chapter 4. It guarantees that there is a continuity not only from
life to life but even from one cosmic creation to another. Unlike the
subtle body, the causal body is not destroyed at the moment of cosmic
dissolution (*pralaya*) but serves as the template for the creation of
the next semipermanent subtle body. It is eliminated only upon full
liberation, when the individual drops all bodies and is present purely
as the transcendental Reality, or Self. Presumably, the combined karmic seeds of all unliberated beings are responsible for the renewed
sprouting of the tree of conditioned existence at the end of a period
of cosmic sleep, or dormancy. Thus, in concert with all other beings,
we ourselves are responsible for the world we inhabit. Together we
create and maintain it.

The *Siddha-Siddhānta-Paddhati* (chapter 1), to give one more example in illustration of the metaphysical diversity of Tantra, distinguishes six bodies, which are called *pinda* (lump, ball, sphere). These,
again, correspond to ever more subtle levels of existence, beginning

with the "primordial body" (*ādya-pinda*) down to the "embryonic body" (*garbha-pinda*). But, again, these are understood not as strictly separate vehicles but as a hierarchy of interlocking and interdependent structures. They are all manifestations of the singular divine Power (*shakti*), which is refracted in various ways in the multidimensional universe. Above all, these structures relate to levels of consciousness and experience.

In their spiritual ascent to the ultimate One, Tantric *yogins* and *yoginīs* progressively intensify their awareness, thus enabling them to experience ever more subtle realms of existence. At the material level, we experience the body as separate from its environment. In the higher levels of existence, however, the boundaries between body and environment become increasingly blurred, and the primordial body is coextensive with the universe itself. In other words, at the highest level of corporeality, we literally *are* the world. At that level we are truly omnipresent as well as omniscient. The further down we step in the ladder of psychocosmic evolution, the more pronounced the split between consciousness, body, and environment becomes.

Finally, at the material level, we not only experience our body as separate from its environment but even sever our mind from the body. This final split is now proving fatal for the human species as a whole, because it has alienated us from our feelings. We can no longer read the signals from our body, which is our primary source of communication with one another. Thus we have become estranged from ourselves, from our physical environment, and from each other. Consequently we are experiencing a high degree of conflict on these various levels of being in the world, which causes us confusion, uncertainty, and a great deal of unhappiness.

For a long time psychologists sought to remedy this situation by awareness-enhancing methods. More recently, they have come to recognize that something more is needed, because greater awareness does not automatically empower a person to make the necessary changes. Thus they have begun to focus on the body as a medium of behavioral change. The "Somatic Yoga" developed by Eleanor Criswell, a professor of psychology, is an inspired attempt to combine the knowledge of body-oriented therapy and biofeedback with the wisdom of traditional Yoga.[2] By furthering the integration between body and mind, Somatic Yoga endeavors to tap into our potential for deeper meditative experience and spiritual growth. Tantra, too, works closely with the body, though it focuses on the body's subtle energetic template. Because the subtle body is senior to the physical body, the Tantric approach would seem to be more direct and also takes into account the still more fundamental karmic factors responsible for our energetic and physical patterns.

HEALING THE SPLIT: *Tantric Medicine*

The subtle body is the energetic mold of the physical body. It is more accessible to the mind and conscious control. On the subtle level, change is instantaneous but also somewhat fragile, demanding powerful intention. Once change on the subtle level has filtered down to the physical level, however, it tends to become more stable. Conversely, it is difficult to make and maintain change purely on the physical level. This is best seen in the area of health maintenance. A person may eat the right diet and exercise regularly yet be handicapped by ill health. By examining that person's karmic conditions and making adjustments in the subtle energy field, a Tantric adept can bring about healing efficiently and sometimes very quickly, if not instantly. More importantly, this kind of intervention can put a person firmly on the spiritual path by removing blockages in the subtle body that previously caused confusion, doubt, lack of will, and impatience.

Tantra has evolved its own form of therapy, which is little known in the West. It is based on the idea of self-purification not only at the physical and mental level but also on the energetic (or subtle) level. Physical purification has been greatly elaborated in Hatha Yoga, which is a Tantric Yoga. Mental purification consists primarily in meditation and visualization, especially visualizing oneself as one's chosen deity (*ishta-devatā*). Energetic purification, which is the forte of Tantra, proceeds by means of visualization and breath control or, strictly speaking, *prāna* energization and harmonization. *Prāna* is on the subtle level what the breath is on the physical plane. Physical illness is foreshadowed by obstructions in the flow of life energy in the subtle body. Conversely, damage to the physical body has its subtle energetic consequences. These, in turn, affect the functioning of the mind. Since the mind is the principal tool by which Tantric practitioners strive to realize their goal, it must be diligently kept in a state of equanimity that allows for the spiritual process to become increasingly subtle.

By removing energetic blockages and correcting damage on the level of the subtle body, Tantric practitioners prevent physical disease and mental imbalance. They understand, however, that health is not a permanent achievement. Both the subtle vehicle and the physical body are constantly influenced by their respective environments. Moreover, the karmic seeds planted through our previous and present volitions are continuously ripening and seeking manifestation. Illness may also be caused by carelessness in the execution of the yogic practices, as Cidghanānanda Nātha points out in his *Sat-Karma-Samgraha*. This scripture prescribes various cleansing practices in cases where ordinary yogic techniques and medicinal substances fail to correct the problem.

In the embodied state, there can be no perfect equilibrium. Everything, including our health, is in a continuous state of flux. We cannot know how our karma or our environment will affect us. Yet from the Tantric viewpoint, a strong, healthy body is a definite asset, because the spiritual process is demanding, and a debilitated body may not be able to withstand the fire of spiritual self-transformation. Therefore Tantric practitioners are keen to maintain their physical well-being.

To this end, they avail themselves of the techniques of Hatha Yoga and the many naturopathic remedies of Āyurveda (Life Science)—from herbs to dieting to fasting. They even make use of alchemical concoctions said to promote health and longevity. From earliest times, there has been a close link between Tantra, medicine, and alchemy. All three were developed through experimentation and personal experience over many centuries. A number of adepts have

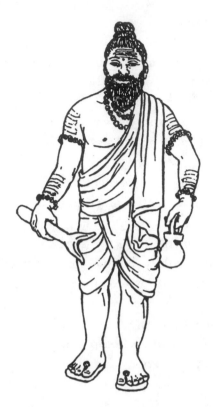

Agastya, an enlightened master and healer who is traditionally credited with articulating the principles and practices of cittar *medicine, "The Science of Mind."* (DRAWING © COPYRIGHT MARSHALL GOVINDAN)

authored texts on Yoga and on medicine. Thus Patanjali, the composer of the *Yoga-Sūtra*, is credited with the authorship of works on medicine and grammar as well.

In South India the Tantric *cittars* developed their own distinct brand of medicine, which makes extensive use of inorganic substances (notably salts, metals, and even toxic compounds).[3] They claim to have developed their system independently of Āyurveda, the naturopathic tradition of the North. But, like their Northern counterparts, the Tantric adepts of the South also have emphasized the superlative importance of the mind and *prāna* in the healing process.

Cittar medicine—known as *citta-vaittiyam* or "science of the mind"—is traditionally traced back to the great master Agastya

(Tamil: Akattiyar). Agastya, whose date is uncertain, was not only an enlightened master but also a healer and miracle worker. A seer (*rishi*) by that name composed several hymns of the ancient *Rig-Veda* and was married to Lopāmudrā, the daughter of the ruler of the Videha tribe. The *Rig-Veda* (1.179.4) has preserved a fascinating conversation between them, which is relevant here. Lopāmudrā, conscious of aging, grew weary of sexual abstinence. Her husband had taken to asceticism and chastity to engender vigor for the spiritual process. She confessed her overwhelming sexual desire for him, and Agastya reminded her that ascetic fervor is pleasing to the deities and that this endeavor is never in vain. But then he added, "We shall overcome a hundred adversities if we unite as a couple (*mithuna*)." This seems to hint at sexual intercourse as an opportunity for higher union through self-transcendence. Yet, as the hymn continues, after Agastya had conceded to sexual congress, Lopāmudrā merely "sucked dry the panting sage." In other words, instead of harnessing the extra energy produced during sexual congress, the seer lost his focus momentarily and spilled his semen. But the story has a happy ending, for we are told that Agastya "found fulfillment of his real hopes among the deities."

According to Indian tradition, Agastya brought the Vedic heritage to the south of the subcontinent. It is possible that he is indeed the Agastya remembered in the Tantric scriptures of the Tamil-speaking South, but there may also have been other great adepts bearing this name, which is often mentioned in many texts and genres of Hindu literature.

Tantric medicine, whether of North or South India, was developed in the context of spiritual practice and was meant to assist those who sought to scale the Himalayas of their own psyche. Its discoveries about the interplay between body and mind via the medium of subtle energy currents are valid even today. A few Western physicians have started to explore this hidden dimension of bodily existence and are confirming some of the findings of the Tantric adepts and healers. Undoubtedly, the contemporary pioneers of "energy medicine," or "vibrational medicine," would benefit greatly from a deeper practical study of Tantric medicine, which has a long history.[4]

OF LOTUSES AND SUBTLE TENDRILS

The energy of the subtle body is called *prāna* meaning "life" or "life force." This is a very old Sanskrit term found already in the *Vedas*. In the *Rig-Veda* (10.90.13) it stands for the "breath" of the macranthropos, or Cosmic Person, and elsewhere is used for the breath of life in general. According to the *Atharva-Veda* (11.4.11), the life force clothes a person as a father would clothe his dear son. This scripture (15.15.2) also refers to seven *prānas* (in-breaths), seven *apānas* (out-breaths), and seven *vyānas* (through-breaths), thus anticipating the pneumatological speculations of the later *Upanishads* and *Tantras*. We can see from this that the sages of India from the beginning have correlated the breath with the vital energy itself, which is thought to spread throughout the universe, enlivening everything. In its deeper meaning, then, the Sanskrit word *prāna* expresses the same reality that is also captured in the Latin term *spiritus*, which is contained in breath-related words like *inspiration* and *expiration*. The connection between spirit and breath is similarly preserved in the Greek word *pneuma* and the Hebrew word *ruah*. This connection is of great significance and suggests an early understanding of the function of the breath in spiritual experience.

Prāna is discontinuous vital energy, which pools to form currents (*nādī*) and vortices (*cakra*). Sometimes these currents are understood as "conduits" analogous to blood vessels, while the *cakras* are confused with nerve plexuses. One of the first Westerners to write about the serpent power and its ascent through the *cakra* system was Vasant G. Rele.[5] He straightforwardly equated the *cakras* with the major nerve plexuses, arguing that the powers (*shakti*) associated with the psychoenergetic centers of the subtle body are the same as the efferent impulses that inhibit nervous activity. He overlooked the fact that these powers are characterized in the Sanskrit scriptures as divine energies of consciousness rather than unconscious neurophysiological forces. Some Western medical authorities even went so far as to suggest that the *cakra* system is merely a poorly conceived anatomical model.

It is true that there are certain correspondences between the structures of the subtle body and the anatomical organs and endocrine system of the physical body, but these are parallel or analogous rather than identical. Most significantly, while the nerve plexuses are located outside the spinal column, the *cakras* are described as being inside the central channel, which is situated inside what on the physical level would be the spinal column. Obviously, the *cakras* cannot be found by dissecting the body but by entering a meditative state and experiencing the energy field from within or by adjusting one's external perception to a higher frequency (namely, that of clairvoyance).

To clairvoyant vision, the subtle body appears as a radiant, shimmering energy field that is in constant internal motion and is crisscrossed by luminous filaments, or tendrils. Unlike the physical body, which appears solid and stable, it is neither compact nor rigid. Although it contains regions of relative stability, the subtle body is highly responsive to the mind and reflects a person's changing mental states quite faithfully.

The most stable structures of the subtle body are known as "wheels" (*cakras*) or "lotuses" (*padma*) because of their circular form and whirling motion and also because of the way in which the *prāna* currents terminate at or issue from them.[6] These major configurations of our "subtle anatomy" are especially responsive to mental manipulation and therefore are often made the focal points of meditation and visualization. Many Tantric teachers speak of seven principal psychoenergetic centers, but some schools list five, and others name nine, ten, eleven, or very many more.[7] Some writers have interpreted this divergence as a sign that the *cakras* are purely imaginary. This is contradicted by most Tantric texts themselves, quite apart from the fact that Eastern and Western clairvoyants have independently provided similar descriptions of these subtle "organs." Furthermore, the Japanese master and researcher Hiroshi Motoyama has been able to objectively demonstrate the existence of *cakras* by means of an apparatus measuring the body's bioenergetic currents.[8]

In contrast to this, some Tantric works treat the *cakras* as creations of intense yogic visualization; one such work is the *Ānanda-*

Laharī, ascribed to Shankara. However, it is possible to reconcile both interpretations insofar as concentration on the *cakras* energizes them, making them more luminous and hence also more visible to clairvoyant sight. In the ordinary person, as most Tantric authorities would agree, the *cakras* are functioning at a minimal level and therefore have been compared to drooping, closed lotus flowers. From a yogic point of view, they can be said barely to exist. Through inner work, however, they automatically become more active, opening like lotuses in full bloom and extending upward toward the Light (which is really omnipresent).

Moreover, in the average individual, the *cakras* function below par and are not harmonized with each other. In the course of spiritual practice, they are increasingly harmonized until they vibrate in unison. It is then that the subtle sound *om*, which is reverberating throughout the cosmos, can be heard in the state of ecstasy. This also coincides with the balanced functioning of the body-mind.

The fact that different authorities have mentioned diverse numbers of *cakras* need not be taken as a sign of disagreement between them. The *cakra* models are just that: models of reality that are designed to assist the Tantric practitioners in their inward odyssey from the Many to the One. As will have become evident by now, this subject matter is extremely intricate. In their excellent book *Yoga and Psychotherapy*, Swami Rama and two of his students and collaborators rightly noted:

> The chakras provide a sort of central point, an underlying framework, in which a multitude of factors intersect and interact. It should be clear that the experience of these centers is a highly intricate and complex affair. Any attempt to express it in words is certain to prove to be only partially successful.[9]

The most common *cakra* model recognizes the following seven psychoenergetic centers in descending order:

1. *Sahasrāra-cakra*[10] (thousand-spoked wheel), which is located at the crown of the head, is also known as the "brahmic fissure" (*brahma-randhra*) because at the moment of libera-

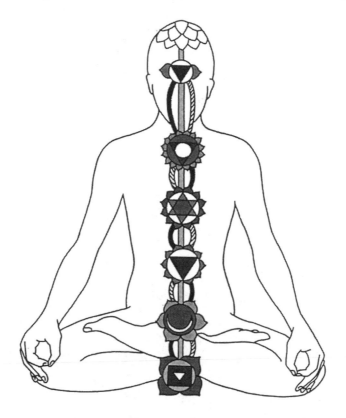

The seven cakras.

tion, while still embodied, consciousness leaves the body through this exit point to merge with the Absolute (*brahman*). This psychoenergetic center is a luminous structure composed of a seemingly endless number of filaments that extend from the head upward into infinity. It corresponds to the level of ultimate Reality on the one hand and to the brain on the other. Symbolically, it is the peak of Mount Meru (corresponding to the spinal column), which is Shiva's divine seat. The Tantric practitioners aim at reuniting the Goddess Power (Shakti) with Shiva, thus bringing about the enlightened state overflowing with bliss. This unification, manifesting in ecstasy and ultimately enlightenment, depends on the arousal of the serpent power (*kundalinī-shakti*) dormant in the lowest psychoenergetic center. In the ordinary person, the *sahasrāra-cakra* is responsible for the higher mental functions, especially

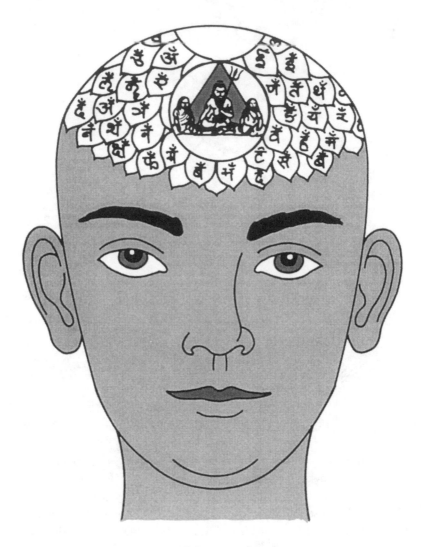

1. Sahasrāra-cakra

discernment (*buddhi*). In the *yogin* and *yoginī*, its full potential manifests in the form of mystical experience and illumination.

2. *Ājnā-cakra* (command wheel), which is situated in the middle of the head, is commonly indicated by the dot (*bindu*) worn on the forehead by Hindu women. This is the subtle organ that acts as a transmitter and receiver of telepathic communi-

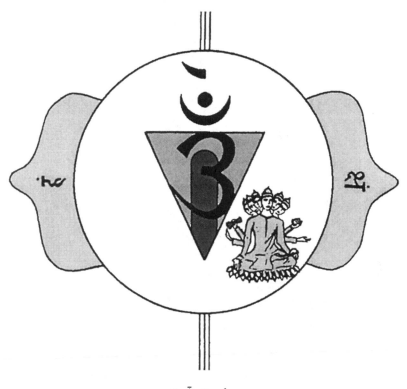

2. *Ājnā-cakra*

cations, especially those between the *guru* and the disciple.
Popularly called the "third eye," it is often depicted as such
on the foreheads of deities (notably Shiva) and Yoga masters.
This points to its function as an "organ" of clairvoyance,
remote viewing (*dūra-darshana*), and other similar paranormal
abilities. It is typically depicted as a two-petaled lotus, the
two petals being related to the natural polarization of the
human mind (and brain), which is organized as an on/off
computer. The lower mind, called *manas* in Sanskrit, has traditionally been defined as that function of consciousness
which oscillates between yes/no, either/or. Most basically, the
ājnā-cakra can be used to either serve the lower functions of
the body-mind (the activities of the first three *cakras*) or the
higher functions of the crown center, which facilitates self-
transcendence, wisdom, and enlightenment. Because the
ājnā-cakra is the meeting place of the three principal channels

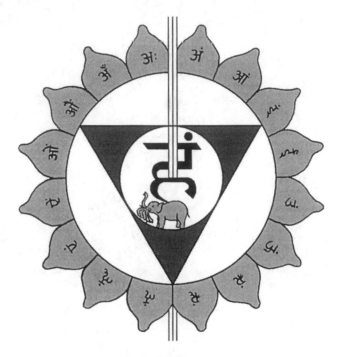

3. Vishuddha-cakra

(i.e., *idā, pingalā*, and *sushumnā*), it is also called "triple confluence" (*tri-veni*).

3. *Vishuddha-cakra* (pure wheel), or *vishuddhi-cakra* (wheel of purity), is found at the throat and hence is also called "throat wheel" (*kantha-cakra*). It is especially connected with the fifth element, ether (*ākāsha*), and thus also with sound and hearing. Its name presumably refers to the purity of the ether, which is the source of the other five elements (air, fire, water, and earth). According to Kālīcarana's commentary on the *Shat-Cakra-Nirūpana* (28), this psychoenergetic center is deemed pure because one attains purity upon seeing the *hamsa* when contemplating this *cakra*. Here *hamsa* refers to the divine metabolism of Shiva-Shakti, which on the physical level manifests as the rhythm of inhalation and exhalation. The hidden significance of this *cakra* seems to be that of balance (which would explain its association with hearing), especially the balance between giving and receiving, as manifested in inhalation and exhalation, speech and silence,

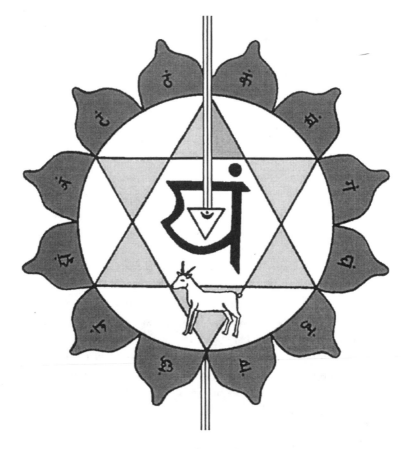

4. *Anāhata-cakra*

as well as metabolism. This center stands midway between the elemental (material) body and the immaterial mind. Its sixteen petals are linked with Sanskrit vowel sounds only, which hints at the status of this *cakra* as a matrix for speech, the vowels being more primitive than the consonants.

4. *Anāhata-cakra* (wheel of the unstruck [sound]), located at the heart, is also widely known as the "heart lotus" (*hrit-padma* or *hridaya-kamala*). Ever since the time of the *Rig-Veda*, the heart rather than the head has been considered the true bridge between consciousness and the body. Later scriptures like the *Dhyāna-Bindu-Upanishad* (50) describe the individuated consciousness as whirling round and round in the twelve-spoked wheel of the heart, impelled by its good and

bad karma. This incessant motion of consciousness (or attention) is stopped only with the realization of the Self as one's
true identity.

Many teachers prefer to work with this *cakra*, as its
energization is thought to lead to the harmonious development of all the other psychoenergetic centers. Without the
awakening of the heart center, activation of any of the other
centers can cause physical and emotional problems. The Tantric adepts seek to raise the serpent power (*kundalinī-shakti*)
from the lowest center as quickly as possible to the heart
center in order to bypass the dangers in activating the first
three centers (in ascending order). These centers are related
to lower bodily functions (notably elimination, sexuality, and
digestion) and their corresponding emotional-mental impulses in the form of desires, if not obsessions. The centers
above the heart are comparatively safe, yet without prior activation of the heart center, they too can cause problems, such
as mental imbalance, psychic hypersensitivity, or extreme
susceptibility to mystical states (as opposed to genuine enlightenment) or even to hallucination. The heart center can
be opened indirectly by cultivating kindness, compassion,
dispassion, calmness, and other similar virtues, which are
fundamental to the spiritual path. Being firmly grounded in
them helps avoid or at least minimize the negative side effects
of activating the three lower *cakras*.

When the heart center is activated, it is possible to
hear the subtle inner sound called *nāda*, which is "unstruck"
because it is not produced by any mechanical means and is
not propelled through space but is a fundamental omnipresent vibration—the sound *om*. This idea has its parallel in the
Gnostic notion of the "music of the spheres," first mentioned by Pythagoras.

5. *Manipūra-cakra* (wheel of the jewel city) is also known as the
   nābhi-cakra (navel wheel), which indicates its location in the
   body. It corresponds on the physical level to the solar plexus,
   which has been called our "second brain" because it represents such a well-developed structure of the nervous system.
   This ten-petaled lotus is associated with the fire element.
   According to the *Shat-Cakra-Nirūpana* (21) of the sixteenth-

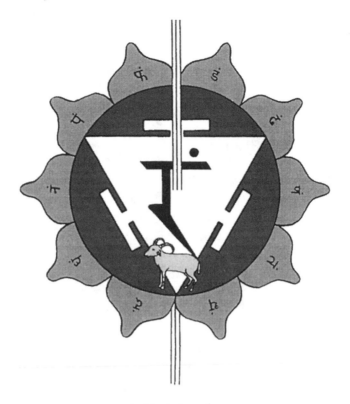

5. *Manipūra-cakra*

century Bengali master Pūrnānanda, by contemplating this *cakra* one acquires the paranormal power to destroy and create the elemental world. Each psychoenergetic center is associated with a specific presiding feminine deity, and in the case of the *manipūra-cakra* this is Lākinī, who is said to be fond of meat and blood. This points to the *cakra*'s connection, on the physical level, with the digestive process. It gets its curious name from the fact that it is "lustrous like a gem" (*Gautamīya-Tantra,* chapter 34).

6. *Svādhishthāna-cakra*[11] (wheel of the self-base), located at the genitals, is associated with the water element and the sense of taste. As Swami Sivananda Radha has pointed out in her pioneering book *Kundalini Yoga for the West,* taste here comprises not only our gustatory sense but taste in the metaphoric sense as well: our hankering for particular experiences

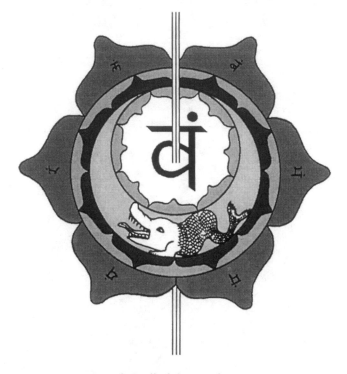

6. *Svādhishthāna-cakra*

and our basic approach to life (which may be tactful or taste-
less).[12] More than any other center, this *cakra* relates to desire, especially the sexual urge. According to the *Rudra-Yāmala*
(27.58), this center gets its name from the fact that it is the
place of the *para-linga* (supreme symbol)—expressed in the
word *sva* (own). It is depicted as a six-petaled lotus whose
petals are connected with the six afflictive emotions of lust
(*kāma*), anger (*krodha*), greed (*lobha*), delusion (*moha*), pride
(*mada*), and envy (*mātsarya*). These factors, which all arise
from the ego sense (*ahamkāra*), can be overcome by contemplating this psychoenergetic matrix.

7. *Mūlādhāra-cakra*[13] (root-prop wheel), located at the base of
the spine, is the counterpole to the crown center. If the
sahasrāra-cakra represents transcendence, divine omnipresence (heaven), and freedom, the *mulādhāra-cakra* symbolizes
immanence, physical limitation, and bondage. It has in fact
been traditionally connected with the earth element, as is

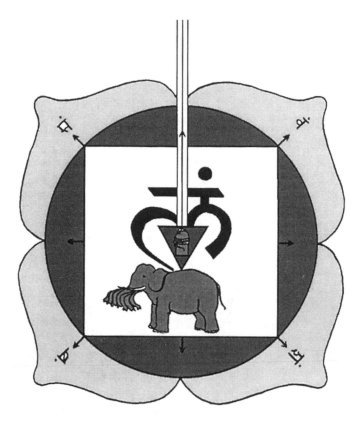

7. *Mūlādhāra-cakra*

symbolically captured in its four petals (representing the four directions of space). It is the root (*mūla*) and support (*adhāra*) of the other *cakras*, because it serves as the resting place of the divine energy in the human body, called *kundalinī-shakti*. Although this is the lowest center—both spatially and functionally—without it liberation would not be possible. Here we have again a clear expression of the high value placed in Tantric philosophy on material embodiment, the lower realms of existence, and the shadow side of life. Far from being redundant or merely defiled or "evil," the earth element (and everything it stands for) is instrumental in our personal growth and ultimate enlightenment. Therefore we must not neglect but embrace it, though without becoming attached to it.

The awakening of a given *cakra* corresponds to a particular state of energy and consciousness, with the crown center as the acme of the entire series. When the divine energy is raised from the lowest center to the thousand-petaled lotus at the top of the head, a radical shift in consciousness occurs: the barrier between subject and object is lifted and the adept experiences a state of perfect unity and wholeness. The divine or serpent power is conducted to the crown center along the axial pathway that connects all *cakras*, as some scriptures put it, like beads on a string. This axial pathway, or *sushumnā-nādī*, is one of numerous such filaments of vital energy that compose the tapestry of the subtle field, or subtle body (*sūkshma-sharīra*). This network is called *nādī-cakra*.

Some *Tantras* speak of 72,000 conduits (*nādī*), though the *Shiva-Samhitā* (2.13) gives the figure 350,000, while the *Tri-Shikhi-Brāhmana-Upanishad* (2.76) insists that they are really countless. The *Shiva-Svaro-daya* (31, 35) declares:

> In the body exist many kinds of channels, which are very extensive. The sage must understand them in order to understand his own body.

> Running transversely, up, and down, they all exist in the body joined together like a wheel, dependent on the life force and linked to the breath of the body.

Even in the Sanskrit literature, the *nādīs* are sometimes treated—with misplaced concreteness—as passageways through which the life force circulates. More accurately, they are *currents* of vital energy. For the sake of convenience, I will switch freely between these two metaphors, asking the reader to bear the preferred interpretation in mind.

The oldest tradition, as recorded for instance in the *Brihad-Āranyaka-Upanishad* (4.2.3), knows of 101 such currents of psychoenergy, of which only one is said to pass all the way to the crown of the head, where it leads to immortality. This special current is none other than the axial pathway, which holds special significance in all schools of Tantra Yoga, as is obvious from such alternative technical terms for it as *moksha-mārga* (way to liberation) or "unsupported interior" (*nirālam-*

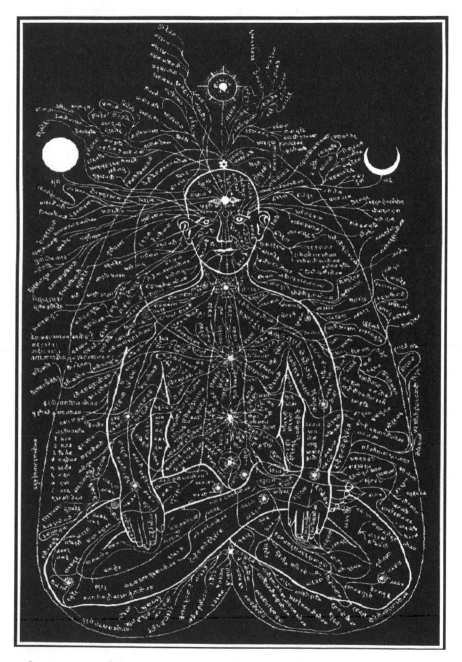

Representation of the subtle channels (nāḍī) through which the life force circulates.

bana-antara). Significantly, its most common name, *sushumnā-nādī*, means "most gracious current"—gracious because it is the royal road to freedom.

According to the *Shat-Cakra-Nirūpana* (2), the axial pathway is composed of several layers, each subsequent layer being more subtle than the previous one. The innermost current is called *citrā-* or *citrinī-nādī*, and between it and the *sushumnā-nādī* is the adamantine current (*vajrā-nādī*). The innermost current, also known as the brahmic current (*brahma-nādī*), is the conductor for the awakened serpent power.

All these luminous filaments of vital energy originate at the egg-shaped "bulb" (*kanda*), which is situated at the perineum. Its size is often specified as being nine or twelve digits long and four digits wide, which would make it reach just below the navel. This position roughly corresponds to the *hara* spoken of in the Japanese Zen scriptures.

The more important currents of the life force terminate at the "command wheel" in the midbrain, but only the central pathway extends all the way to the center at the crown of the head and from there opens into infinity. Many Tantric scriptures list the following fourteen principal currents: *sushumnā, idā* (comfort), *pingalā* (tawny), *sarasvatī* (she who flows), *pūshā* (nourisher), *varunā* (encompassing), *hasti-jihvā* (elephant tongue), *yashasvinī* (splendid), *ālambusā* (or *ālam-bushā*, both meaning "plenteously misty"), *kuhū* (new moon), *vishva-udārā* ("world belly," written *vishvodārā*), *payasvinī* (watery), *shankhinī* (mother-of-pearl), and *gāndhārā* (or *gāndhārī*, "princesslike" or "redolent"). These names are common but not invariable. Some scriptures speak of only ten principal conduits, which they link to the ten openings or "gates" (*dvāra*) of the body: eyes, ears, nostrils, mouth, urethral opening, anus, and either the navel or the "brahmic fissure" (*brahma-randhra*) at the crown of the head.[14]

Twisting around the central pathway in helical fashion and crossing at each *cakra* are the *idā-nādī* and the *pingalā-nādī*. The former is said to be on the left side of the *sushumnā-nādī*, and the latter on the right side. On the physical level, they are related to the left and right nostril and to the parasympathetic and sympathetic nervous system respectively. Symbolically, the former is associated with the cooling moon and the latter with the heating sun. Here we must again remember that in Tantric metaphysics, the macrocosm is faithfully mirrored in the microcosm of the individual body-mind. Thus sun and moon stand for important phenomena in the psychoenergetic system. Through the activities of the lunar and solar channels and the dynamics between them, consciousness (awareness) is kept in constant cyclic motion, causing sleep and waking, as well as inner-directedness and outer-directedness. They are responsible for the fundamental tension inherent in the ordinary mind.

The lunar and solar channels, however, are different from the microcosmic sun and the moon. The former is thought to be placed in the stomach, where it consumes the nectar (*amrita*) oozing from the moon stationed in the head. The *yogin* or *yogini* must gain control over this natural process and augment it, so that the ambrosial fluid is distributed over the entire body rather than wasted in the stomach. This is said to lead to vigor, health, and longevity. In Hatha Yoga the inverted postures such as shoulder stand and headstand are deliberately employed to reverse the position of the microcosmic sun and moon, so as to prevent the wastage of the lunar nectar.

As David Gordon White has shown in some detail, the microcosmic luminaries also play a central role in alchemy, which anyway is closely related to both Yoga and Āyurveda.[15] The microcosmic moon is described as having sixteen digits or units (*kalā*), which correspond to the lunar phases. The sixteenth digit, which makes the macrocosmic moon into a full moon, is associated with immortality and the path of cessation (*nivritti-mārga*), that is, the yogic process of reversal, introspection, renunciation, and recovery of one's true nature.

Only when the life energy flows through the median pathway, which it does periodically for short periods of time throughout the day, is there relative balance in our body-mind. The flow of psychoenergy in the *sushumnā* is the way to immortality, that is, to the full use of the transformative ambrosial nectar dripping from the microcosmic moon located in the head. In most cases, however, the flow through the axial pathway is a mere trickle and thus does not manifest its positive effects fully. Some people are *idā* dominant; others are *pingalā* dominant. Only adepts are *sushumnā* centered, which expresses itself in inner peace, harmony, and lucidity. Tradition relates these three principal pathways and their response systems to the three primary qualities of nature: *tamas* (principle of inertia), *rajas* (principle of dynamism), and *sattva* (principle of clarity).

Before the serpent power can ascend the axial pathway all impurities must be removed from the network of *nādīs*. In the ordinary individual the currents exist in a polluted state, preventing the free flow of vital energy and therefore causing physical and mental imbalance, as well as spiritual blindness. This is yet another way of understanding the human condition, and it reveals the esoteric aspect of the yogic process of self-purification. I will say more about this in the next chapter.

Awakening the Serpent Power

The *yogin* who stirs the [*kundalinī-*]*shakti* comes to
enjoy paranormal abilities. What more need be said?
Like [child's] play he conquers time/death (*kāla*).
  —*Hatha-Yoga-Pradīpikā* (3.120)

CLEANSING THE DOORS OF PERCEPTION

The way we see the world depends on who we are. On the simplest level, a child walking down the street will readily spot all the toy stores; a pennywise shopper will see all the bargains displayed in shop windows; an architect will notice unusual buildings; and a taxi driver will be quick to locate house numbers. In each case, perception is selective, depending on the person's interest and attention. This extends to more significant aspects of life as well, such as our attitude toward relationships, morality, work, leisure, health, sickness, pain, death, and the great beyond. These attitudes are shaped by all kinds of factors, of which karmic conditioning, as the Tantric scriptures would insist, is the most influential one.

We are shaped by our past choices, which is the same as saying that we are creatures of habit. In yogic terms, our thoughts and actions for the most part follow the path of least resistance. That is to say, they are overdetermined by the energetic template of the subtle body. This explains why it is so difficult to change our behavior even when we have realized that our old patterns are wrong, unproductive, or damaging. Hence in addition to behavioral change, Tantric practitioners attempt to modify the pathways of the life force directly. This modification is a matter of cleansing the *nādīs*, a practice called *nādī-shodhana*.

As noted in the previous chapter, in the ordinary individual the energy currents exist in a state of relative defilement. They are not fully functional and therefore impede physical well-being and spiritual growth. The Tantric adept's specific goal is to open the central channel so the life force can flow freely through it and, in due course, entice the far greater energy of the *kundalinī* to follow suit.

Without prior cleansing of the *nādī* system, raising the serpent power (*kundalinī-shakti*) along the axial pathway is not only impossible but also very dangerous to attempt, for instead of entering the central channel (*sushumnā-nādī*) it is likely to force itself into the *idā*- or the *pingalā-nādī*, on either side of the central channel, causing immense havoc in the body and mind. This is what happened to Gopi Krishna during his spontaneous *kundalinī* awakening, and his gripping account of the physical pain and mental anguish resulting from it stands as a timeless warning to all neophytes dabbling with the serpent power, or *shakti*. He wrote:

> My face became extremely pale and my body thin and weak. I felt a distaste for food and found fear clutching my heart the moment I swallowed anything. . . . My restlessness had assumed such a state that I could not sit quietly for even half an hour. When I did so, my attention was drawn irresistibly towards the

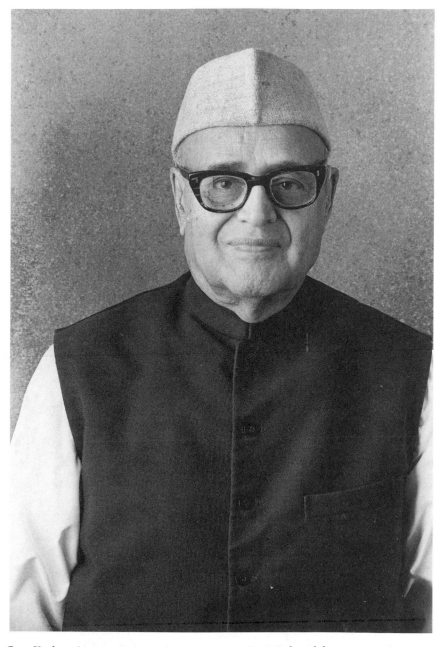

Gopi Krishna (1903–1984), whose writings on his own kundalinī *experiences substantially broadened the awareness about* kundalinī-yoga *in the West.* (Photograph © copyright by Chuck Robinson)

strange behaviour of my mind. Immediately the ever-present sense of fear was intensified, and my heart thumped violently.[1]

He further described how the *kundalinī* generated tremendous heat in his body, "causing such unbearable pain that I writhed and twisted from side to side while streams of cold perspiration poured down my face and limbs."[2] He continued:

> There were dreadful disturbances in all the organs, each so alarming and painful that I wonder how I managed to retain my self-possession under the onslaught. The whole delicate organism was burning, withering away completely under the fiery blast racing through its interior.
>
> I knew I was dying and that my heart could not stand the tremendous strain for long. My throat was scorched and every part of my body flaming and burning, but I could do nothing to alleviate the dreadful suffering. If a well or river had been near I would have jumped into its cold depths, preferring death to what I was undergoing. . . . I racked my distracted brain for a way of escape, only to meet blank despair on every side. The effort exhausted me and I felt myself sinking, dully conscious of the scalding sea of pain in which I was drowning.[3]

Other similar cases have been reported in the literature. The American psychiatrist Lee Sannella, one of the first members of the medical establishment to make an unprejudiced attempt at understanding the *kundalinī* phenomenon, has suggested that the blockages in the energetic field are "stress points." As he explained in his widely read book *The Kundalini Experience*:

> In the course of its upward motion, the kundalini is held to encounter all kinds of impurities that are burned off by its dynamic activity. . . . In particular, the Sanskrit scriptures mention three major structural blockages, known as "knots." . . . We can look upon these blockages as stress points. Thus, in its ascent, the kundalini causes the central nervous system to throw off stress. This is usually associated with the experience of pain. When the kundalini encounters these blocks, it works away at them until they are dissolved.[4]

Sannella's statement holds true only in cases where the *kundalinī* has been prematurely or wrongly aroused, that is, in the absence of adequate preparation. The Tantric scriptures emphasize the need for thorough groundwork before adopting any practices that aim at awakening the serpent power directly. As the fourteenth-century master Svātmarāma states, the *kundalinī* "bestows liberation on *yogins* and bondage on the ignorant."[5] A sharp knife in the hands of a skilled physician can save a life but in the hands of a fool can do irrevocable harm. The *kundalinī* in itself is neither good nor bad. It simply is the Goddess energy as it manifests in the human body. Unless we consciously collaborate with it, it remains on the most subtle level of existence, sustaining us through the agency of the life force (*prāna*) but never entering our field of awareness. Through self-purification and an appropriate course of disciplines, we can benefit from it more immediately by inviting it into our life as a powerful transformative force. In its hidden state, the *kundalinī* is said to be sheer potentiality. This is only relatively correct, for the Goddess energy is always active on our behalf, maintaining all the subtle energetic processes that underlie our physical and mental structures and functions. In its awakened state, however, the *kundalinī* is an incredible agency of transformation, spiritual growth, and at last enlightenment. As the *Rudra-Yāmala* (2.26.41) affirms: "The *kundalinī* is ever the master of Yoga." In the same scripture (2.26.21–22) the serpent power is called the "mother of Yoga" and the "bestower of Yoga."

Various postures (*āsana*) are said to effect the purification of the conduits or channels (*nādī*). The *Hatha-Yoga-Pradīpikā* (1.39) singles out the adept's posture (*siddha-āsana,* written *siddhāsana*) as being particularly suited for this purpose, but other scriptures favor different postures. The adept's posture is practiced by placing the left heel at the rectum and the right heel above the genitals, while resting the chin on the chest and gazing at the spot between the eyebrows. Sometimes the position of the legs is reversed. The potency of this popular posture derives from the fact that it balances the subtle energies and thereby awakens the serpent power.

While postures like the *siddha-āsana* are important, the principal means of cleansing the channels is controlled breathing, as has been elaborated in great detail in the scriptures of Hatha Yoga. The *Gheranda-Samhitā* (5.36) distinguishes between two basic types of purification practices: *samanu* and *nirmanu*, which denote "mental" and "nonmental" respectively. As the text explains, the latter consists in physical cleansing processes called *dhauti,* comprising the following techniques:

1. *Antar-dhauti* (inner cleansing) consisting of the following four techniques:
   (a) *vāta-sāra* (air process), inhaling through the mouth and expelling the air through the lower passage
   (b) *vāri-sāra* (water process), sipping water until the stomach is completely filled and expelling it through the lower passage
   (c) *vahni-sāra* (fire process), pushing the navel one hundred times back toward the spine, which increases the "gastric fire"
   (d) *bahish-krita* (external action), sucking in air through the mouth until the stomach is filled, retaining it for ninety minutes, and then expelling it through the lower passage; this is followed by standing in navel-deep water and pushing out the lower intestinal tract for cleansing

2. *danta-dhauti* (dental cleansing), which includes cleaning the teeth and the tongue, as well as the ears and frontal sinuses

3. *hrid-dhauti* (lit. "heart cleansing"), which consists of:
   (a) introducing the stalk of a plantain, turmeric, or cane into the throat to clean it out
   (b) filling the stomach with water and then expelling it through the mouth
   (c) swallowing a long strip of thin cloth and then pulling it out again (a process called *vāso-dhauti,* "cloth cleansing")

4. *mūla-shodhana* (rectal cleansing), which is done by means of turmeric, water, or the middle finger

The *samanu* type of purificatory practice consists in breath control "with seed" (*sabīja*), that is, with silent *mantra* recitation. As the *Gheranda-Samhitā* (5.38–44) explains:

Seated on a seat, the *yogin* should assume the lotus posture. Next he should place the *guru*, etc. [in his heart],[6] as instructed by the *guru*, and commence with the purification of the channels for purification through breath control.

Contemplating the seed syllable (*bīja*) of the air element, which is energetic and of the color of smoke, the sage should inhale the air through the lunar [channel, i.e., the left nostril], repeating the seed syllable sixteen times.

Then he should retain it for sixty-four repetitions [of the seed syllable] and exhale the air through the solar channel [i.e., the right nostril] over thirty-two repetitions.

Raising the fire from the root of the navel [i.e., the *kanda*], he should contemplate the glow associated with the earth element. Then, while repeating the seed syllable of the fire element sixteen times, he should inhale through the solar channel [i.e., the right nostril].

Next, he should retain the air for sixty-four repetitions and then exhale it through the lunar channel [i.e., the left nostril] over thirty-two repetitions.

Contemplating the luminous reflection of the moon at the tip of the nose, he should inhale the air through the *idā* [i.e., left nostril] for sixteen repetitions of the seed syllable *tham*.

Then, while contemplating the nectar oozing [from the moon at the tip of the nose], he should retain the air for sixty-four repetitions of the seed syllable *vam* and thereby cleanse the channels. Finally, he should firmly exhale for thirty-two [repetitions] of the *la* sound.

The seed syllables mentioned in the above passage are the root sounds associated with the four elements: *yam* for air, *ram* for fire, *lam* for earth, and *tham* for the visualized moon, which stands for the water element in its higher aspect as the nectar of immortality (*amrita*). The common seed syllable for water is *vam*. The fifth element, "quintessence," is ether, whose seed syllable is *ham*. Although this is not mentioned in the quoted passage, oral transmission takes the ether element into account as well.

Thus the renowned contemporary Hatha Yoga master B. K. S. Iyengar has explained the connection between breath control and the elements as follows:

> In our body we have five elements. The element responsible for production of the elixir of life (prāna) is earth. The element of air is used as a churning rod, through inhalation and exhalation, and distribution is through the element of ether. Ether is space, and its quality is that it can contract or expand. When you inhale, the element of ether expands to take the breath in. In exhalation, the ether contracts to push out toxins.
>
> Two elements remain: water and fire. If there is a fire, water is used to extinguish it. This gives us the idea that fire and water are opposing elements. With the help of the elements of earth, air, and ether, a friction is created between water and fire, which not only generates energy but releases it, just as water moving turbines in a hydroelectric power station produces electricity. To generate electricity, the water has to flow at a certain speed. An inadequate flow will not produce electricity. Similarly, in our system, normal breathing does not produce that intense energy. This is why we are all suffering from stress and strain, causing poor circulation, which affects our health and happiness. The current is not sufficient so we are merely existing, not living.
>
> In the practice of prānāyāma, we make the breath very long. In this way, the elements of fire and water are brought together, and this contact of fire and water in the body, with the help of the element of air, releases a new energy, called by yogīs divine energy, or kundalinī śakti, and this is the energy of prāna.[7]

Other texts recommend similar procedures in which the left and the right pathway of the life force are alternately activated. According to the *Shiva-Samhitā* (3.26–28), alternate breathing should be performed twenty times, four times a day—at dawn, midday, sunset, and midnight. If done regularly for three months, this procedure, we are told, will definitely cleanse the channels. It is only then that the practitioner should turn to breath control proper.

The *Shiva-Samhitā* (3.31–32) also states that when the *nādīs* have been purified, certain signs will manifest: The body becomes harmonious (*sama*) and beautiful and emits a pleasant scent, while the voice becomes resonant and the appetite increases. Also, the *yogin* whose subtle pathways are thoroughly cleansed is always "full hearted," energetic, and strong. The *Hatha-Yoga-Pradīpikā* (2.19) mentions leanness and brightness of the body as indications of a purified *nādī* system, though there have been adepts with an awakened *kundalinī* who were corpulent. The Hatha Yoga texts and *Tantras* also mention that the inner sound (*nāda*) becomes audible to the practitioner, manifesting in progressively subtler form.

Now the *sādhaka* is like a finely tuned instrument and ready to engage the higher processes of Tantra, leading to the activation of the serpent power. As outlined in the previous chapter, these processes range from breath control to complex rituals and visualizations. Before describing the Tantric repertoire in more detail, we must understand the concept of the serpent power, which is at the core of Tantra Yoga.

AWAKENING THE GODDESS ENERGY

As we have seen, the universe is a manifestation of the play, or transcendental polarization, between Shiva and Shakti, God and Goddess, Being and Becoming, Consciousness and Energy. In the human body, which microcosmically replicates all cosmic principles and levels of existence, the divine Energy expresses itself in two principal forms—the life force (*prāna*) and the serpent power (*kundalinī-shakti*).

The life force is universally present in the cosmos and as such is known as *mukhya-prāna*, or "primary life force." It assumes the following five functional aspects in connection with the human body, which the ancient *Chāndogya-Upanishad* (2.13.6) styles the "gatekeepers of the heavenly world":

1. *Prāna,* in the sense of the ascending vital energy that is chiefly located in the area between the navel and the heart, is linked

particularly with inhalation but can stand for both inhalation
and exhalation.

2. *Apāna* (down-breath) is the descending vital energy associated
   with the lower half of the trunk and with exhalation.

3. *Vyāna* (through-breath) is the vital energy circulating in all
   the limbs.

4. *Udāna* (up-breath), which is connected with physiological
   functions such as speech and eructation, also denotes the
   ascent of attention into higher states of consciousness.

5. *Samāna* (mid-breath) is localized in the abdominal region,
   where it is connected with the digestive process.

In addition to the above principal types of life force, some scriptures also know of five secondary types (*upaprāna*), namely *nāga* (serpent), *kūrma* (tortoise), *kri-kara* (*kri* maker), *deva-datta* (God-given),
and *dhanam-jaya* (conquest of wealth), which are respectively associated with vomiting or eructation, blinking, hunger or sneezing, sleep
or yawning, and decomposition of the corpse.

From a yogic perspective, the two most important forms of the
vital energy are *prāna* and *apāna*, because they are the subtle realities
underlying the ebb and flow of breathing. Breath control directly
affects the ascending and descending current of the life force, which
naturally alternates—roughly every eighty minutes—between the
channel on the left (called *idā*) and the one on the right (called *pingalā*) of the central pathway.[8] The ultimate purpose of breath control
is to effect the flow of *prāna* through the central passage, which then
draws the much more powerful energy of the *kundalinī* into it.

What exactly is the *kundalinī*? In answering this question, I will
take my cue from Sir John Woodroffe, who pondered it as long ago
as 1918.[9] As he noted, the divine Energy is polarized into a static or
potential form (called *kundalinī*) and a dynamic form (called *prāna*).
The latter is responsible for maintaining all the life processes that
make embodiment possible. The former is the infinite pool of Energy
coiled into potentiality at the base of the central pathway, in the

lowest psychoenergetic center. This *cakra* is the normally closed plug hole to the infinite storehouse of Energy (and Consciousness).

In his voluminous work *Tantra-Āloka* (chapter 3), the great Tantric master Abhinava Gupta distinguishes between the *pūrna-kundalinī, prāna-kundalinī,* and *ūrdhva-kundalinī.* The first is the divine power as the Whole or Plenum (*pūrna*); the second is the divine power in its manifestation as life energy; the third is the divine power as the awakened serpent moving upward (*ūrdhva*).

By means of the kinetic energy of *prāna,* which is freely available in the body and its environment, the *yogin* or *yoginī* can tap into the energetic matrix, the Goddess Power, itself. The psychoenergetic center at the base of the axial channel corresponds to the lowest level of manifestation. It is the terminal point of cosmic evolution, as powered by Shakti. Here the Goddess comes to rest in the earth element. Far from having exhausted itself, this supreme Power now simply exists as sheer potentiality awaiting its reawakening through conscious action. The Sanskrit texts speak of the *kundalinī* as being "coiled up" three and a half times around the *linga,* the "sign" of Shiva. The coils have been taken to refer to the ground of nature (*prakriti*) and its three primary constituents or qualities—*sattva, rajas,* and *tamas.*[10] This notion may be related to the Vedic teaching of Vishnu's three steps by which he crossed the entire universe. Only a being greater than the universe can traverse it in this manner. In the case of the serpent power, this transcendence is suggested by the extra half coil. The name *kundalinī* means "she who is coiled" and is related to the word *kundala,* earring, perhaps as worn by the Pashupatas and later by some practitioners of Hatha Yoga, notably members of the Kānphata sect. Some texts shorten the word to *kundalī,* while others use the term *kutilāngī* (crooked bodied). The coils of the *kundalinī* graphically convey the notion of potentiality. For the same reason, the *Shāradā-Tilaka-Tantra* (15.62) refers to the serpent power as a "lump" (*pinda*).

We can understand the evolutionary process from the transcendental plane to the earth realm through an analogous model furnished by modern cosmology. At the "time" of the Big Bang, the world existed in a state that can be described as an unimaginably condensed ball of energy, sometimes called "quantum vacuum." Suddenly (and for no known reason), some fifteen billion years ago, a chain reaction occurred in this original high-energy soup that led to the creation of hydrogen atoms. This event coincided with the emergence of space and time and the gradual formation of our spatiotemporal universe, with its billions of galaxies, supernovas, black holes, and quasars and the cold dark matter interspersed between them. Within this unimaginable vastness are the planet Earth and the human species—both products of the original flash from chaos to cosmos or, in yogic terms, of Shiva's ecstatic dance.[11]

Now scientists are busy exploring ways of freeing up the energy stored in matter by smashing high-energy subatomic particles into protons. *Yogins* and *yoginīs* are engaged in a parallel operation in the laboratory of their own body-mind. They use the vital energy to repeatedly "smash" against the blocked opening of the central pathway of the *nādī* system. The *Goraksha-Paddhati* (1.47–51) describes this process clearly:

> The serpent power, forming an eightfold coil above the "bulb" *(kanda)*, remains there, all the while covering with its face the opening of the door to the Absolute.

> Through that door the safe door to the Absolute can be reached. Covering that door with her face, the great Goddess is asleep [in the ordinary individual].

> Awakened through *buddhi-yoga*[12] together with [the combined action of] mind and breath, she rises upward through the *sushumnā* like a thread through a needle.

> Sleeping in the form of a serpent, resembling a resplendent cord, she, when awakened by the Yoga of fire [i.e., mental concentration and breath control], rises upward through the *sushumnā*.

> Just as one may forcibly open a door with a key, so the *yogin* should break open the door to liberation by means of the *kundalinī*.

Vimalananda, a contemporary master of the Aghorī branch of Tantra, similarly remarked that to arouse the *kundalinī*, one must put pressure on it, and it will ascend only so long as this pressure is maintained.[13] Perhaps tongue in cheek, he blamed gravity for its inclination to rest in or, if awakened, return as quickly as possible to the lowest psychoenergetic center of the body. In the *Hatha-Yoga-Pradīpikā* (3.111–12), we find the following stanzas:

> One should arouse that sleeping serpent by seizing its tail. Then that *shakti*, awakening from her slumber, forcefully rises upward.

> One should seize the reclining serpent by means of *paridhāna*[14] and, while inhaling through the solar channel, every day cause her to stir for about ninety minutes, both morning and evening.

The practice mentioned here is known as *shakti-cālana* (stirring the power). It is done by contracting the sphincter muscle and by applying the throat lock (*jālandhara-bandha*) while holding the breath, which causes the *prāna* and *apāna* to mix and "combust," thereby driving the life force upward into the central channel. *Manthana* (churning) is another term used in the texts to describe the process of forcing *prāna* and *apāna* to "combust" by means of breath retention (*kumbhaka*) and most intense concentration. The Kashmiri *yoginī* Lallā hints at this process in one of her mystical poems:

> Closing the doors and windows of my body,
> I seized the thief, *prāna*, and shut him in.
> I bound him tightly inside the chamber of my heart,
> And lashed him hard with the whip *om*.[15]

> I pulled the reins of the steed of the mind;
> I compressed the life force circulating through the ten channels;
> Then, indeed, did the lunar particle (*shashi-kalā*) melt and
>   dissolve,
> and the Void merged with the Void.[16]

> Concentrating on the *om*-sound,
> I made my body like blazing coal.
> Leaving behind the six crossroads,
> I travelled the path of Truth.
> And then I, Lallā, reached the Abode of Light.[17]

The earlier image of seizing the serpent by the tail is characteristic of the forceful (*hatha*) approach of Hatha Yoga. Some traditional authorities might find it disrespectful to speak of the divine Shakti in this manner, while others would object to the idea that one can coerce the Goddess and obtain her liberating grace by mechanical means.

All are agreed, however, that the serpent energy must ascend along the central pathway, which is also called the "great path" (*mahā-patha*) and "cremation ground" (*shmashāna*) because it alone leads to liberation. In keeping with this typically Tantric symbolism, the *Gheranda-Samhitā* (3.45) specifies that the *yogin* engaged in this esoteric practice should besmear his body with ashes, an outward sign of his internal renunciation of all worldly things and desires. The adept who seeks to arouse the *kundalinī* must be prepared to die, because this process quite literally anticipates the death process. As the serpent power rises along the central passage, the *yogin*'s or *yoginī*'s microcosm is gradually dissolved. I will deal with this process shortly, though first I want to mention Abhinava Gupta's concept of *prāna-danda-prayoga*, or the "process of making the life force like a rod (*danda*)."

A cobra is dangerous only when it is coiled, ready to strike in an instant; when its body is completely erect it is quite harmless. Similarly, the *kundalinī* is dangerous only in its form of the diffuse life energies, which fuel the unillumined person's hankering for sensory and sensual experiences, entangling him or her ever more in worldly *karma*. When the serpent power is erect, however, it is not poisonous but a source of ambrosia, because it is erect only when it has entered the central pathway leading to liberation and bliss. As Jayaratha explains in his commentary on the *Tantra-Āloka* (chapter 5, p. 358), when one strikes a serpent it draws itself up and becomes stiff like a rod. Similarly, through the process of "churning," the *kundalinī* stretches upward into the perpendicular pathway of the *sushumnā,* reaching with its head for the topmost psychoenergetic center.

The ascent of the Goddess power in the body is associated with the progressive dissolution of the elements, a process that is called *laya-krama* (process of dissolution) or *laya-yoga* (discipline of dissolution). In the present context, the technical term *laya* refers to the resorption of the elements into the pretemporal and prespatial ground of nature (*prakriti-pradhāna*). That this esoteric process has often been misunderstood can be gathered from the following comments in the *Hatha-Yoga-Pradīpikā* (4.34):

> They say "*laya, laya,*" but what is the nature of *laya*? *Laya* is nonremembrance of the sense objects because the tendencies (*vāsanā*) do not arise again.

This stanza from the pen of the adept Svātmārāma indicates that the yogic process of microcosmic dissolution brings about a dramatic change in the mind, for it wipes clean karmic seeds stored in the subconscious. This is the purpose of all higher processes of Yoga, for only when the karmic seeds are burned completely is their future germination rendered impossible and liberation ensured. But Svātmārāma's comments do not tell us how this Tantric process actually occurs. The *Tantras* are little more communicative on this point, which is one of the many experientially based truths of Tantra Yoga.

In principle, *laya* is effected as the *kundalinī* rises from center to center. Its arrival causes each center to vibrate intensely and to function fully, but as it goes to the next higher psychoenergetic center, the departure of the Goddess power leaves the previous center or centers as if void. The reason for this is that at each center Shakti works the miracle of a profound purification of the elements (called *tattva*), rendering them extremely subtle. More precisely, their vibration is speeded up to the most subtle level of nature (*prakriti*), and hence they are said to have become reabsorbed into the cosmic matrix. The intelligent Goddess power henceforth—or at least for the period of *kundalinī* arousal—takes over their respective functions.

This esoteric process is the basis for the *bhūta-shuddhi* ritual, in which the elements are visualized as being purified through their progressive absorption into the divine Shakti. This practice, which is discussed in detail in the *Bhūta-Shuddhi-Tantra*, is done prior to visualizing oneself as one's chosen deity (*ishta-devatā*) and doing ritual worship. The earth element governs the area between the feet and the thighs; the water element has authority over the area between the thighs and the navel; the fire element rules the zone between the navel and the heart; the air element reigns over the section between the heart and the forehead; the ether element governs the area above the forehead. The practitioner visualizes earth dissolving into water, water into fire, fire into air, air into ether, and then ether into the higher principles (*tattva*), until everything is dissolved into the Goddess power itself.

Thus the *yogin* or *yoginī* starts out as an impure being (*pāpa-purusha*) and through the power of visualization recreates himself or herself as a pure being, a worthy vessel for the divine Power. Through the *kundalinī* process, this visualized pure body-mind then becomes actuality, for the ascent of the serpent power through the axial pathway of the body recapitulates the mental process of *bhūta-shuddhi*, literally changing the body's chemistry. Through repeated practice of *kundalinī-yoga*, Tantric adepts succeed in speeding up the vibration of their body permanently, leading to the creation of the much-desired "divine body" (*divya-deha*).

The language of vibration is by no means modern but is integral to the vocabulary of Tantra, particularly the Tantric schools of Kashmir. The idiom of vibration has been developed in great detail by the philosopher-*yogins* of the Spanda school. According to them, everything is vibration—the elements, their subtle templates, the sense objects, the life force, the *cakras*. Even the ultimate Shakti itself is vibratory in nature, though its vibration is, in contemporary terms, "translocal." The Spanda masters speak of this as a "quasi-vibration." But they insist that we must assume the transcendental Shakti to be dynamic, as otherwise there is no plausible explanation for the existence of the world or the fact that it is constantly changing. An analogous concept, which it might be helpful to evoke here, is physicist David Bohm's "holomovement," which is essentially undefinable and immeasurable.[18] This coinage refers to the ultimate foundation of all "implicate orders," that is, the multiply enfolded reality mirrored in each of its parts.

Similarly, the *kundalinī* is the ultimate, translocal vibration—Shakti—affecting the space-time continuum more directly in the form of the *yogin*'s or *yoginī*'s localized body-mind. Its supervibration radically transmutes the constituents of the body-mind, ultimately creating a transubstantiated or divinized body (*divya-deha*) endowed with extraordinary capacities that transcend the laws of nature as we know it.

The earth element, which is connected with the lowest psychoenergetic center, is dissolved into its energetic potential of smell (*gandha-tanmātra*). This is conducted by the rising *kundalinī* to the second psychoenergetic center, where the Goddess power next dissolves the water element into its energetic potential of taste (*rasa-tanmātra*). This subtle product is elevated to the level of the psychoenergetic center at the navel. Here the *kundalinī* transmutes the fire element into its energetic potential of sight (*rūpa-tanmātra*). This distillate is then taken to the level of the heart center, where the *kundalinī* effects the transmutation of the wind element into its energetic potential of touch (*sparsha-tanmātra*). This subtle form of the wind element is next raised to the level of the throat center, where the *kundalinī* refines the ether element into its energetic potential of sound (*shabda-tanmātra*). This product of yogic alchemy is conducted to the level of the *ājnā-cakra*, in the middle of the head, and here the lower mind (*manas*) is dissolved into the higher mind (*buddhi*), which, in turn, is dissolved into the subtle matrix of nature (*sūkshma-prakriti*). The final phase of dissolution occurs when the serpent power reaches the topmost psychoenergetic center, where the subtle matrix of nature is dissolved into the *para-bindu,* which is the supreme point of origin of the individuated body-mind. Dissolution (*laya*) is fundamental to Tantra Yoga. Hence we can read in the *Kula-Arnava-Tantra* (9.36):

> Ten million rituals of worship equal one hymn; ten million hymns equal one recitation [of a *mantra*]; ten million recitations equal one meditation; ten million meditations equal a single [moment of] absorption (*laya*).

Thus, in its ascent toward the crown center, the *kundalinī-shakti* invigorates the various *cakras* and then causes them to shut down again. But this shutdown differs from the earlier state of minimal function in the ordinary person, for the *cakras* of the adept are no longer closed down because of impurities (or karmic obstructions) but because their energy has been transmuted. Hence when the *kun-dalinī* returns to its resting place at the base of the spine, the *cakras* resume their respective functions but in a far more integrated or harmonious way.

As soon as the *kundalinī* pierces the center in the midbrain—the *ājnā-cakra*—it assumes a new form of existence and becomes *cit-kun-dalinī*, or the "serpent of Consciousness." This event is accompanied by the great bliss of nondual realization. This bliss, arising from the union of the Shakti with Lord Shiva, extends throughout the body while yet transcending it.

Along the route, the ascending *kundalinī* may produce all kinds of physiological and mental phenomena, which are all the result of incomplete identification with the Goddess power and a certain attachment to the body. The *Tantras* mention startled jumping (*udbhava* or *pluti*), trembling (*kampana*), a whirling sensation (*ghūrni*), sleepiness (*nidrā*), as well as ecstatic feelings (*ānanda*) that are not, however, of the same magnitude or significance as the supreme bliss of transcendental realization. The texts also speak of all kinds of auditory phenomena, increasingly subtle manifestations of the inner sound (*nāda*).

The ascent of the serpent power through the six principal "wheels" of the body is technically called *shat-cakra-bhedana*, or "piercing the six centers." This curious expression is explained by the fact that in the ordinary individual the *cakras* are undeveloped and more like knots (*granthi*) than beautiful lotus flowers. The awakened *kundalinī* breaks them open, disentangles their energies, and vitalizes and balances them. Three of the *cakras* represent a particular challenge to the *yogin* and *yoginī*. Thus the Tantric and non-Tantric scriptures mention three knots, at the base of the spine, the throat, and the "third eye." They are called *brahma-, vishnu-,* and *rudra-granthi* respectively, after the deities Brahma, Vishnu, and Rudra (= Shiva).

There are other places at which the life force is "knotted," causing constrictions. Blockages can occur particularly at the sensitive spots called *marmans* (junctions), which are distributed over the whole body. Yoga, Tantra, and Āyurveda generally recognize eighteen such spots. The *Shāndilya-Upanishad* (1.8.1f.) mentions the following twenty-five locations for them: the feet, big toes, ankles, shanks, knees, thighs, anus, penis, navel, heart, throat, jugular notch (called *kūpa*, "well"), the palate, nose, eyes, middle of the eyebrows, forehead, and head. Hatha Yoga, which is a Tantra based discipline, includes practices designed to discharge blocked energy in these *marmans*. These involve guiding the life force through focused visualization to each *marman* and then retaining the breath, which activates them. Upon exhalation, the blocked energy is released. This is also an excellent way of aiding the healing process where disease is present.

The goal of Tantra is to have the *kundalinī* remain permanently elevated to the topmost psychoenergetic center, which state coincides with liberation. At the beginning, however, the *kundalinī* will tend to return to the *cakra* at the base of the spine because the body-mind is not yet adequately prepared. Therefore the practitioner must repeatedly invite the Goddess power to unite with her divine spouse, Shiva, at the top of Mount Kailāsa, that is, in the *sahasrāra-cakra*. This will gradually remove the karmic inclination toward identifying with the body-mind rather than Shiva-Shakti as one's ultimate identity. In Kashmiri Tantra, this ever-blissful transcendental identity is called *aham* ("I") versus the finite ego (*ahamkāra*, "I-maker"), which is driven by the desire to maximize pleasure and minimize pain and yet continuously sows the seeds of suffering.

Tantra Yoga aims at dissolving the illusion of being a separate finite entity, and it does so by means of the union of the *kula-kundalinī* with the transcendental principle of *akula*, or Shiva. When this is accomplished there is nothing that is not realized as utterly blissful. Even the body, previously experienced as a material lump (*pinda*), is seen to be supremely conscious and suffused with the invigorating nectar of bliss and at one with all other bodies and with the universe itself.

Under the influence of Shakti, the body's chemistry starts to change and the practitioner looks transfigured to the eyes of outside observers. He or she becomes increasingly radiant, manifesting the supreme Consciousness-Bliss (*cid-ānanda*). The Tantric adept literally becomes a beacon of Light in the world.

Mantra

THE POTENCY OF SOUND

> The mind is transfixed by the beautiful inner sound (*nāda*),
> as a snake in a hole is [caught] because of the scent [of a
>   decoy]
> and drops its fickleness. Completely forgetting the world,
> where could it run to?
> —*Nāda-Bindu-Upanishad* (43)

THE SONIC UNIVERSE

Modern science and ancient Tantra agree: the universe is an ocean of energy. Where they differ is in how this fact should be understood. The Tantric approach affirms that this finding has very personal implications. If matter can indeed be resolved to energy, then the human body, as a product of the material cosmos, is likewise energy at a more primary level. As the *Tantras* further insist, energy and consciousness are ultimately conjoined as the two poles of the same Reality, Shiva-Shakti. Therefore the human body is, in the final analysis, not merely unconscious matter but a stepped-down version of superconscious Energy. This insight has far-reaching practical ramifications for each person. For if the body is not merely the sarcophagus of an immaterial soul but a vibrant, living reality suffused with the same Consciousness that also animates the mind, then we must cease to regard the body as an external object radically distinct from our conscious selves. The habitual split between body and mind is not only unwarranted but detrimental to the wholeness to which spiritual seekers aspire. To put it in traditional terms, the body is a temple of the Divine. It is the foundation for realizing the essential oneness of everything; it is the springboard from which we can attain enlightenment—an enlightenment that for it to be true must necessarily include each of the physical body's thirty billion billion billion cells.

The Tantric position is clear: existence is One, and we are it. All division and divisiveness is a subsequent mental construct (*vikalpa*). However, the *Tantras* do not deny differentiation as such. The Many appears within the One but without ever becoming isolated from it. The Tantric adepts merely reject the notion of duality and the accompanying ego-driven attitude of separativeness. Existence is continuity "stretching from the Radical Potential to its actualisation as the crust of matter."[1]

All this is beautifully contained in the concept of the serpent power (*kundalinī-shakti*), which is the ultimate Energy, or Shakti, as it manifests at a suitably stepped-down degree in the human body. The *kundalinī* is the power of Consciousness (*cit-shakti*), and as such is the superintelligent force sustaining the body and the mind through the agency of the life energy (*prāna*). Upon full awakening, the *kundalinī*'s fundamental role in the maintenance of our physical and mental structures and functions is witnessed directly. Gopi Krishna has expressed this vividly as follows:

> I searched my brain for an explanation and revolved every possibility in my mind to account for the surprising develop-

ment as I watched attentively the incredible movement of this intelligent radiation from hour to hour and day to day. At times I was amazed at the uncanny knowledge it displayed of the complicated nervous mechanism and the masterly way in which it darted here and there as if aware of every twist and turn in the body.[2]

That the *kundalinī* is a cosmic—even a supracosmic—intelligent energy is borne out by its traditional name *sarasvatī,* meaning "she who flows." Originally, this was the name of North India's mightiest river, which flowed through the heartland of the Vedic civilization, now lying buried under the sand dunes of the Thar Desert. A memory of the former cultural greatness of that region has survived in the figure of Sarasvatī, the goddess of learning, who is typically portrayed holding a lute (*vīnā*). Shakti is indeed the source of all knowledge and wisdom, for in the absence of the Goddess power, neither the mind nor the brain would exist.

Moreover, in the Tantric scriptures, *vīnā-danda* or "fiddlestick" is an esoteric designation for the spinal column and, by extension, the central channel. When the central channel is activated through the ascent of the life force (*prāna*) followed by the serpent power itself, all kinds of subtle sounds can be heard inwardly. Connected with this is the idea that the body of the divine serpent is composed of the fifty basic letters of the Sanskrit alphabet, which corresponds to the fifty skulls worn by the goddess Kālī as a garland (*mālā*). The alphabet is called "garland of letters" (*varna-mālā*), suggesting the higher purpose envisioned for human language by the Vedic sages, namely, to appropriately honor and express divine Reality.

Sanskrit, as the word itself indicates, is a purposely constructed (*samskrita*) language. According to tradition, it is the language of the gods—*deva-vānī.*[3] The script itself is known as *deva-nāgarī* (city of the gods), which hints at the Tantric (and Vedic) notion that each letter of the alphabet represents a particular type of fundamental energy, or deity power. Together these matrix energies weave the web of cosmic and hence also bodily existence. Here we have again the idea, quintessential to Tantra, that the microcosm mirrors the macrocosm. The body and the universe at large are produced by the same energy equations that the Tantrics have expressed in the form of the fifty principal sounds of the Sanskrit alphabet, which was developed in the context of spiritual practice and sacred vision.

As the *Shārada-Tilaka-Tantra* (1.108) states, the *kundalinī* is the sonic Absolute (*shabda-brahman*). The sonic Absolute is the soundless Absolute (*ashabda-brahman*) stepped down to the level of cosmic sound (*shabda*), corresponding to the hermetic "harmony of the spheres" and the gnostic *logos:* "In the beginning was the Word." The *Mantra-Yoga-Samhitā* (3) offers this explanation:

> Wherever there is activity, it is inevitably connected with vibration. Similarly, wherever there is vibration witnessed in the world it is invariably associated with [audible or inaudible] sound.

> Owing to the differentiation occurring at the initial moment, creation is vibratory as well. The sound produced then is the *pranava*, which has the form of the auspicious *om-kāra*.

The *Shārada-Tilaka-Tantra* (1.108) describes the cosmogonic process in terms of the production of sound as follows: From the supreme Shakti—pure Consciousness combined with the factor of lucidity (*sattva*)—comes the most subtle sound (*dhvani*), which is marked by a preeminence of the factors of lucidity and dynamism (*rajas*). Out of the *dhvani* develops the subtle sound (*nāda*), characterized by a mixture of the factors of lucidity, dynamism, and inertia (*tamas*). This subtle sound, in turn, gives rise to the energy of restriction (*nirodhikā*), which has an excess of the factor of inertia. This ontic principle emanates the "half-moon" (*ardha-indu*, written *ardhendu*), which at this lower level again shows a predominance of the factor of lucidity. Out of it comes the vibratory source point (*bindu*), the immediate source of all letters and words. These form *mantras*, which are thus manifestations or vehicles of Shakti. This scripture (1.8) further explains that the *bindu* is itself composed of three parts: *nāda, bindu,* and *bīja* (seed). The first part has a predominance of Consciousness (i.e., Shiva), the second a preponderance of Energy (i.e., Shakti), and

the third an equal presence of Consciousness and Energy. Such esoteric accounts of the evolution of sound remain relatively unintelligi-
ble outside of Tantric practice. However, they become increasingly
meaningful as the practitioner makes progress on the path of *mantra-
vidyā*, or "mantric science."

Unlike the sounds we can hear with our ears, the cosmic sound
is uncaused. It is an infinite vibration (*spanda*) that is coextensive with
the universe itself and is realizable only in deep meditation when the
senses and the mind have been deactivated. The primordial sound
is symbolically represented by the sacred syllable *om*. Although not
mentioned directly in the *Rig-Veda*, the *om* sound—also called *pranava*[4]
and *udgītha*—is hinted at in various hymns. It is first mentioned by
name in the *Shukla-Yajur-Veda* (1.1). Later on, in the era of the *Upanishads*, it came to be explained as consisting of the three constituent
sounds *a, u,* and *m*. According to the *Māndūkya-Upanishad* (9–12),
these represent the three states of waking, dreaming, and sleeping
respectively. Beyond these is the "fourth" (*turīya*), which is the condition of utter wakefulness throughout all states of consciousness. It is
the ultimate Being-Consciousness itself. Subsequent scriptures have
elaborated on this symbolism, adding the elements of *nāda* (subtle
sound) and *bindu* (zero-dimensional seed point).[5] I will address these
and other metapsychological refinements in the next section.

The Tantric speculations about sound and transcendence are extremely ancient and were foreshadowed by the Vedic notion of *vāc*,
divine speech. In the *Rig-Veda* (10.125.3–5), *vāc* is personified as the
Goddess by that name, who utters the following sacred words:

> I am the queen, gatherer of riches, the wise one, chief among
> those worthy of sacrifice. The deities have placed me in many
> places, and so I abide in many stations and enter into many
> [forms].

> Through Me alone, he who eats food sees, breathes, and hears
> what is said. Dwelling in Me, they perish [ignorant of this fact].
> Listen who can hear, I tell you that in which you should have
> faith.

> Verily, I declare of myself that which is congenial to deities
> and humans. Whomsoever I desire I render him formidable
> (*ugra*), a seer, a sage, a brahmin.

Another hymn of the *Rig-Veda* (10.71.4) states that "one who
looks does not see Vāc, and another who listens does not hear her."
She reveals herself, the text continues, as a loving wife reveals her
body to her husband. In other words, Vāc is extremely subtle and
self-revealing—an agent of grace. As the opening verse declares, it
was through affection that Vāc first revealed herself to the Vedic seers.
Then, continues verse 3, wise bards traced Vāc's path through their
sacrifices and found her hidden within the sages. There can be no
question that this Vedic goddess stands for the same divine Power
that in later times came to be venerated as Shakti and evoked as the
serpent power.

What the various models describing the evolution of sound or
vibration have in common is the idea that there are at least three levels
at which sound exists. The Tantric scriptures distinguish between the
following:

1. *Pashyantī-vāc* (visible speech)—the most subtle form of sound
   visible only to intuition

2. *Madhyamā-vāc* (intermediate speech)—sound at the subtle
   level of existence, which is the voice of thought

3. *Vaikharī-vāc* (manifest speech)—audible sound transmitted
   through vibration of the air

Beyond these three is the transcendental level called *parā-vāc*, or "supreme speech," which is Shakti in perfect union with Shiva. It is
soundless sound, hinted at in the *Rig-Veda* (10.129) in the phrase "the
One breathed breathlessly."

The three levels of sound correspond to the three forms or levels
of the serpent power:

1. *Ūrdhva-kundalinī* (upper serpent), the *kundalinī* primarily active in the *ājnā-cakra* and tending to ascend toward the thousand-petaled lotus at the crown of the head[6]

2. *Madhya-kundalinī* (middle serpent), the Goddess power active in the region of the heart and capable of ascending or descending

3. *Adhah-kundalinī* (lower serpent), the psychospiritual energy primarily associated with the three lower *cakras*

In its divine aspect, the serpent power is known as *parā-kundalinī,* or Shakti per se. From the perspective of Tantric philosophy, every single form or aspect of the universe is a manifestation of that ultimate Power and a symbol for it. In light of contemporary quantum physics, the "energy language" of Tantra makes more sense than perhaps it did to outsiders at the time of its creation two thousand and more years ago.

In its upward passage through the body's axial pathway, the Goddess power dissolves the *cakras* step by step. This can also be understood in sonic terms. According to almost identical descriptions found in various *Tantras*, when the *kundalinī* leaves the bottom *cakra*, it gathers in the fundamental energies captured in the four letters inscribed in the four petals of the *mūlādhāra* lotus. It then proceeds to the second *cakra*, where it gathers the six letter energies from there, and so on. Finally, the letter energies of the *ājnā-cakra* are dissolved into the transcendental seed point together with the *cakra* itself. When all fifty letters of the alphabet, or basic vibrations, are thus dissolved, enlightenment occurs. The *Shārada-Tilaka-Tantra* (5.121–132) describes a form of initiation (*dīkshā*) in which the teacher enters the disciple's body and performs this process himself or herself. This has been described in chapter 7 as *vedha-dīkshā*, or "initiation by penetration."

THE NATURE OF MANTRAS

The fifty letters (*varna*) of the Sanskrit alphabet, which in a way represent the body of the *kundalinī*, are called "matrices" (*mātrikā*), a term that can also mean "little mothers." They are the wombs of all sounds that make up language and are embedded in the subtle sound (*nāda*). These letters produce not only secular words but also the sacred sounds called *mantras*. A *mantra* can consist of a single letter, a syllable, a word, or even an entire phrase. Thus the vowel *a,* the syllable *āh,* the word *aham* ("I"), or the phrase *shivo'ham* ("I am Shiva," consisting of *shivah* and *aham*) can serve in a mantric capacity. In addition, the four Vedic hymnodies (*Rig-Veda, Yajur-Veda, Sāma-Veda,* and *Atharva-Veda*) have traditionally been held to consist of *mantras* only, because the hymns have all been revealed by seers (*rishi*).

The word *mantra* is composed of the verbal root *man* (to think) and the suffix *tra,* indicating instrumentality. Thus a *mantra* is literally an instrument of thought. In his *Vimarshinī* commentary on the *Shiva-Sūtra* (1.1.), Kshemarāja explains that a *mantra* is "that by which one secretly considers or inwardly reflects on one's identity with the nature of the supreme Lord." This interpretation focuses on the connection between *mantra* and *manana* (thinking, considering, reflecting). According to another traditional etymology, *mantra* gets its name from providing protection (*trāna*) for the mind (*manas*).

Far from being nonsense syllables, as an earlier generation of scholars has claimed, *mantras* are creative forces that act directly upon consciousness. But for a sound to have mantric potency it must have been transmitted by an initiate. In other words, the famous *om* sound on its own is no more a *mantra* than the word *dog.* It acquires mantric value only when it has been empowered by an adept and transmitted to a disciple. This is a vitally important point that is generally unknown to Western seekers. The reason why *mantras* can be thus potentized at all is that they have the Goddess power for their essence. "Without Her," declares the *Tantra-Sadbhāva,* "they are as unproductive as clouds in autumn."[7] But only an adept in whom the *kundalinī* is awake can empower a sound—*any* sound—so that it is transmuted into a *mantra.* As Shiva tells his divine spouse in the *Mahānirvāna-Tantra* (5.18a), "O Beloved, your *mantras* are countless."

Successful *mantra* practice depends not only on proper initiation but also on realizing the essence behind the sound. This is made clear in the *Shrī-Kanthīya-Samhitā* (as quoted in the *Vimarshinī* 2.1.), which states:

> So long as the *mantrin*[8] is distinct from the *mantra,* he cannot be successful. Wisdom alone must be the root of all this; otherwise he is not successful.

A *mantra* must be awakened (*prabuddha*) in order to unleash its inherent power. This is also known as "mantric consciousness" (*mantra-caitanya*), which goes beyond the audible sound to the level of psychospiritual power itself. As the Western adept Swami Chetanananda explains:

> Ultimately, our practice of any mantra is intended to refine our awareness to the point where we experience that pulsation going on within us all the time. When we can do that, we forget about the mantra itself because we are now aware, instead, of the dynamic event going on within and around us. As a result, the total vibration of what we are is changed. In the process, we transform ourselves.[9]

A *mantra* lacking in "consciousness" is just like any other sound. As the *Kula-Arnava-Tantra* (15.61–64) states:

> *Mantras* without consciousness are said to be mere letters. They yield no result even after a trillion recitations.

> The state that manifests promptly when the *mantra* is recited [with "consciousness"], that result is not [to be gained] from a hundred, a thousand, a hundred thousand, or ten million recitations.

> Kuleshvarī, the knots at the heart and throat are pierced, all the limbs are invigorated, tears of joy, gooseflesh, bodily ecstasy, and tremulous speech suddenly occur for sure . . .

> . . . when a *mantra* endowed with consciousness is uttered even once. Where such signs are seen, the [*mantra*] is said to be according to tradition.

To charge up or "strengthen" a *mantra*, one should repeat it thousands of times—a technique called *purashcarana* (preliminary practice). As the *Shrī-Tattva-Cintāmani* (20.3–4) states:

Just as the body is incapable of action without the psyche, so also is said to be a *mantra* without the preliminary practice.

Therefore the foremost of practitioners should first undertake the preliminary practice. Only through such application can the deity [of a *mantra*] be brought under control.

The last stanza contains an explanation for the difference between a *mantra* and an ordinary sound. While all sounds are ultimately manifestations of the divine Power, *mantras* are especially concentrated expressions of Shakti. This gives them their particular potency and usefulness on the spiritual path. The idea of bringing a deity under control may sound strange or even offensive to Western ears, but according to Tantra these deities (*devatā*) are in the final analysis simply higher types of psychospiritual energy. Because they are intelligent forces and appear to have a personal center, the Tantric practitioners are mindful to relate to them with appropriate respect and devotion. They understand, however, that these deity-energies are their own true nature, the Self. To bring a deity under control means to be able to use his or her specific energy for the spiritual process or even for worldly ends. The Tantric practitioners must constantly juggle the twofold recognition that there is only the One and that this Singularity (*ekatva*) appears differentiated at the level of phenomenal existence. Thus they know that they are both devotee and the ultimate object of devotion.

The *Mantra-Yoga-Samhitā* contains detailed information about selecting a *mantra* for a disciple, auspicious and inauspicious days for imparting a *mantra*, and the various fruits of mantric practice. *Mantras* can be employed both for liberation and other secondary purposes, such as combating illness or evil influences, or gaining wealth and power. Most high-minded practitioners are reluctant to use *mantras* for anything other than the greatest human goal (*purusha-artha,* written *purushārtha*), which is liberation. In Tantric rituals, *mantras* are used to purify the altar, one's seat, implements such as vessels and offering spoons, or the offerings themselves (e.g., flowers, water, food), or to invoke deities and protectors, and so on. Yet the science of sacred sound (*mantra-shāstra*) has since ancient times been widely put to secular use as well. In this case, *mantras* assume the character of magical spells rather than sacred vibrations in the service of self-transformation and self-transcendence.

The *Kula-Arnava-Tantra* (15.65–70) mentions sixty defects that can render *mantra* practice futile. To list only some of these: a *mantra* can be "blocked" (by duplicating a syllable), "wrongly syllabled," "broken," "lifeless," "defiled," "unstable," "fear-instilling," "powerless," and "deluded." In order to remedy these shortcomings, the *Shāradā-Tilaka-Tantra* (2.111) recommends the practice of *yoni-mudrā*.[10] This technique, which is well known from Hatha Yoga scriptures, is performed by contracting the muscles of the perineum, which causes the vital energy to rise. In addition, however, the Tantric practitioner should visualize the fifty letters of the alphabet ascending from the psychospiritual center at the base of the spine to the *cakra* at the crown of the head. This text (2.112ff.) also gives an alternative to this practice, which can be found in the *Kula-Arnava-Tantra* (15.71–72) as well. These are the following ten remedial practices (*samskāra*):

1. Creating (*janana*)—extracting a *mantra*'s constituent syllables from the alphabet

2. Enlivening (*jīvana*)—reciting each syllable separately with the *om* sound prefixed to it

3. Hammering (*tādana*)—sprinkling each written syllable of a *mantra* with water while reciting the seed syllable *yam* (for the air element)

4. Awakening (*bodhana*)—touching each written syllable with a red oleander flower while reciting the seed syllable *ram* (for the fire element); the number of flowers should correspond to the number of syllables

5. Consecrating (*abhisheka*)—sprinkling each written syllable with water containing the twigs of the *ashvattha* tree (the sacred fig tree); the number of twigs should correspond to the number of syllables

6. Cleansing (*vimalī-karana*)—visualizing a *mantra*'s impurities being burned by reciting *om hraum*, which is the *mantra* for light

7. Strengthening (*āpyāyana*)—sprinkling each written syllable with water containing *kusha* grass

8. Offering water (*tarpana*)—offering water to the *mantra* while saying, "I satiate *mantra* so-and-so"

9. Offering light (*dīpana*)—prefixing the seed syllables *om hrīm shrīm* to a *mantra*

10. Concealing (*gupti*)—keeping one's *mantra* secret

Mantras of concentrated potency are known as "seed syllables" (*bīja*). *Om* is the original seed syllable, the source of all others. The *Mantra-Yoga-Samhitā* (71) calls it the "best of all *mantras*," adding that all other *mantras* receive their power from it. Thus *om* is prefixed or suffixed to numerous *mantras*:

Om namah shivāya. "*Om.* Obeisance to Shiva."

Om namo bhagavate. "*Om.* Obeisance to the Lord [Krishna or Vishnu]."

Om namo ganeshāya. "*Om.* Obeisance to [the elephant-headed] Ganesha."

Om namo nārāyanāya. "*Om.* Obeisance to Nārāyana [Vishnu]."

Om bhūr bhuvah svah tat savitur varenyam bhargo devasya dhīmahi dhiyo yo nah pracodayāt. "*Om.* Earth. Mid-region. Heaven. Let us contemplate the most excellent splendor of Savitri, that he may inspire our visions." (This is the famous Vedic *gāyatrī-mantra*.)

Om shānte prashānte sarva-krodha-upashamani svāhā. "*Om.* At peace! Pacifying! All anger be subdued! Hail!" (Note pronunciation: *sarva-krodhopashamani*)

Om sac-cid-ekam brahma. "*Om.* The singular Being-Consciousness, the Absolute." (The word *sac* is a euphonic variant of *sat*, meaning "being.")

The *Mahānirvāna-Tantra* (3.13) calls the last-mentioned *brahma-mantra* the most excellent of all *mantras*, which promptly bestows not only liberation but also virtue, wealth, and pleasure. It is suitable for all practitioners and does not require careful computations before it is given. "Merely by receiving the *mantra*," this scripture (3.24) claims, "the person is filled with the Absolute." And, this *Tantra* (3.26) continues, "guarded by the *brahma-mantra* and surrounded with the splendor of the Absolute, he becomes radiant like another sun for all the planets, etc."

Over many centuries, the Vedic and Tantric masters have conceived, or rather envisioned, numerous other primary power sounds besides *om*. These seed syllables (*bīja*), as they are called, can be used on their own or, more commonly, in conjunction with other power sounds, forming a mantric phrase. According to the *Mantra-Yoga-Samhitā* (71), there are eight primary *bīja-mantras*, which are helpful in all kinds of circumstances but which yield their deeper mystery only to the *yogin:*

1. *Aim* (pronounced "I'm")—*guru-bīja* (seed syllable of the teacher), also called *vahni-jāyā* (Agni's wife)

2. *Hrīm*—*shakti-bīja* (seed syllable of Shakti), also called *māyā-bīja*

3. *Klīm*—*kāma-bīja* (seed syllable of desire)

4. *Krīm*—*yoga-bīja* (seed syllable of union), also called *kāli-bīja*

5. *Shrīm*—*ramā-bīja* (seed syllable of delight); because Ramā is another name for Lakshmī, the goddess of fortune, this seed syllable is also known as *lakshmī-bīja*

6. *Trīm*—*teja-bīja* (seed syllable of fire)

7. *Strīm*—*shānti-bīja* (seed syllable of peace)

8. *Hlīm*—*rakshā-bīja* (seed syllable of protection)

Other schools or texts furnish different names for these eight primary *bījas* or even altogether different schemas. Some other well-known seed syllables are *lam, vam, ram, yam, ham* (all associated with the five elements and the lower five *cakras*), *hum, hūm* (called *varman*, or "shield"), and *phat* (called *astra*, or "weapon").

THE ART OF RECITATION

When a practitioner has received a *mantra* from the mouth of an initiate, he or she can be confident of success in mantric recitation (*japa*), providing of course all the instructions for proper recitation are followed as well. Mindfulness, regularity, and a large number of repetitions of the *mantra* are the three most important requirements. Also, there are certain sacred places where *mantra* practice is considered particularly auspicious. According to the *Kula-Arnava-Tantra* (15.25), *japa* near one's teacher, a brahmin, a cow, a tree, water, or a sacred fire is particularly promising. This text (15.46–47) additionally prescribes the practice of "infusion" (*nyāsa*) for mantric recitation, which will be discussed in the next chapter.

Japa can be performed in three fundamental ways: verbalized (*vācika*), whispered (*upāmshu*), and recited mentally (*mānasa*). The first style, audible recitation, is considered inferior to the other two styles. In whispered recitation only the lips move but no audible sound escapes them. Superior to this style is mental recitation, where attention is fixed exclusively on the inner meaning of the *mantra*.

Twenty-one, 108, or 1,008 repetitions are considered auspicious. But for the *mantra* to unlock its potency (*vīrya*), hundreds of thousands of repetitions may be necessary. Once this has occurred, however, even a single pronunciation of the *mantra* will make its power available to the *mantrin* or *japin*, the reciter of *mantras*. In practice, after a while the *mantra* recites itself spontaneously, and its intrinsic power can be felt as a steady charge of energy present in one's body. This is *ajapa-japa*, or "unrecited recitation"—also known as the *hamsa-mantra*—which is more than the mental "echo" that occurs when we repeat a word over and over again. It is not simply a mental groove caused by verbal repetition but a mind-transforming energetic state of being.

It is thought important to keep a record of the number of repetitions. This is generally done by means of a rosary (*mālā*). Rosaries may consist of 15, 24, 27, 30, 50, or most commonly, 108 beads, plus one "master bead," representing one's *guru* or Mount Meru, a symbol for the central channel. The number 108 has been held sacred and auspicious in India since ancient times. Various interpretations have been offered for this highly symbolic number, but the most likely explanation lies in astronomy. Already in the Vedic era, the sages were aware that the moon's and also the sun's average distance from the earth is 108 times their respective diameters. As the American Vedic researcher Subhash Kak has shown, this number was crucial in the construction of the Vedic fire altar.[11] Symbolically speaking, 108 is the number signifying the midregion (*antariksha*), the space between heaven and earth. Thus the 108 beads can be taken to represent an equal number of steps from the material world to the luminous realm of the divine Reality—India's version of Jacob's ladder.

The rosary is often referred to as *aksha-mālā*, which corresponds to the *varna-mālā* or "garland of letters" of the Sanskrit language. The Sanskrit word *aksha* means "eye," but in the present context refers to the letters *a* and *ksha,* the Sanskrit equivalents of the Greek *alpha* and *omega*. Thus the rosary (of fifty beads) represents the entire alphabet. The *Kula-Arnava-Tantra* (15.48) distinguishes between an actual and an imaginary rosary. The former is composed of the fifty letters of the Sanskrit alphabet. The beads of the latter can be made from sandalwood, crystal, shell, coral, or most commonly *rudra-aksha* ("Rudra's eye," written *rudrāksha*), which is the multifaced seed of the blue marble tree sacred to Shiva. The *Mantra-Yoga-Samhitā* (76) mentions all kinds of other materials that can profitably be used to make a rosary. Like any ritual object, the rosary too must be purified before use. The *Mahānirvāna-Tantra* (6.171b–172a) furnishes the following mantric utterance for this purpose:

> O rosary! O rosary! O great calculator! You are the essence of all power.
>
> In You are found the four goals [i.e., material prosperity, pleasure, morality, and liberation]. Therefore grant me all success.

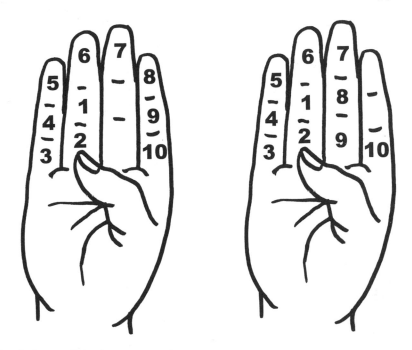

The phalanxes of the fingers are used to count mantra recitations, sometimes in specific sequences.

Another traditional way of keeping track of the number of repetitions is by counting with one's fingers. Various methods are known, and some are specific to certain *mantras*. It is considered inauspicious to count merely with the tip of one's fingers, and instead one should, according to the *Mantra-Yoga-Samhitā* (75), use the other phalanxes as well, shown in the figure.

A *mantra* should be recited with the right intonation, as learned from one's teacher, and also at the proper pace. If, as the *Kula-Arnava-Tantra* (15.55) makes clear, it is repeated too fast, there is the danger of disease. If it is recited too slowly, however, it will diminish one's energy. In either case, *japa* will be "useless like water in a broken vessel." This *Tantra* (15.57–58) furthermore points out the natural impurities at the onset and the closing of recitation, which must be countermanded by a special mantric practice, namely, by reciting the *mantra* 7 or 108 times with *om* at the beginning and the end.

Because *mantras* must be recited numerous times over many hours every day before they can bear fruit, it is easy for a practitioner to get tired. In that case the scriptures typically recommend shifting from *japa* to meditation. Then again, when the mind is exhausted from meditation, switching back to reciting one's *mantra* can bring renewed vigor and enthusiasm.

Mantras may not only be spoken or mentally recited but also written out on paper, metal, cloth, or other materials. This technique is known as *likhita-japa*, which, in the words of Swami Sivananda Radha, "brings peace, poise and strength within."[12] The same is of course true of other forms of *japa* as well. As with all yogic practices, the success of *mantra* recitation depends to a large degree on the practitioner's motivation and dedication.

Creating Sacred Space 🕉

NYĀSA, MUDRĀ, YANTRA

A love offering from a striving soul that is offered
to Me with love—be it a leaf, flower, fruit,
or water—I will eat.
  —*Bhagavad-Gītā* (9.26)

RENDERING THE BODY SACRED

The fundamental Tantric teaching that the corporeal world is in
fact the divine Reality must be not merely believed but personally
realized. Only then can we be liberated from the constraints of the
changeable reality of finite forms. But in order to realize—in Buddhist Tantric terms—the nirvanic essence of the world and of our
own body, we must anticipate or recreate as it were the purity or
flawless integrity of *nirvāna* here and now. This is the famous theological principle of *imitatio Dei*, the emulation of the Divine in our present

life. As the ancient sages of India recognized, we become whatever we contemplate with sufficient intensity and hence ought to choose our objects of contemplation carefully.

This esoteric principle is illustrated in the traditional story of the untalented disciple who could not follow the simplest instruction for meditation. He was unable to read or study any scriptures or even to memorize a single *mantra*. In a final attempt to help this backward disciple, his *guru* inquired what he would find pleasing to think about. The boy smiled from ear to ear and told his teacher that he always thought of his favorite cow and that this brought him much joy. Promptly the *guru* locked the boy in a room and told him to do nothing else but think about his cow. When the teacher checked up a couple of days later, he found the lad in deep contemplation. He had not even touched the food that had been pushed under his door. The teacher waited a few more days and then called out to his disciple to awaken him from his meditative abstraction. The response was a loud moo coming from the room. The *guru* realized that his disciple had contemplated his cow companion with such furious intensity that he had *become* it. He knew that it would be easy now to teach him to focus his every thought on the Divine so as to realize it equally swiftly.

Tantric practitioners aid their contemplation of the ultimate Reality by inviting their chosen deity (*ishta-devatā*), whether male or female, into their own body. First, however, they purify and sanctify themselves and their practice environment by visualizing the inner and outer space clear of all impurities and obscurations. Their vivid visualization is accompanied by the recitation of special *mantras* and the performance of symbolic gestures (*mudrā*). Part of this process is the ritual of elemental purification (*bhūta-shuddhi*) mentioned in chapter 11.

Equally important are the various forms of what is called the ritual of "placement" (*nyāsa*), which may well go back to the early post-Vedic era, when the *Brāhmana* texts were composed. This ritual consists in creating a divine imaginal body infused with higher aspects of reality. According to the *Kula-Arnava-Tantra* (15.46), practitioners who create for themselves an "armor" out of *nyāsa* do not need to worry about any obstacles in their path; these take flight like "elephants who have seen a lion." The *Vīnā-Shikha-Tantra* (72–73) recommends a meditation practice in which the *sādhakas* visualize their mortal body being burned to ashes and a new "wisdom body" (*vidyā-deha*) being created from the ambrosial shower (*amrita-dhārā*) that continuously irrigates their head. This elaborate process is accompanied by the downward flow of the mantric energy of the sacred syllable *om* visualized above the head.

Tantra knows a great variety of *nyāsas*. The *Mantra-Yoga-Samhitā* (48) states that only seven are considered important. This text singles out *kara-nyāsa* and *anga-nyāsa* for ordinary worship and *rishi-nyāsa* and *mātrikā-nyāsa* for more elaborate worship. The following are the most common forms.

1. *Jīva-nyāsa*, or "placement of life," is generally done immediately after the purification of the elements (*bhūta-shuddhi*) and is also called *prāna-nyāsa* or "placement of vital energy." According to the *Mahānirvāna-Tantra* (5.5), it is performed by touching the heart with the right hand while uttering *am, hrīm, krom, hamsah so'ham* and visualizing one's chosen deity's life force entering the imaginal body.

2. *Mātrikā-nyāsa*, or "placement of the alphabet," follows upon *jīva-nyāsa*. The body of the Goddess is thought to be composed of the fifty letters of the Sanskrit alphabet. The letters are to be placed in the six *cakras* as follows: *ha* and *ksha* in the *ājnā-cakra* at the forehead; the sixteen vowels in the petals of the lotus at the throat; the consonants from *ka* to *tha* in the twelve petals of the heart lotus; the next series of consonants up to *pha* in the ten spokes of the *cakra* at the navel; the consonants from *ba* to *la* in the center at the genitals; the consonants *va, sha* (= *śa*), *sha* (= *ṣa*), and *sa* in the lowest psychoenergetic center. The *Mantra-Yoga-Samhitā* (50–51) distinguishes between an "external" (*bāhya-*) and an "internal placement" (*antar-nyāsa*) version of alphabetic placement. The latter has been described above. The former is done by placing the right hand on various parts of the body as shown in table 2.

The sequence can be from the head downward or from the heart upward and downward and is often combined with breath control

TABLE 2. *MĀTRIKA-NYĀSA*, OR "PLACEMENT OF THE ALPHABET."

BODY PART	THUMB	INDEX FINGER	MIDDLE FINGER	RING FINGER	LITTLE FINGER	PALM
Heart						X
Forehead			X	X		
Face			X			
Head			X			
Mouth		X	X	X		
Lips			X			
Upper/lower teeth				X		
Mouth (inside)			X	X		
Cheeks		X	X	X		
Eyes	X			X		
Ears	X					
Nostrils	X		X			
Nape of the neck			X	X	X	
Hands			X	X	X	
Upper arms			X	X	X	
Forearms			X	X	X	
Elbows			X	X	X	
Thighs			X	X	X	
Lower legs			X	X	X	
Knees			X	X	X	
Sides			X	X	X	
Back			X	X	X	
Navel	X		X	X	X	
Stomach	X	X	X	X	X	
Various places on the chest						X
Shoulders						X
Place between the shoulders						X

(*prāṇāyāma*). With each touch, one letter of the alphabet is pronounced together with *om* in front and *namaḥ* (obeisance) at the end.

3. *Rishi-nyāsa,* or "placement of the seer," consists in installing the seer (*rishi*) associated with a given *mantra* in the head corresponding to the celestial region. After the seer has been placed in the head and duly saluted there, the poetic measure must be placed in the mouth, and the presiding deity in the heart. Moreover, the "seed" (*bīja,* standing for the consonants collectively) is placed in the genitals, while the "powers" (*shakti,* here meaning the vowels), are placed in the feet.

4. *Kara-nyāsa,* or "placement on the hand," consists in touching the fingers and the front and back of the palms while uttering *mantras.*

5. *Anga-nyāsa,* or "placement on the limbs," is usually performed on six parts of the body and hence is known as *shad-anga-nyāsa* (from *shat,* or "six," and *anga,* or "limb"). It is done as follows: touch the heart with the palm while reciting *aim hridayāya namah;* the forehead with four fingers while uttering *om klīm shirasi svāhā;* the crown of the head with the tip of the thumb while reciting *om sahuh shikāyai vashat;* the shoulders with hands crossed on the chest while saying *om sahuh kavacāya hūm;* the closed eyes with the index finger and middle finger while reciting *om bhuvah netra-trayāya vaushat*; the left palm with the index finger and middle finger of the right hand while uttering *om bhur bhuvah phat.* Some texts speak of eight places: crown of the head, forehead, midpoint between the brows, throat, heart, navel, genitals, and perineum.

6. *Pītha-nyāsa,* or "placement of the sacred sites," consists in assigning to the body the various "seats" (*pītha*) recognized by Tantra as specially empowered sites (see chapter 9).

The *Kula-Arnava-Tantra* (4.19ff.) particularly recommends *mahā-shodhā-nyāsa*, which yields *devatā-bhāva*, the state of identification with one's chosen deity. As the name indicates, this consists of a series of six "placements" (*prapanca-, bhuvana-, mūrti-, mantra-, daivata-,* and *mātrikā-nyāsa*) combined with the uttering of mantric formulas. Those who practice this ritual are said (4.120, 122) to attain self-control, grace, victory, fame, and fortune, as well as the *ājnā-siddhi* (4.128), which is the power of seeing all one's orders carried out to the letter; nor, the text continues (4.124–25), do they ever need to fear demons or the influence of the planets. The text further explains (4.121) that wherever this *nyāsa* is performed, an area with a radius of up to ten *yojanas* (about ninety miles) is rendered sacred.

By means of *nyāsa,* Tantric practitioners sanctify and simultaneously "cosmicize" their own body. As stated repeatedly in this book, Tantra acknowledges the interconnectedness of all things: *sarvam sarva-ātmakam,* "everything is the essence of everything else." The bodily microcosm enshrines within itself the entire macrocosm, because everything that exists comes out of the same One. Taking this insight seriously, the *sādhakas* symbolically reenact and empower it through the ritual of *nyāsa* and the meditative identification with their chosen deity. Inevitably this procedure yields not only a higher state of consciousness (corresponding to the Shiva principle) but also a higher level of energetic presence (corresponding to the Shakti principle). Hence the imaginal body of the initiate is also called *shākta-deha* (power-charged body) or *sakalī-karana* (complete instrument). With this specially empowered vehicle, the Tantric adept seeks to realize the sublime condition of perfect unity between Shiva and Shakti as Parama-Shiva—beyond all differentiation, yet not separate from the multiplicity of creation.

This cosmicized or divinized body is essentially a mantric body, *mantra* being the very essence of the deity. As the opening stanza of the *Vāmakā-Īshvarī-Mata,* an important *Tantra* of the South Indian Shrī-Vidyā school, has it:

> I bow to the goddess Mātrikā fashioned from *mantras*, consisting of Ganeshas, Yoginīs, planets, star configurations, and zodiacal signs.[1]

Not surprisingly, *nyāsa* entails complex mantric recitations that are meant to fortify the process of spiritual metamorphosis from ordinary worldling to deity. This ritual requires direct instruction and transmission from a qualified *guru*. Although some texts disclose the *mantras* for specific deities, they remain unproductive without proper empowerment. The same is true of the performance of the hand gestures (*mudrā*) associated with those deities, to which I shall turn next.

SYMBOLIC HAND GESTURES (MUDRĀ)

Tantric practitioners charge the universe with a profusion of symbolic significances, even though their ultimate goal is to go beyond all concepts and meanings. For the purpose of *sādhanā,* however, the world of the ordinary worldling is too flat and must be completely reconceptualized to accommodate the rich experiences awaiting the traveler on the road of Tantra. Thus the world of the *tāntrikas* is, to say the least, quite distinct from the world inhabited by the uninitiated. One aspect of Tantric ritual particularly rich in symbolism is the numerous hand gestures known as "seals" (*mudrā*). This practice undoubtedly originated with the priesthood of the Vedic era but was vastly elaborated with the rise of Tantra around the middle of the first millennium CE. The term *mudrā* also is used to denote certain bodily postures in Hatha Yoga;[2] the female partner in the Tantric sexual ritual; the large earrings worn by members of some Tantric sects, notably the Kānphatas (veterans of Hatha Yoga); and parched grain (which is thought to have aphrodisiacal properties).

Symbolic hand gestures (*hasta-mudrā*) are employed in iconography, dance, worship (*pūjā*), recitation (*japa*), and meditation (*dhyāna*), as well as in magical rites. According to traditional etymology, the term *mudrā* is related to the verbal root *mud,* meaning "to rejoice." The seals are said to delight the deities because they seal the relationship between deity and adept. As the *Mantra-Yoga-Samhitā* (53) states, "The sages call it *mudrā* because it delights all deities and it removes all sins."[3] The American scholar Douglas Renfrew Brooks, who has studied the Shrī-Vidyā tradition in depth, observes that by doing the *mudrā* or *mudrās* specific to a deity, the practitioner "creates a physical manifestation and visual display of divine form."[4] This is both an expression of, and a way of deepening, the *tāntrika*'s identification

with the chosen deity. A *mudrā* is "finger play," as one scholar translated the term, only in the profound sense of mirroring on the human
level the divine play (*līlā*) itself, which is the play of infinite Consciousness and Energy. The fingers are related to the five elements,
hinting at the cosmic significance of the hands. As Brooks also points
out, by performing a *mudrā,* the practitioner acquires the power associated with the particular aspect of the deity a given hand gesture
seeks to express symbolically.[5] *Mudrās* are not mere creations of an
inventive mind but originally came to adepts spontaneously. This is
captured in a telling observation found in Kshemarāja's *Vimarshinī*
commentary on the *Shiva-Sūtra* (3.26). He quotes an earlier work, the
Trika-Sāra:

> The sage is always characterized (*mudritah*) by seals (*mudrā*)
> arising [spontaneously] in his body. He alone is said to be a
> holder of seals (*mudrā-dhara*). Others are just holders of bones
> [i.e., their bony fingers].

Symbolic hand gestures are known outside India as well, and
they belong to the grammar of ritual. In India they have been employed since time immemorial. Later, hand gestures entered the
realm of art. They were sculpted and painted as part of the icono-
graphic representation of deities and higher beings, characterizing
specific aspects of their cosmic or terrestrial functions. Subsequently
artistic imagination in turn enriched ritual practice. In this connection
we must recollect that the artist has traditionally been regarded as a
yogin or *yoginī,* and the act of creation was pursued with all the dedication and single-mindedness of a spiritual practitioner. Traditional
Indic art can thus be seen as a form of Yoga.

Tantra knows a large number of hand gestures. The Jaina *Mudrā-
Avadhi* mentions 114 *mudrās,* and the Buddhist *Manjushrī-Mūla-Kalpa*
(chapter 35) mentions 108, of which 55 are said to be in common
use. The *Jayākhya-Samhitā* (chapter 8) mentions 58, and the *Tantra-
Rāja-Tantra* (chapter 4) mentions 25, whereas the *Shāradā-Tilaka-Tantra* (23.106–14) describes only 9 seals. The number of *mudrās* em-

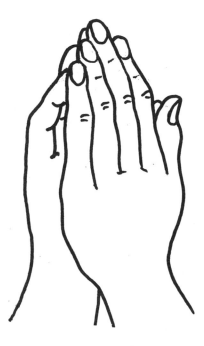

1. Anjali-mudrā

ployed during worship varies from deity to deity. Thus, according to the *Mantra-Yoga-Samhitā* (53), 19 seals are necessary in the worship of Vishnu, 10 for Shiva and the goddess Tripurā Sundarī, 9 for Durgā, 7 for Ganesha, 5 for Tārā, 4 for Sarasvatī, 2 for Rāma and Parashu-Rāma, and only a single *mudrā* for Lakshmī.

Common ritual hand gestures are:

1. *Anjali-mudrā* (seal of honoring). Bring the palms of your hands together in front of the heart, with the extended fingers pointing upward. Particularly when done at the level of the forehead, this prayerful gesture is used to welcome the deity.

2. *Āvāhani-mudrā* (seal of invitation). Bring your hands together, palms up and forming an offering bowl, with thumbs curled and the other fingers fully extended. This gesture is used, for instance, when offering a flower to the deity.

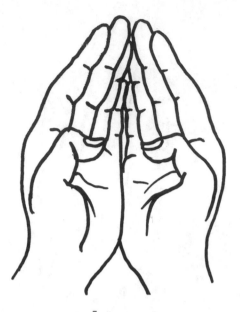

2. Āvāhani-mudrā

3. *Sthāpana-karmanī-mudrā* (seal of fixing action). Bring your
   hands together, palms down, with thumbs tucked under-
   neath. This is essentially the same gesture as the one above,
   but in reverse.

4. *Samnidhāpanī-mudrā* (seal of bringing close). Bring your
   closed fists together, with thumbs placed on top.

5. *Samnirodhanī-mudrā* (seal of full control). Same as the preceding gesture but with thumbs tucked into the fists.

6. *Dhenu-mudrā* (cow seal), also called *amritī-karana-mudrā* (seal
   creating the nectar of immortality). Place the tip of the right
   index finger on the tip of the left middle finger, the tip of
   the right middle finger on the tip of the left index finger,
   the tip of the right ring finger on the tip of the left little
   finger, and the tip of the right little finger on the tip of the
   left ring finger.

7. *Matsya-mudrā* (fish seal). Place the palm of the left hand on
   top of the right hand with the fingers fully extended and
   the thumbs pointing outward at right angles.

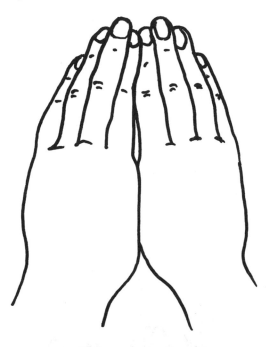

3. Sthāpana-karmanī-mudrā

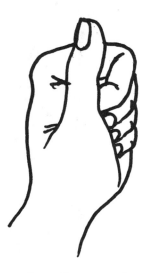

4. Samnidhāpanī-mudrā

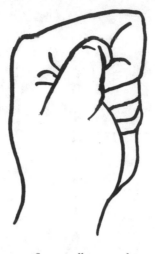

5. *Samnirodhanī-mudrā*

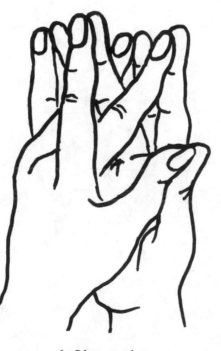

6. *Dhenu-mudrā*

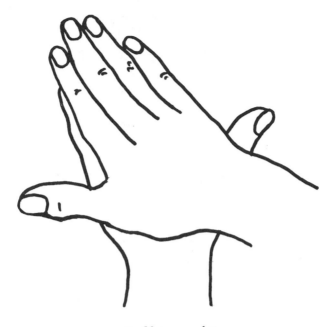

7. *Matsya-mudrā*

8. *Kūrma-mudrā* (tortoise seal). Place the palms together in such a way that the right thumb rests on the left wrist, the right index finger touches the tip of the left thumb, and the tips of the right little finger and left index finger touch.

9. *Padma-mudrā* (lotus seal). Bring the wrists together, with the fingers forming the petals of a lotus blossom. The fingertips do not touch.

10. *Yoni-mudrā* (seal of the womb/vulva). Bring your hands together, palms facing. Interlace the little fingers, and cross the ring fingers behind the fully extended middle fingers, which touch at the tips. The ring fingers are held down by the index fingers. This is the classic symbol of the Goddess.

In the Shrī-Vidyā tradition, the goddess Tripurā Sundarī is invoked by means of ten hand gestures, which are symbolically related to the nine sets (called *cakra*) of subsidiary triangles composing the famous *shrī-yantra* (or *shrī-cakra*), with the tenth *mudrā* representing the *yantra* and goddess as a whole.

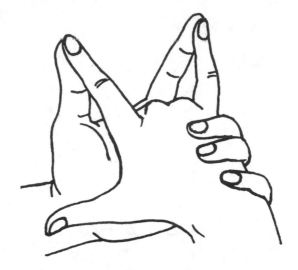

8. *Kūrma-mudrā*

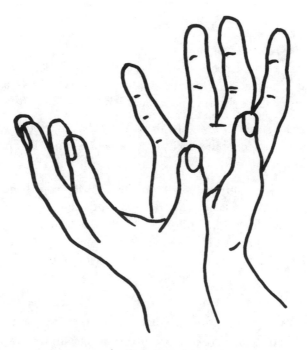

9. *Padma-mudrā*

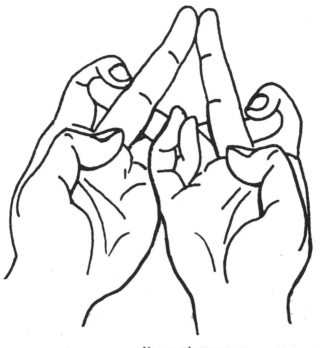

10. Yoni-mudrā

These hand gestures are also associated with the ten Yoginīs: Sarva-Samkshobhinī, Sarva-Vidrāvanī, Sarva-Ākarshinī (written Sarvā-karshinī), Sarva-Vashankarī, Sarva-Unmādinī (written Sarvonmādinī), Sarva-Mahānkushā, Sarva-Khecarī, Sarva-Bījā, Sarva-Yoni, and Sarva-Tri-Khandā. These are thought of as not only entities but also energies. They are called "deities of obstruction" (*āvarana-devatā*) because they represent specific limitations that the adept must transcend. The Shrī-Vidyā tradition acknowledges twenty-eight Yoginīs in all, each of which is connected with a particular power (*siddhi*) and has its seat in the *shrī-yantra*. This subject matter is enormously complex and makes little sense to the uninitiated.

In addition to hand gestures, in some rituals the posture of the whole body is significant as well. Various such postures are referred to in the Tantric literature and are sometimes called *sakali-kriti* (complete performance).

Mudrās are also prescribed for therapeutic purposes—one of

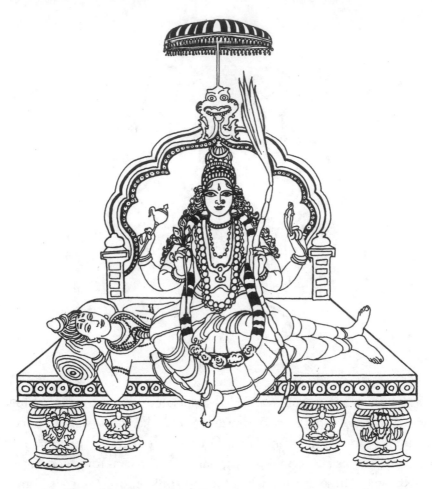

The goddess Tripurā Sundarī. (ILLUSTRATION BY MARGO GAL)

many areas of overlap between Tantra and Āyurveda.[6] The *prāna-mudrā* (seal of life), for instance, is used to stop a heart attack or bring relief from one. It is performed by bringing the thumbs in contact with the tips of the middle and ring fingers and by tucking the index fingers into the mounds of the thumbs.[7]

Deafness is thought to be helped by bending the middle fingers down on the mounds of the thumbs while pressing the middle fingers lightly with the thumbs. This technique is called *shūnya-mudrā* (seal of the void), perhaps because hearing is associated with the ether (which is the void in which all the other elements arise) or perhaps because middle finger and thumb form a zero.

For those feeling heaviness in the body, the Tantric adepts recommend *sūrya-mudrā* (solar seal). This gesture is done by pressing the ring fingers against the mounds of the thumbs while being seated in the lotus posture (*padma-āsana*). The thumb is associated with the sun and the ring finger with the water element. The juncture between them is said to stimulate the energy flow in the body.

The practice of *jnāna-mudrā* (seal of wisdom) can help with insomnia, stress, poor memory, and other undesirable conditions of the mind. It is performed by bringing the tips of the index fingers and thumbs together, forming a loop, while leaving the other fingers extended. The hands rest on the knees. This gesture, which is also called *cin-mudrā* ("seal of consciousness," *cit*), is frequently used for meditation while seated in the lotus posture (*padma-āsana*) or heroic posture (*siddha-āsana*).

Various other *mudrās* are considered suitable for meditation as well. The most common hand gesture is *dhyāna-mudrā* (meditation seal), which is done by placing the left hand in one's lap and the right hand on top of the left. Both palms are turned up.

SACRED GEOMETRY: *Yantras and Mandalas*

If *mantra* is the soul of the initiate's chosen deity, *yantra* is the deity's body. *Yantra* is also a drastically reduced image of the universe, since the universe is a theophany, a manifestation of the Divine. As a receptacle or vehicle for the deity invoked during the Tantric ritual, the *yantra* is a sacred area charged with numinous power. The word *yantra* means literally "instrument," "device," or "contrivance" and is explained in the *Kula-Arnava-Tantra* (17.61) as that which saves (*trāy-ate*) all beings from fear and from Yama, Lord of Death, himself.[8] The *yantra* is indeed employed in Tantric rituals as an instrument of concentration and visualization. It is a graphic representation of the psychocosmic energies associated with a given deity.

In addition to *yantras* used for worship, there are also portable *yantras* that serve the purpose of amulets. They protect or cure the person wearing them. I will be concerned here with *pūjā-yantras* (instruments of worship) rather than *raksha-yantras* (protective instruments).

Yantras can be drawn in sand or on paper or wood or engraved in metals or other hard substances. They consist mostly of simple geometric forms, such as point, triangle, square, rectangle, pentagon, hexagon, circle, and spiral, as well as lotus petals and Sanskrit letters. Sometimes more pictorial elements are employed in their design. The most pictorial versions are called *mandalas*, which are based on a circular arrangement and are most common in Tibetan Tantric Buddhism. Jayaratha, in his commentary on Abhinava Gupta's *Tantra-Āloka* (37.12), explains *mandala* as that which yields *manda,* meaning the essence (*sāra*) of Shiva. "Some *mandalas,*" noted Mircea Eliade, "look like labyrinths, other like palaces with ramparts, towers, gardens; we find floral patterns side by side with crystallographic structures, and sometimes the diamond or the lotus blossom seems to be discernible."[9] *Mandalas* have been made popular in the West by Carl Jung and his school. He saw in them "archetypes of wholeness."[10]

Mandalas best demonstrate the profound symbolism underlying all such geometric constructions used in Tantric rituals. The *mandala* has a fiery surround that protects the initiate against outside interferences and also is symbolic of the fire of wisdom that burns the initiate's ignorance and karma. Inside the fiery surround is the adamantine circle, symbolizing enlightenment. Next often comes a circle depicting eight graveyards, esoterically symbolizing eight forms of world-enmeshed consciousness. The third circle is fashioned from lotus petals, representing spiritual regeneration or rebirth. Inside this last circle is the "palace" (*vimāna*), the square area that contains the various deities associated with the *mandala*. This area has four gateways at which terrifying protector deities are stationed.

The *yantra,* which can be regarded as a simplified representation of the "palace" of the pictorial *mandala*, also has four gates. Within this outer ring, called *bhū-pura* (earth city), is often a circle made of lotus petals. The inner section varies from deity to deity. Almost invariably there is a dot (*bindu*) in the middle of the entire design. This is the matrix of creation and the source point of the *yantra*.

Like *mantras, yantras* can in principle be countless. The *Yantra-Uddhāra-Sarvasva,* a recent Sanskrit text, speaks of as many as 10,000 *yantras*.[11] A better-known classic text listing 103 *yantras* is the supplement to the *Saundarya-Laharī,* attributed to Shankara. The *Mantra-Mahodadhi* describes around 79 *yantras*, and relatively late works like the *Yantra-Prakāsha* and *Yantra-Pūjana-Prakāra* contain illustrations of many of them.

Some well-known *yantras* are the *yantra-rāja* (king of instruments), *mukti-yantra* (instrument of liberation), *ganapati-yantra* (instrument of the Lord of hosts), *vishnu-yantra* (instrument of Vishnu), and *kālī-yantra*. By far the best known *yantra* is the *shrī-yantra* or *shrī-cakra,* which is a symbolic representation of Shrī, one of the many female forms of the Divine. This is the most sacred symbol of the Shrī-Vidyā tradition, still flourishing in South India and other parts of the subcontinent. This *yantra* is composed of five equilateral triangles, of progressively larger size, representing the female or power (*shakti*) aspect of the Divine and four equilateral triangles, also of progressively larger size, representing the male or consciousness aspect, or Shiva. Most commonly the *shakti* triangles point downward and the *shiva* triangles point upward. The intersection of these nine major triangles (called *yonis*, or "wombs") creates forty-three small triangles. This complex figure is enclosed by the square design of the *bhū-pura*, made of three parallel lines, and also is often surrounded by three concentric circles, called *tri-vritta*. The first circle stands for twenty-nine Mā-trikās, or mother deities; the second circle represents another sixteen Mātrikās; the third circle symbolizes the sixteen eternal beings called Nityās (who are related to the fifteen phases, or *tithis*, of the moon in the outer cosmos, the sixteenth signifying completion and the lunar ambrosia). Next comes a sixteen-petaled lotus, each of whose petals accommodates one of the Kala deities. This is followed by an eight-petaled lotus, each of whose petals contains one of eight divinities.

The forty-three interlaced triangles form a fourteen-corner

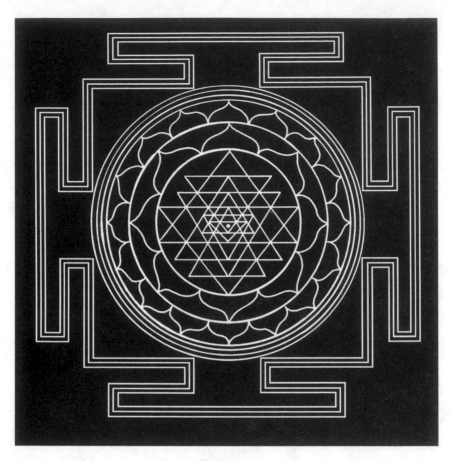

Shrī-yantra.

structure, and the fourteen corners also house one deity each. In fact, each of the triangles is the dwelling place of a deity. The central point (*bindu*), which is also called the "wheel entirely made of bliss" (*sarva-ānanda-maya-cakra*), represents the great goddess Tripurā Sundarī herself, to whom the *yantra* as a whole is dedicated.

The various parts of the *shrī-yantra* are said to correspond to the various parts of the human body. Thus the three lines composing the outer square correspond to the feet, knees, and thighs respectively; the three concentric circles correspond to the abdomen; the sixteen-petaled lotus to the lower half of the trunk; the eight-petaled lotus to the navel; and the various triangles to different parts of the upper

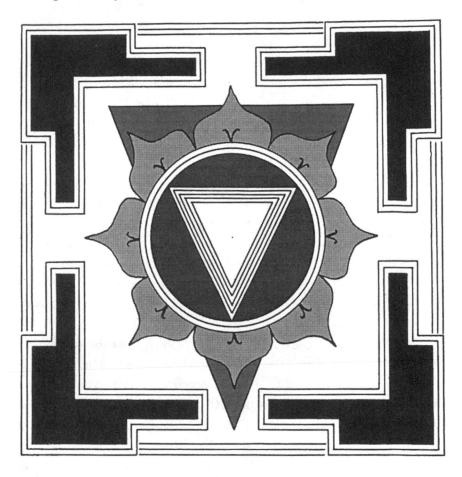

Kālī-yantra.

body, particularly the head. The central point is correlated to the thousand-petaled lotus at the crown of the head, which contains the opening to the divine dimension. In this way, the *shrī-yantra* is a geometric representation of the cosmic *purusha* or macranthropos.

The *shrī-yantra,* which has been found to have a fascinating mathematical structure, is a good indicator of the metaphysical sophistication of the Shrī-Vidyā tradition, which is the most influential Tantric branch still active today. It contains many aspects of the Kaula branch of Tantra, but also includes more conservative schools and teachers grouped under the heading of *samaya* (conventional).

In the typical Tantric ritual, the *yantra* is constructed after the initial ablution (*ācamana*), the various *nyāsas* combined with breath control, and meditation on the chosen deity. The most important aspect of *yantra* construction is the *prāna-pratishthā* ritual, by which the deity is invoked into the design. Without this, the *yantra* remains an inanimate object. The deity is the very life (*prāna*) of the *yantra* and through invocation, prayer, and other means must be established (*pratishthā*) in it. Afterward the initiate internalizes the *yantra* by picturing it within the body together with the deity. This is followed by further external ritual acts such as making invocations and offerings to the deity and his or her spirit attendants. At the end of the ceremony, temporarily constructed *yantras* are destroyed, and also the mental *yantra* is dissolved back into the central dot. Through this ritual, inner and outer—or microcosmic and macrocosmic—realities are inextricably intertwined, in keeping with the extraordinarily complex symbolism of Tantra.

Through *mantra, mudrā, nyāsa, yantra,* and all the other numerous elements of Tantric ritual, the initiates carve a sacred niche for themselves out of ordinary reality. In this sacred space into which deities and other higher beings are invoked, they relentlessly pursue the great challenge of self-transformation. To the outsider, who is busy with work and family and not driven by the impulse for liberation, the lifestyle of the *tāntrikas* looks difficult and obsessive. From the initiatory point of view, however, it is the lifestyle of the ordinary person that seems obsessive and pointless, for the worldling (*samsārin*) is constantly looking for self-fulfillment and happiness without understanding that these cannot be achieved by conventional means. Whatever pleasure the ordinary person may chance upon, it is always short-lived and ultimately unfulfilling. The Tantric path, by contrast, is the quest for the everlasting bliss, the "great delight" (*mahā-sukha*), that remains undiminished in all circumstances. As the scriptures repeat over and over again, the Tantric adepts enjoy both *yoga* and *bhoga,* or *mukti* and *bhukti*, that is, spiritual realization and enjoyment in the world. For they directly experience the identity of *nirvāna* and *samsāra*. Having found their true center, they do not get lost in the sensory world but know how to enjoy it as a manifestation of the Divine. As the Kashmiri adept Utpaladeva sings in one of his hymns to Shiva:

> Like worldly people, O Lord, may I thirst *more* for sense objects,
> but may I see them as Your body, without any notion of
> difference![12]

Initiates know that the energy and time they invest in complicated rituals and long meditations are not wasted but are the shortest route to the kind of self-fulfillment that transcends the ego and all its fears and limitations that merely keep others bound to the spatiotemporal universe. As the *Bhagavad-Gītā* (3.5) taught long ago, everyone is destined to be active, for life itself is action. The challenge is to be active in such a way that our actions are not dictated by ignorance or delusion but by liberating wisdom. Far from being merely superstitious, ritual is a potent means of purifying the mind so that it can recognize its true nature, which is pure Consciousness. Tantra does not regard action to be diametrically opposed to wisdom, as is the doctrinal stance of Advaita Vedānta, for instance. The ultimate Reality, which is pure Consciousness, also is thought to be pure Energy. Thus *jnāna* and *kriyā*—knowledge and action—are merely two aspects of the same reality. This important notion is one of the great contributions of Tantra to philosophical discourse in India.

The Tantric adepts enjoy the beauty of the spiritual path because all the while they are traveling toward the sublime goal of Self-realization, or liberation, they are certain of the fact that they are always already liberated and merely have to rediscover, remember, or recognize this eternal verity. As the adept-poetess Lallā sang:

> If your desires have snapped the threads of the web of time,
> You may live at home or take your abode in a forest;
> Knowing that the Pure Self is all-pervading,
> As you will know, so shall you be.[13]

*The Transmutation
of Desire*

One should cultivate desire (*kāma*) by means of desire.
One should cast desire into desire. Desiring by means
of desire, abiding in desire, one should stir the world.
—*Vāmakā-Īshvara-Tantra* 4.46

THE CULTIVATION OF DESIRE

If the Divine is everywhere, as the Tantric adepts affirm, it must
also be present in and as the body. This crucial insight in fact led to
the creation of Tantra, which favors an inclusive, integral approach
embracing embodiment as a manifestation of the Divine. India's more
ascetic—verticalist—traditions have typically looked upon the body
as an inconvenience, even an obstacle, to the bliss of freedom. The
body and bodily functions fill ascetics of whatever provenance with

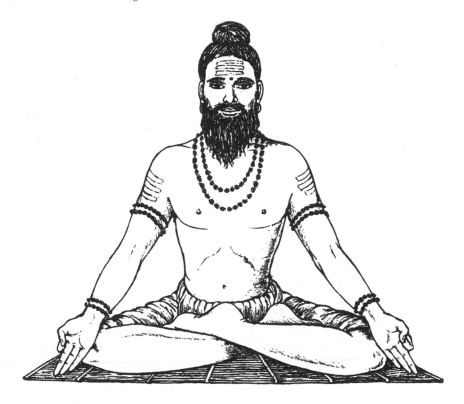

Tirumūlar (7th century CE), a great tantric adept. (DRAWING © COPYRIGHT BY MARSHALL GOVINDAN)

disgust and horror. The notion that the body is a bag of filth is as much at home with the ascetics of India as it is with the Gnostics of the Mediterranean.

The Tantric masters assumed an altogether different attitude, which is captured in the words of Tirumūlar, one of Tantra's most famous representatives:

> Those who let the body decay, destroy the spirit;
> and they won't attain the powerful knowledge of truth.
> Having learned the skill of fostering the body,
> I fostered the body, and I nurtured the soul.
>
> Formerly I thought that the body was foul.
> I saw that there was Ultimate Reality within the body.

The Perfect One has entered the temple of the body.
I protected and preserved my body.[1]

It was this body-positive orientation among *tāntrikas* that also
prompted them to adopt a new attitude toward sexuality, emotions,
and the female gender. Instead of seeing in them a danger or handicap, the initiates of Tantra welcomed them as an opportunity to attain
liberation more quickly. More than that, it looks increasingly likely
that the main initiators into the esoteric world of Tantra were originally not male but female adepts. This helps us understand why the
tāntrikas should have held women in high esteem ever since. They are
seen as manifestations of the divine Shakti, Shiva's consort, the feminine aspect of the ultimate Reality.

The ascetic stream of Indic teachings operated on the basis of a
whole series of philosophical/cosmological equations, namely, "Nature (*prakriti*) $\neq$ Spirit (*purusha*)," "Nature $=$ Suffering (*duhkha*),"
"Spirit $=$ Bliss (*ānanda*)," "Suffering $=$ Undesirable (*akāmya*),"
"Bliss $=$ Desirable (*kāmya*)," and "Man (*pums*) $=$ Spirit," "Woman
(*strī*) $=$ Nature," arriving at the unfortunate and fateful equation
"Woman $=$ Suffering $=$ Undesirable." Tantra turned this widespread ascetic view upside down. Although it continued to equate the
female gender with nature, it no longer saw in nature an illusion
(*māyā*) or aberration but a manifestation of Shakti, which was in itself
desirable.

This new orientation is expressed in a nutshell in the *Kula-
Arnava-Tantra* (2.23–24):

> The *yogin* cannot be a *bhogin*, and a *bhogin* cannot be a knower
> of Yoga. However, O Beloved, [the path of] Kaula, which is
> superior to everything, is of the essence of *bhoga* and *yoga*.

> O Mistress of the *kula*! In the *kula* teaching, *bhoga* is directly
> conducive to *yoga*, sin is conducive to good karma, and the world
> is conducive to liberation.

Here *bhoga* stands for "enjoyment," specifically worldly pleasure,
and a *bhogin* is a "pleasure seeker," representing the typical worldling
caught in the web of the senses. Yoga is introduced as the exact

opposite of this tendency. On the Kaula path, we are told, both these extremes are brought together in a third, integral approach. The *tāntrikas* neither neurotically embrace nor anxiously avoid sensory pleasure, and they neither reject nor desperately strive for mystical union (*yoga*) to the exclusion of the world. Rather, they see the world as a display of Shiva-Shakti and so are free to delight in all its myriad activities. Everything truly depends on one's point of view. Hence the ancient sages declared the mind to be the real cause of either bondage or liberation.[2] For those pure in mind, everything is pure. For those whose mind is defiled with misconceptions and base emotions, even the pure is polluted. As we can read in the *Vijnāna-Bhairava* (1 2 3):

> What is called purity by those of little understanding is impurity in the view of Shambhu [i.e., Shiva]. But [in truth] there is neither purity nor impurity. Therefore he who is free from [such] notions is happy.

Everything that the conventional mind, which is burdened by all kinds of illusions, delusions, misjudgments, and negative emotions, rejects as undesirable or reprehensible, the disciplined mind of the Tantric initiate welcomes openly as a form of the Divine.

For the *tāntrikas,* the world is the body of the ultimate Being; women are Shakti in human guise; sex is the love play between Shiva and Shakti; pleasure is a modification of supreme bliss. The Tantric practitioners cultivate not only pure motivation and pure thought but also pure desire (*kāma*). As the *Kula-Arnava-Tantra* (9.76–77) affirms:

> Like the sun, which dries up everything, or like fire, which consumes everything, so the *yogin* enjoys everything but is not stained by sin.

> Like the wind, which touches everything, or like space, which is everywhere, or like those immersing themselves completely in rivers, the *yogin* is always pure.

The *tāntrikas* are not afraid to dive deep into matter to recover the very principle of consciousness, the spirit. Those on the left-hand path or those following certain Kaula schools endeavor to go all the way to the base of material existence, which is symbolically expressed in the functions associated with the two lowest psychoenergetic centers. In particular, they do not shy away from human sexuality, which they understand as one of the manifestations of the Goddess, Shakti, who is all desires. In her microcosmic form, as the *kundalinī-shakti,* she is the driving force behind all bodily and mental processes. This includes natural bodily urges such as defecation (linked with the *mūlādhāra-cakra*), urination, and sexual desire (connected with the *svādhishthāna-cakra*).

These are taboo subjects that especially in the Judeo-Christian civilization are associated with numerous behavioral rules, laws, and a great deal of repression. Sigmund Freud pointed out to us the extent to which civilization is "built upon a renunciation of instinct, how much it presupposes precisely the nonsatisfaction (by suppression, repression or some other means?) of powerful instincts."[3] Tantra faces squarely the instinctual life.

This involves going even beyond the ideal of sublimation recommended by Freud. I have elsewhere coined the neologism *superlimation* to describe the Tantric approach.[4] Whereas sublimation is largely driven by external standards imposed on us by society, superlimation is based on bringing the light of consciousness to the actual psychosomatic process that makes sublimation possible: the process of activating *prāna* and the *kundalinī*. This allows Tantric initiates to appreciate the larger context in which the sexual drive is embedded, for the sexual impulse is merely one expression—at the level of the second *cakra*—of the psychospiritual power that extends over the entire spectrum of human and superhuman possibilities.

According to the psychoanalytic theory of sublimation, whenever we disallow the sexual impulse to express itself in sexual terms and instead focus our attention, for instance, on the creation of a work of art, we rechannel the sexual energy (or libido) to our creative activity. For most people, this is an unconscious and quite haphazard process, as many famous artists who have consciously pursued sublimation have revealed in their autobiographies. The *tāntrikas* understand that the energy that goes into the creative process is not sexual libido but the far more fundamental energy of the *kundalinī-shakti,* which can manifest as basic bodily functions, the sexual urge, the need to dominate others, the creative impulse, the desire to communicate, the need to understand, and finally, the impulse to transcend all possible urges and desires. These seven forms of desire are associated with the seven psychoenergetic centers of the body, the seventh being a special case because it actually exceeds the body-mind.

The impulse for total transcendence, or what the transpersonal psychologist Ken Wilber has called the "Atman Project," is considered the apex of the hierarchy of needs and desires.[5] The reason for this is that upon full transcendence of all partial desires (based on illusory limited ego identities), we recover our true nature, the Self, which is the repository of *all* desires and their fulfillment. As the *Bhagavad-Gītā* (2.70) declared:

> Just as the waters enter the ocean, full and of unmoving ground, so all desires enter him who attains peace, but not the desirer of desires.

Unenlightened individuals have many desires and pursue their fulfillment with greater or lesser eagerness. But the more desires are fulfilled, the more new desires will arise. This is the stuff of which *samsāra* is made. The enlightened being, however, floats in the infinity of all desires and therefore does not have to cling to any one desire but can remain in the world, at peace, fulfilled, unattached, and yet at the same time with a relish for life in all its countless forms.

LOVE, PHYSICAL AND SPIRITUAL

The Tantric position, which regards desire and spiritual life as perfectly compatible, is beautifully illustrated in the mythological figure of the god Shiva. In the *Purānas,* Shiva is portrayed not only as the archetypal *yogin* and *tapasvin* (ascetic) but also as a deity of insatiable desire, especially of the sexual variety. In her masterful study on

the enigmatic figure of Shiva, Wendy Doniger O'Flaherty brought out
the inherently paradoxical character of this ancient deity.[6]

Shiva is the naked ascetic whose penis is chronically erect, who
plunges so deeply into meditation that he can threaten the universe
with extinction and who yet is overcome by passion whenever he sees
a beautiful maiden, who is the ultimate renouncer (indicated by his
ashen body) but who simultaneously preaches that one ought to practice austerities (*tapas*) to magnify pleasure (*kāma*),[7] who is a model
ascetic capable of patiently enduring the most severe discipline for a
thousand years and who also unhesitatingly makes love to his spouse,
Pārvatī, for an entire millennium.

O'Flaherty observed that "Śiva embodies *all* of life, in *all* of
its detail, at every minute. He alone need make no choice; through
him all of the conflicting challenges are accepted at once."[8] This
accurately describes the approach of the Tantric adept, who identifies
completely with Shiva-Shakti. Even prior to enlightenment, the *tāntrikas* strive to live from the integral vantage point of enlightenment,
with great passion but without attachment, always remembering the
omnipresence of the Divine. "Bliss is the Absolute (*brahman*)," states
the *Kula-Arnava-Tantra* (80), "and that [bliss] exists in the body." Almost three thousand years earlier, the *Brihad-Āranyaka-Upanishad*
(2.4.11) pointedly referred to the genitals as the "single locus of
pleasure (*ānanda*)."

Nonattachment in the exercise of one's mental and physical capacities is tested to the maximum in the sexual ritual of *maithunā,* or
"twinning," which is at the core not only of the left-hand schools but
also of many schools of the widespread Kaula branch of Tantra. The
synonym *mithuna* ("twinning" or "coupling") is used many times in
the *Rig-Veda* and other ancient Vedic texts. In fact, the idea of sexual
polarity is a preeminent symbolic motif in the Vedic era and can be
said to be a foundation stone for later metaphysical developments
such as Tantra.[9]

This aspect of Tantra, which brings spiritual love down to earth
and elevates physical love to a higher dimension as it were, has been
a principal cause of Tantra's decline in India and of its popular revival

in the West. According to David Gordon White, a second important stimulus came from within its own ranks. This was the purging of offensive Tantric practices by the influential adept-scholar Abhinava Gupta, who introduced an incredibly sophisticated intellectual mysticism—too sophisticated for most.[10]

There can be no question that the Tantric tradition has had its share of excesses and aberrations, which naturally fueled the long-standing suspicion and criticism of Tantra by the conservative section of Hindu society. There is a fine line between free action and libertinism, transcendence of the norms of the moral majority and plain immorality, passionate worship of the Goddess in human form and mere self-indulgence. The Tantric authorities themselves have been well aware of this, and many *Tantras* contain warnings to the hypocritical practitioners who turn to the Tantric practices not in order to transcend the self, or ego-personality, but to indulge it and gratify their every whim. For instance, the *Kula-Arnava-Tantra* (2.112–19) declares:

> Drinking wine, eating meat, and gazing at the face of one's beloved are not [in themselves] behaviors leading to the supreme state.

> Only your devotees [O Goddess] and none other know this vision of *kula,* which bestows enjoyment and liberation and is obtainable through the *guru*'s compassion.

> Lacking instruction from a *guru* and being thoroughly confused themselves, such people confuse everyone else.

> Some rogues who are fond of wrong conduct hold forth, but how can such a person be a master (*svāmin*) or his disciples (*sevaka*) not be of the same sort?

> Many who lack transmission (*paramparā*) and are duped by false knowledge imagine the *kaulika* teaching according to their own mind.

> If men could attain perfection (*siddhi*) merely by drinking wine, all the wine-bibbing rogues would [readily] attain perfection.

If the mere eating of meat would lead to a meritorious state, all the meat eaters of the world would [effortlessly] enjoy merit.

If mere intercourse with a woman (*shakti*) would lead to liberation, all creatures in the world would be liberated by cohabiting with females.

The text (5.99, 111–12) continues:

One who drinks the unprepared substance [i.e., wine], consumes [unprepared] meat, and commits forcible intercourse [i.e., rape] goes to the *raurava* hell.

Shakti is fast asleep in the beast [i.e., in the person of worldly disposition] but is wide awake in the *kaulika*. He who serves that Shakti is [known as] a servant of Shakti.

He who is filled with the bliss of the union or intercourse between himself and the supreme Shakti engages *maithunā* [in the true spirit]; others are womanizers.

The Precious Substance of Love

Tantric ritual coition is surrounded by all kinds of esoteric notions that are fundamental to Tantra and without which this particular practice makes little or no sense. As David Gordon White has shown, one of the conceptual pivots of Tantric spirituality is the notion of *rasa*, a term that lends itself to various translations. It denotes essential life-sustaining fluid, and as such has been known since Vedic times. The bodily fluids—notably semen and vaginal secretion[11]—early on came to be viewed as power-charged substances that the aspirant on the path to freedom and immortality needs to harness carefully. The Vedic seers spoke of *soma,* the divine draft, which brought them into the company of the deities. This concept was assimilated into the idea of *amrita,* the nectar of immortality, which has its cosmic counterpart in *retas,* the divine seed. In the *Kaula-Jnāna-Nirnaya* (14.94), for instance, *amrita* is described as the true condition of *kaula*. It is the crux of Tantric practice and realization.

Tantra fully exploited this archaic imagery, which also fertilized the conceptual frameworks of Āyurveda and alchemy. In the former system, *rasa* stands for plasma as one of the somatic constituents (*dhātu*), together with blood, flesh, fat, bone, marrow, semen, and, in women, menstrual blood. In the latter system, *rasa* denotes mercury—Shiva's semen. The parallels between Tantra, Āyurveda, and alchemy all have their origin in a philosophy that conceptualizes the universe in sexual or erotic terms, as the creation of Shiva and Shakti. In medieval Indic alchemy, the sexual fluid of the Goddess was equated with mica, her menstrual blood with sulfur. Together with Shiva's semen, in the form of mercury, it was supposed to produce gold. In the left-hand and some Kaula schools of Tantra, menstruating women are considered especially desirable—another major breach of Hindu morality. The *Yoga-Shikhā-Upanishad* (1.138) explains the compound *rāja-yoga* as the union of menstrual blood (*rajas*) with semen (*retas*). While some (left-hand) schools of Tantra encouraged the literal mixing of menses and semen, most teachers understood these either completely metaphorically (as the union of feminine and masculine energies) or as subtle forces emanated by the female and male practitioner respectively.

The literalist interpretation has, among other things, led to the invention of Hatha Yoga practices like *vajrolī-mudrā*. The *Hatha-Yoga-Pradīpikā* (3.86–91) gives the following description:

> Blow carefully and gradually into the opening of the penis (*vajra*) by means of a prescribed tube so as to allow the passage of air.

> The semen that is about to fall into the woman's vagina should be drawn back up by this practice. If already fallen, [the *yogin*] should draw up his own semen [together with the woman's secretions] and preserve it.

> Thus the knower of Yoga should fully preserve his semen. Thus he conquers death. When the semen drops, death ensues. By holding the semen, there is life.

> By holding the semen, a pleasant smell arises in the body of the *yogin*. As long as the semen is retained in the body, how can there be fear of death?

> The semen of men is dependent on the mind, and life is dependent on the semen. Therefore both semen and mind should be carefully preserved.

> The knower of Yoga who has completely mastered this practice should draw up [the secretions] through the penis and thus preserve his own semen and that of the sex partner.

In Tantric terms, the alchemical "gold" mentioned above is the state of ecstasy deriving from the marital bliss of God and Goddess filtering down from their celestial abode into the duly prepared body of the *tāntrika*. The *yogin*'s rapture is the conscious experience of, or direct participation (*sākshātkāra*) in, the fundamental erotic nature of existence, polarized as it is into feminine and masculine potencies. The eternal love play (*līlā*) between God and Goddess became a cardinal image especially among the adherents of the Vaishnava Sahajiyā tradition, the Tantric worshipers of Vishnu in the form of Krishna and his beautiful spouse, Rādhā. This tradition, which flourished in Bengal from the sixteenth to the nineteenth century, gave fullest expression to the Tantric spirit of inclusiveness. Most *Tantras* read like manuals written in dry, formulaic language—which is basically their function. However, the Sahajiyā masters communicated their thoughts and sentiments in animated, metaphor-rich poetry composed in the vernacular. Their poems, which were meant to inspire and elevate rather than merely record the teachings, express a lifestyle that embraces the emotional realm so largely downplayed in other traditions, especially those favoring the ideal of world renunciation.

The Sahajiyās typically lived like love-crazed people. True to their ideal of "reversed discipline" (*ultā-* or *ujāna-sādhanā*), they identified with Shiva (if male) and Shakti (if female) and sought to express the divine union and accompanying love bliss in their own practice of *maithunā*. They called it "enjoyment" (*sambhoga*), which involves a return to the state of spontaneity (*sahaja*). They employed prolonged devotional singing and chanting of the divine names of Krishna to secure this lofty state, which they also conceptualized as the very essence (*rasa*) of devotion or love (*bhakti*). In the natural state, all

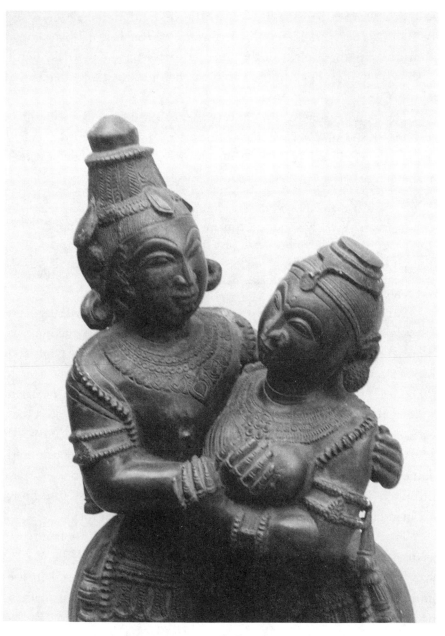

The eternal love play of Krishna and Rādhā.

male devotees are Krishna, the "Dark Lord," and all female devotees are Rādhā. They anticipated this realization through ritual playacting, often dressing themselves in the modest garb of a shepherdess (with Krishna as the lover) or, more rarely, a shepherd (with Rādhā as the beloved).

The famous nineteenth-century Bengali saint Sri Ramakrishna, the *guru* of Swami Vivekananda, is known to have worshiped the Divine for a period of time by dressing and behaving as a female devotee, or shepherdess (*gopī*). He said about this unusual practice:

> I spent many days as the handmaid of God. I dressed myself in women's clothes, put on ornaments, and covered the upper part of my body with a scarf, just like a woman. With the scarf on I used to perform the evening worship before the image. . . . I cannot speak of myself as a man.[12]

For a period of time, when in the grip of divine madness, Sri Ramakrishna would also ceremoniously worship his own genitals as the mark (*linga*) of Shiva.[13] Clearly, Sri Ramakrishna was through and through a *tāntrika*, though he is today mostly remembered as a holy master of Advaita Vedānta. It is true that he regarded the *brahman* alone as real and everything else as illusory. Yet he also remarked that *brahman* and *shakti* are identical, "like fire and its power to burn."[14] It is, therefore, all the more surprising that he should have considered Hatha Yoga as "not good," because it requires the practitioner to pay too much attention to the physical vehicle.[15] Nevertheless, the body is a manifestation of the Divine, like all other material forms.

The Sahajiyās, like Sri Ramakrishna, took their lead from the celebrated *Bhāgavata-Purāna,* the most sacred scripture of the Vaishnava tradition. In this monumental Sanskrit work, composed in the ninth or tenth century CE, the god-man Krishna is depicted as frolicking with the love-stricken wives of the local villagers. Orthodox Vaishnava interpreters understand this episode in purely allegorical terms, as the dance between God and human souls. Historians of religion, however, are bound to see in this a clear instance of Tantric influence, which subsequently led to the creation of the Sahajiyā tradition.

The Sahajiyās thought of their divine nature in terms of the "innate person" (*sahaja-mānusha*), who can be realized by tapping into or producing the essential fluid (*rasa*) or, as Glen Hayes translates the term, "divine juice." This immortal and immortalizing liquid becomes accessible through the Tantric process of reversal, particularly the upward motion of the semen (*ūrdhva-retas*) during sexual intercourse. In other words, the very fluid (i.e., the semen) that is ordinarily ejected from the body is carefully preserved and transmuted into *rasa*, which, in turn, brings immortality in the form of the person within the heart, the true man or woman. The Tantric scriptures, leaning on Āyurvedic terminology, speak of the conversion of semen into *ojas,* which is essential food for the spiritual process. Orgasm is thought to waste not only semen but also deplete the store of *ojas* and thus negate the possibility of spiritual growth. According to the *Kaula-Jnāna-Nirnaya* (14.57), by transmuting his semen the initiate gains the eight paranormal powers (*siddhi*). The preservation of semen and the energy for which it stands is an important aspect of Tantra that is almost completely ignored in Western Neo-Tantrism, whose votaries take their lead from the *Kāma-Sūtra* rather than the Tantric heritage.

The term *ojas,* which is one of the key concepts of Indic culture, is derived from the verbal root *vaj,* meaning "to be strong" and denoting "strength" or "vitality." It manifests in the body as *vīrya,* or "virility," which word is related to *vīra,* the Tantric hero. According to native Indic medicine, *ojas* is the quintessence of the somatic constituents (*dhātu*). Some contemporary interpreters identify it as albumen or glycogen, but for the *yogins* it is a subtle substance or force. They regard it as being distributed over the entire body and to be especially concentrated in semen. It is the most subtle form of the life force (*prāna*) sustaining body and mind, and being the energetic motor behind inner growth and the transcendence of the ego-personality (*jīva*).

The term *ojas* first occurs in the *Atharva-Veda* (2.17.1), where the god Agni, who is equated with *ojas,* is invoked to give the worshiper this vital essence. As is clear from other verses in the same hymnody, a worshiper is expected to practice chastity (*brahmacarya,* meaning "brahmic conduct"), which has for many millennia been considered a premium discipline for the preservation and generation of *ojas*. Patanjali, in his *Yoga-Sūtra* (2.38), states that the *yogin* who is firmly established in the practice of chastity (*brahmacarya*) acquires virility, or energy. And, no doubt, this strength is directly due to the accumulation of *ojas,* which is equivalent to *rasa*.

The alchemical fluid, or *rasa*, is also said to reside in *vastu,* meaning "substance" and referring to the building blocks that go into the construction of the divine body. In the words of Krishnadāsa, an early Vaishnava poet:[16]

> One who understands the principles of cosmic substance (*vastu*)
>   will receive the treasure of that cosmic substance.
> Without the cosmic substance, you'll never reach the Dark Lord
>   in his pastoral heaven.
>
> No one understands that the principles of the cosmic substance
>   are found within the divine juice (*rasa*).
> Without the divine juice, there can be no cosmic substance
>   in the three regions of the universe.
>
> Within the glowing divine juice, there is a singular cosmic
>   substance.
> If you do not experience that cosmic substance, you will never
>   reach the Dark Lord.
>
> The delectable experience of the erotic state is the embodiment
>   of divine juice.
> While in that erotic state, the Dark Lord has command of that
>   cosmic substance.

The Sahajiyās fully embraced the emotional and aesthetic capacities of the psyche, which is reflected in their lyrical poetry. Their allegorical descriptions of the divine body created by *sādhanā* stand apart from the mostly static psychocosmographies of other Tantric traditions. They speak of a lotus pond (*sarovara*) that is filled with flowers. The pool's water is none other than the juice of immortality, which oozes from a single blue lotus. The pond itself is to be found in a most beautiful garden in a place called the "Eye of the Great

Lord" (*mahā-īsha-locana,* written *mahesha-locana*). There also flows a mighty river through the blessed garden, which comes from distant mountains where it forms a whirlpool containing precious substances—perhaps a reference to the walls of the vagina yielding the *rasa* of transmutation and most certainly a classic example of Tantric intentional language.

Dynamic imagery like this expresses very well the Tantric penchant for using *rajas,* the active quality of nature, in spiritual practice. This is also behind Tantra's positive regard for desire, which is simply a high state of energy, which can be mobilized to achieve the desired spiritual goal. The same principle is at work in the recommendation to use extreme anger, a state of utter frustration, or even hatred to get in touch with what is prior to all emotions—the creative pulsation (*spanda*) of the ultimate Being itself.[17]

THE FIVE *M*'S

At the core of the left-hand branch and some schools of the Kaula branch of Tantra is the ritual of the *panca-ma-kāras,* or "five m's." It is so called because the names of the five "ingredients" or "substances" (*dravya*) in the ritual all start with the letter m: *madya* or *madirā* (wine or liquor), *matsya* (fish), *māmsa* (meat), *mudrā* (parched grain), and *maithunā* (sexual intercourse). These are also referred to as the "five principles" (*panca-tattva*).

The first four are all thought to have an aphrodisiacal effect. It is easy enough to see how even a drop of alcohol in an abstinent society can break down inhibition and stimulate the sex drive.[18] Consuming fish and meat can have a similar effect on an individual who is normally a strict vegetarian with strong moral injunctions against a nonvegetarian diet. The alleged aphrodisiacal property of the fourth ingredient, however, is not readily apparent, and scholars have speculated a great deal about it.

In a Tantric context, *mudrā* generally refers to symbolic hand gestures. In Hatha Yoga the term denotes special bodily postures. In

Buddhist Tantra *mudrā* is one of the designations of the female partner in the sexual ritual. They all are "seals"—the primary meaning of this Sanskrit term—which in some fashion seal in or retain the life force of the body. It is not known in what sense parched grain can be considered such a seal or even a sexual stimulant. Some scholars have translated this term as "kidney beans," which does not add to our understanding; others have rendered it as "fermented grain," which makes somewhat more sense.

The *Kula-Arnava-Tantra* (5.29–30) names twelve kinds of wine; the twelfth type, called *surā*, is said to have three subtypes and to be "appreciated by the deities" (*devatā-priyā*). The *Shakti-Sangama-Tantra* (9.46) mentions thirteen kinds. But as this *Tantra* makes clear, any type of wine can be rendered suitable when purified by *mantras*. According to the *Kula-Arnava-Tantra* (5.79), wine represents Shakti and meat symbolizes Shiva. In the right-hand schools this and the other ingredients are understood symbolically and are completely internalized. In middle-of-the-road approaches, milk or sweet juice can be substituted for wine. The *Kula-Arnava-Tantra* (5.85–86) affirms:

> Goddess! After worshiping the deities and ancestors according to the manner prescribed in the *shāstras* and remembering one's *guru,* there is no fault (*dosha*) attached to drinking wine and eating meat.

> One should resort to wine (*madhu*) and meat to satisfy the deities and ancestors and to stabilize one's contemplation of *brahman* but not for [one's own] enjoyment. Otherwise he is a sinner.

And (5.80):

> Bliss (*ānanda*) is a form of *brahman*. And that exists in the body. The wine drunk by *yogins* manifests it.

This scripture (5.107–8) also explains that the real wine is the nectar produced by the ascent of the *kundalinī-shakti* to the crown center and its merging with the "moon of Consciousness" (*ciccandra*).[19] This ambrosia is the loadstone for the external ritual without which the consumption of wine would make no sense.

The *Mahānirvāna-Tantra* (6.8) allows three types of fish for ritual consumption, which can be replaced by cakes made of beans or other similar ingredients. According to the *Prāna-Toshanī* (7.2), *matsya* symbolizes the salvific agent, which cuts all binds.

The *Kula-Arnava-Tantra* (5.44) speaks of three kinds of meat, depending on whether it stems from creatures of the sky, the earth, or the water. This scripture emphasizes that killing animals for sacrificial purposes and in the prescribed fashion is not a sin. If necessary, meat can be replaced by ginger, garlic, or salt. The *Mahānirvāna-Tantra* (6.6) sanctions only the slaughter of male animals, probably because they embody the quality of *rajas* favored in Tantra.

The final ritual "ingredient," *maithunā,* epitomizes the entire Tantric program, which seeks to overcome duality and reinstate the fundamental unity of all things, which is our inalienable nature. The sexual union between male and female practitioner is inwardly experienced as the utterly blissful transcendental identity of Shiva and Shakti, God and Goddess.

WORSHIPING THE GODDESS IN THE FORM OF A WOMAN

The heart of the left-hand and Kaula *sādhanā* is the ritual of twinning, or *maithunā,* in which a male and a female practitioner enact the divine intercourse between Shiva and Shakti. Typically but not invariably this ritual is performed in a group setting and then is called *cakra-pūjā* (wheel worship) or *rasa-cakra* (wheel of essence/juice). The word *cakra* refers to the fact that male and female practitioners engage in ritual sexual intercourse while sitting in a circle around the *guru* and his partner. The *guru* is known as the "lord of the wheel" (*cakra-īshvara*, written *cakreshvara*). He is the steady axis and anchor point for all the energies unleashed during the ritual. The male participant is typically called *bhairava* and the female participant is known as *bhairavī*—in honor of Shiva and Shakti respectively, who are both "terrifying" (*bhīra*) to the ordinary mortal but infinitely beautiful to the initiate. Other common designations for the female partner are *shakti, yoginī,* and *nāyīkā*

Various types of *cakra-pūjā* are distinguished. Thus the *Rudra-Yāmala* speaks of a *rāja-cakra*, which bestows rulership (*rāja*); a *mahā-cakra*, which gives participants prosperity; a *deva-cakra*, which brings happiness; and a *vīra-cakra*, which alone leads to liberation. The *Mahā-nirvāna-Tantra* (8.153) differentiates between a *bhairavī-cakra* and a *tat-tva-cakra* (also called *divya-cakra*). The former is suitable for all kinds of practitioners, but the latter can be formed only by adepts who have attained knowledge of *brahman* and see *brahman* in all beings and things.

The *Kula-Arnava-Tantra* (10.3) deems daily Tantric worship the best but allows monthly worship as a minimum, stating that after a longer lapse the initiate reverts to the beastly (*pashu*) state. It recommends the eighth, fourteenth, and fifteenth days of the dark fortnight, days of the full moon, days on which the sun transitions to another zodiacal sign, and the birthdays of one's *guru* and *guru*'s *guru*. This text (11.8) further stipulates that daily worship should be done during the day, while occasional worship should be reserved for the night.

The actual sexual union is variously called *maithunā, mithuna, samgama, samghatta, yāmala, strī-sevana,* or *latā-sādhanā* (practice of the creeper). The last-mentioned term refers to the fact that during sexual intercourse, male and female practitioners have their limbs intertwined in intimate embrace. This practice is described in Vatsyayana's *Kāma-Sūtra* (2.15) as *latā-veshtitaka,* "that which is twisted like a creeper." Sacred intercourse is preceded by a great deal of preparation and also occurs according to a strict protocol.[20] At least this is the format in theory. Since by no means have all Tantric "families" or "clans" (*kula*) been bona fide spiritual groups, however, it should not come as a big surprise that such events occasionally or perhaps even frequently degenerate into orgies. I am using present tense here because there are still a few Tantric circles in India, although they are as much underground as ever and carefully screen recruits.

Tantra-style teachings meet with hostility in modern India more than they do in the Judeo-Christian Western world. Few teachers are willing to flout mainstream morality openly, as did Bhagwan Shree Rajneesh (now called Osho) to his own detriment. Although he did not belong to any Tantric lineage, claiming to have attained enlightenment of his own accord, he presented his teaching as a form of Tantra. He took Tantra to be diametrically opposed to Yoga:

> Yoga is suppression with awareness; Tantra is indulgence with awareness.[21]

This represents of course a glaring oversimplification, yet it set the stage for Rajneesh's sexual theater with students, whom he sought to liberate from their inhibitions and neuroses. True enough, Rajneesh taught that in Tantra sex must not remain sex but be transformed into love, but he also acknowledged that Tantra is unlikely to be of general appeal and that those who are drawn to it will very likely practice it for the wrong reasons. "Tantra," he said, "is not to help your indulgence, it is to transform it."[22] Alas, few of his devotees seem to have heard this qualifying message, and he merely earned the sobriquet "Sex Guru" for himself.

There is nothing glamorous about Tantric sexual intercourse, even when practiced in a group. Ideally, all participants are spiritual practitioners, but a male initiate may team up with an uninitiated female, who must then be properly guided or, if necessary, controlled. Likewise, if rarely, a female initiate may take an uninitiated male partner, who for the duration of the ritual must be willing or made to comply with the expected role. Brajamadhava Bhattacharya, in his autobiographical book *The World of Tantra*, describes how as a boy he was initiated into the sexual secrets of Tantra by a woman, the mysterious "Lady in Saffron." Together they went to an abandoned temple where the *bhairavī* lit a fire, threw incense into it, and then became deeply absorbed in meditation. Sitting next to her, he too closed his eyes and drifted off. Suddenly he felt her gentle touch and when he looked at her, he found to his utter astonishment that she was now completely naked, lying prone with her legs in the lotus posture, and flower petals scattered over and around her genitals and with her pubic hair and other parts of the body besmeared with ashes and dabs of red and black color. The female genitals (*yoni* or "womb") are the most sacred power spot of a woman's body and must be duly worshiped.

The *bhairavī* in Bhattacharya's autobiographical story looked transfigured and asked him to sit on her lap, as he had done many times before, though never without her wearing a stitch of clothing. He was dumbfounded but obeyed.

> I climbed over the sacred body, and sat over the dark space left by the folding of her legs. At the very first contact I was aware that her skin was burning. The heat was forbidding. But I knew it was not for me to question. I assumed the accustomed lotus posture. . . . Minutes passed; perhaps hours. Who cared? A stream of delight rippled through the 84,000 *nādīs* of which she had always spoken. At the base of my spine I experienced a half-tickling, half-singing urge which ran up and down my spine. I closed my eyes.[23]

The *bhairavī* told him that he was the living flame, time eternal, the sun, *brahman*, while she was a corpse, time-bound, the sky, and the lotus. Then she asked him to recite Sanskrit verses, and soon he lost all sense of her presence and even his own being.

> Something was happening to the mound around my penis. A vibration, thrilling, hot deep throb hammered beat after beat. The more it came in waves the more I was pushing out my spinal base . . . a strange feeling of completeness, fulfilment and ecstasy settled on my nerves.[24]

When he finally came to his senses, he felt exhausted but still asked when they would visit the ruined temple again. She assured him that they would meet there again and again, explaining, "A carpet also hungers for someone to sit on it." Many years later, shortly before her death, she explained to him:

> Of all the emotions man suffers from . . . sex and sex-ori-ented emotions demand the most vital sacrifice. It is the most demanding and the most daring of emotions; it is also the most self-centred, next to hunger. It adores the self most, and hates to share its joy and consummation. It is wanted the most, it is

regretted the most. It is creative; it is destructive. It is joy; it is sorrow. Bow to sex, the *hlādinī* [the power of ecstasy].[25]

Over the years, Bhattacharya learned from this female initiate the various consecrations and other rituals involved in Tantric worship. The *Kula-Arnava-Tantra* (2.134) is very clear that sexual intercourse should be engaged only in the appropriate manner, as part of a carefully orchestrated ritual. Those who fail to do so run the risk of forfeiting their hard-won knowledge. As this text states (2.136), "One should not even pick a blade of [ritual] grass improperly." Thus sacred sexual intercourse, or *maithunā,* is embedded in a complex liturgy that—from the male initiate's point of view—involves much *mantra* recitation, ritual acts of self-purification, symbolic hand gestures, visualizing himself as Shiva and his partner as Shakti, and then ceremonial worship of the Goddess in human form, which itself encompasses a number of ritual acts. Actual intercourse comes after seemingly endless preliminaries that would deter anyone but the most determined and focused practitioner. Besides, as is evident from Bhattacharya's description of his own initiation, *maithunā* is not about sex but energy, specifically the vast psychospiritual force of the *kundalinī.*

Bhattacharya also participated in a Tantric circle amid other initiates in the middle of the night, as is the custom for such rituals. After prolonged chanting, the girl who had been assigned to him took her seat on his lap, and then more chanting and meditation were demanded. There was no sensuality involved at all but the transcendence of the senses through their acute stimulation. One way in which Tantra seeks to prevent emotional bonding and sensual entanglement between participants is by random selection of partners. Any girl or woman can be paired up with any male practitioner.

Maithunā is at the core of what is known as the *yoni-pūjā,* the ceremonial worship of the womb or female genitals. For the author of the *Yoni-Tantra* (8.13), this ceremony is so important that he recommends abandoning all other forms of worship and cultivating only the *yoni-pūjā.* This text (8.2) even goes so far as to state that without it, one cannot attain liberation. One of the great motifs of Tantric and Purānic mythology is the story of Shiva's madness following the death of his divine spouse. He danced madly across the earth, carrying her corpse on his shoulders. Because his dance threatened to destroy all creation, the other deities intervened. Vishnu cut up the Goddess's body piece by piece. Where the fragments fell to the ground, they immediately created power spots that became centers of pilgrimage and worship. The genitals of the Goddess fell at Kāmākhyā in Assam. There is no image of Devī in the shrine dedicated to her, but its innermost sanctum is a rock cleft resembling a *yoni* where the Goddess is worshiped. The rock is perpetually moist from a spring inside the cave, and during the months of July and August the water, rich in iron oxide, even runs red.

Both the *Yoni-Tantra* and the *Brihad-Yoni-Tantra* speak of ten parts of the *yoni*, each of which is assigned a female deity, and these deities are almost completely identical with the ten Wisdom Goddesses (*dasha-mahā-vidyā*). In other words, the *yoni* is a seat of divine presence and power. The female genitals should not be shaven, which may be related to the ancient symbolism found expressed in the *Brihad-Āran-yaka-Upanishad* (4.4.3), where the pubic hair is likened to the sacrificial grass.

The *Yoni-Tantra* (2.3–4) specifies nine types of unmarried women who are deemed particularly suitable for this ceremonial worship, but finds any experienced and wanton woman acceptable. The text (3.25–26) specifically excludes virgins, as they predictably cause a loss of power (*siddhi*). The *Kaula-Āvalī-Nirnaya* (15.7), however, recommends the worship of virgins (*kumārī*), stating that Shiva and Devī both are virgins. They may be worshiped singly or in groups. In the latter case, a favorite ceremony involves nine young girls and an equal number of boys. No sexual activity takes place.

Also the ritual—without coitus—may be performed on one's mother, and we must understand contrary statements in other Tantric scriptures, where incest is recommended, as purely symbolic. The *Vāmakā-Īshvarī-Mata-Tantra* (2.19), moreover, emphasizes that the *yogin* should never use violence toward the female initiate, who must participate of her own free will. Yet there are also texts that describe magical means of subjugating a woman.

The *Mahācīna-Ācāra-Krama-Tantra* (chapter 3) stipulates that the female partner should be a lovely young woman free from shyness, recruited from the ranks of actresses, prostitutes, washerwomen, shepherdesses, hairdressers, or from other members of the *shūdra* estate, but also *brahmin* women, if available. The text does not mention women from the *kshatriya* and *vaishya* estates, but there is no restriction regarding them either. Tantra is egalitarian, and at least for the duration of the ritual banishes all caste distinctions. Some *Tantras*, such as the *Kāmākhyā-Tantra* (chapter 3), emphasize that for successful practice a woman other than one's wife is preferable, presumably because it is easier to see the Goddess in a stranger than an all-too-familiar person to whom one may be emotionally attached. However, the more conservative *Mahānirvāna-Tantra* (8.178) favors one's own wife. The two modes are captured in the terms *svakīyā* (one's own) and *parakīyā* (another's).

Maithunā is preceded by a preliminary ritual in which the *yoni* is anointed with sandalwood paste. This makes it resemble a beautiful flower and also highlights the Tantric interest in menstrual blood (also called *pushpa*, or "flower"). The female initiate, or *shakti*, also is offered hemp (*vijayā*), a mildly narcotic substance. To this day, many *sādhus* are found smoking cannabis (called *bhāng* in Hindi and *bhangā* in Sanskrit). The *Kaula-Avalī-Nirnaya* (2.110–111) mentions hemp as an alternative to wine and also speaks of four classes of hemp and their respective purificatory *mantras*.

Next the *yogin* invites the woman to sit on his left thigh. Then the *shakti*, who is also called *dūti* or "messenger," is given wine to drink, and the male initiate begins to arouse her through fondling and kissing. All the while the *sādhaka* is saying *mantras*, especially the *bīja-mantra* for the *yoni*. The woman in turn anoints the *yogin*'s genitals (*linga*) with sandalwood paste and saffron (*kunkuma*) to prepare them for the great sacrifice of *maithunā*.

Apart from its symbolic significance, ritual coition has the purpose of generating the sacred substance, that is, *yoni-tattva*, which the *yogin* must assimilate. This is done orally or genitally by means of the *vajrolī-mudrā*, which uses the penis as a suction tube. Also, the vaginal secretions duly transformed into a sacred substance are mixed with saffron, and the *yogin* uses this paste to paint a dot (*tilaka*) on his forehead. The similarities between the Tantric *yoni-tattva* and the Vedic *soma* have often been pointed out. Both are described as reddish, are related to the moon, and are a substance of whitish color (in the one case male semen, in the other case milk). As in so many instances, here Tantra harks back to very ancient symbolism and ritual practice.

Maithunā is followed by the concluding rituals, which involve paying homage to the *yoni* and the *guru*, as well as more *mantra* recitation. Thus the *yoni-pūjā* is a sacred process that uses bodily functions that are ordinarily considered profane and even vulgar.

At the climax of the *cakra-pūjā,* the participants will all be in a state of ecstasy, and then any act is permissible. As the *Kula-Arnava-Tantra* (8.63ff.) explains, in this state of self-forgetful intoxication with the deity (*devatā*), the practitioners may walk around in absolute bliss, recite poetry, sing, clap their hands, weep with joy, play musical instruments, dance, stagger, and fall down. They may take food and wine from each other's purified vessels, even feed each other mouth to mouth, and of course randomly engage in coitus with one another. This scripture distinguishes seven degrees of exhiliration (*ullāsa*), and the seventh level is accompanied by the following eight conditions: trembling (*kampana*), hair-raising thrill (*romānca*), throbbing (*sphurana*), shedding tears of love (*prema-ashru,* written *premāshru*), perspiration (*sveda*), laughter (*hāsya*), dancing (*lāsya*), and spontaneous singing (*gāyana*). These are said to arise from the initiate's knowledge of past, present, and future. The *Kula-Arnava-Tantra* (8.75) further assures us that there is no mental perturbation (*vikriti*) despite all this outward display of ecstasy.

Maithunā is perhaps the most precious of the five "family substances" (*kula-dravya*), yet they all are necessary for the successful completion of the core Tantric ritual. Moreover, as the *Kula-Arnava-Tantra* (5.69) stresses, without the "five *m*'s" the other Tantric means remain as barren as sacrificial offerings poured into ashes rather than into the sacred fire. When used correctly, they yield the "vision of the truth of the *kula*" (*kula-tattva-artha-darshana*), that is, the intuition of the ultimate Reality. When Bhairava, or Shiva, is thus intuited, the practitioner gains the "vision of sameness" (*sama-darshana*).[26] This is the spiritual recognition of the Divine in all beings and things, as taught long before the rise of Tantra by the god-man Krishna.[27]

Enlightenment and the Hidden Powers of the Mind

Goddess! The body is the temple of God.
The psyche (*jīva*) is God Sadā-Shiva.
Discard the dross of knowledge!
Worship with the notion "I am He"!
—*Kula-Arnava-Tantra* (9.41)

BLISS BEYOND PLEASURE

There are many ways to look at the Tantric *sādhanā*. One way is to see it as the cultivation of bliss by magnifying pleasure to the *n*th degree. Pleasure and pain—*sukha* and *duhkha*—are the warp and woof of mundane experience. The ordinary person constantly seeks to maximize pleasure and minimize pain. In the verticalist traditions, the worldling's hunt for pleasure, or gratification of the senses, is typically viewed as a by-product of spiritual ignorance (*avidyā*) and as the primary source of pain. As the *Yoga-Sūtra* (2.16) puts it succinctly, pain or suffering is what is to be overcome. The recommended way to accomplish this is by curbing the volatile senses through unwavering mental concentration and inward-mindedness (*pratyak-cetanā*).

While Tantra concurs that suffering is undesirable, it does not subscribe to the simplistic belief of the verticalist traditions that pleasure (*kāma*) is intrinsically wrong or evil. Rather, it views the natural human impetus to avoid painful experiences and encounter pleasurable experiences in a new, broader context. Pleasure, the *tāntrikas* realized, is a manifestation of the ultimate bliss, which is an inalienable part of our true nature. Put differently, our search for pleasure is, in the final analysis, a quest for the bliss of the Self (*ātman*). There is nothing wrong with pleasure as such. It is merely too limited, a minuscule trickle of the delight that is the energy packed into every single atom of existence. Moreover, pleasure is frustratingly temporary, and therefore it tends to make addicts out of us, for we want to recapture pleasurable moments again and again. This pursuit enslaves all of us to one degree or another and thus is a form of suffering all its own. Either we become addicted to pleasure or we become addicted to the struggle for recovering an authentic state free from suffering. In either case we obscure our intrinsic freedom and bliss.

The Tantric path is a genuine middle path that, at least ideally, cultivates the natural (*sahaja*) state lying beyond all naive ideas about pleasure and pain. Tantra seeks to expand into daily life those sacred moments in which we are in touch with a larger truth, a greater sense of being, just as it endeavors to expand ordinary moments of pleasure to the point where they reveal their true face, which is bliss. This is expressed well in the *Vijnāna-Bhairava*, a remarkable Kashmiri text of perhaps the sixth century CE or earlier. In this work (65), which is also called *Shiva-Jnāna-Upanishad* (Secret Teaching on the Wisdom of Shiva), we can read the following instruction:

[The *yogin*] should remember the entire universe or his own body as being filled with his innate (*sva*) bliss. Then by means of his innate nectar (*amrita*) he should simultaneously assume the form of the supreme bliss.

The *Vijñāna-Bhairava* teaches 112 ways of "remembering" one's divine status. It gives methods for all kinds of situations, especially those in which a high amount of psychosomatic energy is mobilized, such as moments of great anger and passion. It is difficult to transform a mind dominated by the principle of inertia (*tamas*), manifesting as lethargy, apathy, and indifference. When the dynamic principle (*rajas*) holds sway, however, the energetic charge inherent in the unstable condition of the agitated mind can be put to positive use. To proceed from *tamas* to *sattva* (the principle of lucidity), one must first establish a presence of *rajas*. The following verses from the *Vijñāna-Bhairava* (69–72) clearly illustrate the Tantric approach.

The delight (*sukha*) associated with the penetration of the *shakti* at the peak of intercourse with the *shakti* is said to be the delight of one's own brahmic Truth.

O divine Mistress, even in the absence of a *shakti*, there is a flood of bliss from the presence of the memory of the delight [one has experienced with] a woman by much licking and churning.

Or when one experiences great joy (*ānanda*) at seeing a relative after a long time, one should contemplate the arising joy and then merge the mind with it.

Upon experiencing an expansion of joy from savoring the pleasure produced by food and drink, one should contemplate the condition of being filled [with joy] from which will come great bliss (*mahā-ānanda*).

The recommendation contained in the first two stanzas of the above quotation has been fully explored by practitioners of the left-hand and Kaula schools. They have used sexuality, which affords the greatest conceivable pleasure for most people, yet without allowing that pleasure to overrun the mind. The *tāntrikas* have always looked for a more profound truth in sex than that of mere orgasm. In fact, the fleeting thrill of orgasm spells the end of pleasure through the sexual organs. It involves an ejection of life force (*prāna*) and characteristically leads to a diminution of awareness. But the preservation of the life force and the careful cultivation of awareness are what the Tantric adepts are most interested in, because they understand that both energy and acute wakefulness, or lucid waking, are the means to bliss.

Our true nature, the transcendental Self, is supreme Being-Consciousness-Energy. It is also innately blissful. This bliss is no mere experience, for experiences come and ago, but bliss (*ānanda*) is stable and eternal. Just as we can taste a semblance of this bliss in the sexual act, we can also discover or rediscover it in any other circumstance so long as we arrest the motion of the mind's conveyor belt.

The *Tri-Pura-Rahasya*, an outstanding scripture of the Shrī-Vidyā tradition of South India, acknowledges that we all at least intermittently experience our true, blissful nature. It speaks of momentary ecstasies (*kshana-samādhi*), in which the Self shines through into our consciousness—if only we can learn to capture those moments. Instants that reveal the Self are the short intervals between waking and sleeping and between one perception and the next, or one thought and the next, or at the height of terror or extreme anger.

These fleeting ecstasies are instances of spontaneous ecstasy or *sahaja-samādhi*, which is highly valued in the *Tri-Pura-Rahasya* (10.1– 23a, 36–40), as the following story bears out.

> Hemalekhā saw that her beloved husband had attained the desired supreme State and did not disturb him. After three hours, he awoke from the supreme Condition. He opened his eyes and saw his beloved and the surroundings. Eagerly desiring to rest in that Condition once more, he closed his eyes.
>
> Quickly grasping his hands, she asked her beloved in a beautiful ambrosial voice, "Tell me, what have you found to be the benefit by closing your eyes or the loss by keeping them open? What happens when they are closed? What happens when they are left open? Tell me this, my dearest. I would like to hear about your experience."

Asked in this manner, he said to her, lazily or reluctantly, as if he were drunk on wine or made slow from idleness, "My dear, I have at last found complete repose. I find no rest in external things, which are filled with suffering. Enough of such activities, which are [habitual] like constantly chewing cattle!

"He who is blinded by misfortune, which lies outside oneself, does not know true joy within himself. Just as someone goes begging for food because he does not know about his own treasure, so did I, ignorant of the ocean of joy within myself, again and again go after the pleasure obtained from things as if they were most excellent, even though they are overflowing with massive suffering and are transient like lightning. I deemed them permanent by force of habit.

"He who is stricken with suffering does not attain repose. So, people unable to discern between joy and sorrow always uselessly accumulate a mass of suffering. Enough of such efforts, which merely enhance the experience of suffering!

"My dear, I beg you with folded hands, be kind to me! I want to find repose in my Self's innate joy again. Oh, you are unfortunate because even though you know this State yourself, you abandon that repose and instead engage in useless activity leading to suffering."

Thus spoken to, the wise woman smiled and said, "My dear, it is you who does not know the supremely holy State, knowing which the learned of pure heart are no longer deluded. That State is as far removed from you as is the sky from the surface of the Earth. You know next to nothing. Realizing that State certainly does not depend on closing or opening one's eyes! Nor is it ever attained by doing or not doing something. Nor is that State realized by any coming or going.

"How can the Whole possibly be attained by doing anything, going anywhere, or closing one's eyes? If it were located inside oneself, then how could that State be the Whole? Myriads upon myriads of universes exist in one corner alone. How can these be made to disappear by the mere opening or closing of an eyelid measuring a digit's width? Oh, what can I say about the amazing magnitude of your delusion?

"Listen, Prince! I will tell you what is the essential truth. So long as the knots [of ignorance] are not cut, [true] joy will escape you. There are myriads of knots, which form a rope of delusion. . . . Get rid of the knots and confine the notion 'I perceive' in your heart. Uproot the very tight knot 'I am not this.' Everywhere behold the undivided, blissful, expansive Self. Behold the whole world in the Self, as if it were reflected in a mirror. Do not think that there is more than the Self that is everywhere and everything. Entering everything, abide as that which also is within by means of the innate Self."

Thus listening to what his beloved said, the brilliant Hema-cūda was rid of his misconception and understood that the Self is the Whole, which is everywhere. Gradually he stably realized this by becoming absorbed into the Whole itself and lived happily ever after with Hemalekhā and a host of other maidens.

Sahaja-samādhi is open-eyed ecstasy in which *nirvāna* is recognized in *samsāra*, or to put it differently, in which both these concepts are transcended. The sage who has attained this level of realization is perpetually happy. In his magnum opus, the *Tantra-Āloka*, Abhinava Gupta speaks of the following seven levels of bliss:

1. *Nija-ānanda* (written *nijānanda*), or "innate bliss," consists in the realization of the Self as totally separate from the objective reality and is due to the *yogin*'s concentration on the subjective side of emptiness (*shūnyatā*) at the heart.

2. *Nirānanda*, or "trans-bliss," arises when the *yogin* focuses on the external reality. It results from the ascent of the life force (*prāna*) to the psychoenergetic center at the crown of the head.

3. *Para-ānanda* (written *parānanda*), or "supreme bliss," is the realization of the Self as containing within its infinite compass all objects, which are grasped individually. It is caused by the descent of the life force in the form of *apāna* from the crown center to the heart.

4. *Brahma-ānanda* (written *brahmānanda*), or "brahmic bliss," is similar to *para-ānanda*, but here objects are grasped as a totality. This state is caused when the life force assumes its *samāna* form at the heart.

5. *Mahā-ānanda* (written *mahānanda*), or "great bliss," consists in the realization of the Self transcending all objective forms

as a result of the ascent of the life force as *udāna* in the central channel.

6. *Cid-ānanda*, or "Consciousness bliss," is the realization of the Self as subject, object, and means of cognition and comes about with the conversion of the *udāna* life force into its *vyāna* aspect.

7. *Jagad-ānanda*, or "world bliss," is the realization of the Self as including absolutely everything within and without. This is the most complete type of enlightenment.

FROM DARKNESS TO LIGHT

India's spiritual traditions are all *moksha-shāstras*, or liberation teachings. In the words of a much-quoted Upanishadic prayer, they seek to guide the aspirant from falsehood to Truth and from darkness to Light. The final goal is conceived differently in the various traditions. In Patanjali's *yoga-darshana*, for instance, liberation is conceived as the irrevocable separation of the eternal principle of Consciousness (called *purusha*) from the eternal principle of unconscious nature (called *prakriti*). For this reason, one of the commentators on the *Yoga-Sūtra,* King Bhoja, even defines Yoga as "disunion" (*viyoga*). In the ordinary, unenlightened state, the *purusha*, or spirit, deems itself entangled in the processes of nature, forgetting its perpetual freedom. The goal of Pātanjala Yoga is, through discernment (*viveka*) and dispassion (*vairāgya*), to separate the unfettered *purusha* from the automatic machinery of nature (including the brain-dependent mind). The final state is called *kaivalya,* or "aloneness," meaning the transcendental isolation of the spirit.

This is not the conceptualization of the spiritual goal in Tantra. The Tantric masters, on the contrary, constantly speak of the ultimate identity of *purusha* and *prakrti,* or Shiva and Shakti. For them, as we have seen, nature is not mere unconscious matter that like a giant rock weighs down the spirit, but a living manifestation of the very same Reality that also includes the principle of Consciousness. Therefore liberation cannot have the same meaning in Tantra as it has in Pātanjala-Yoga.

For Patanjali, liberation depends on the resorption (*pratiprasava*) of the primary constituents of *prakriti*, the *gunas*, back into the transcendental ground of nature, whereupon the entire body-mind in all its levels of manifestation is dissolved. Thus, for him, liberation inevitably coincides with the death of the bodily envelope and the disappearance of the mind associated with it. The individual cosmos ceases to exist, just as in Hindu mythocosmology the entire universe vanishes at the end of a cosmic age, when the Creator-God Brahma falls asleep. The only significant difference is that the universe reemerges when Brahma reawakens, whereas upon liberation the individual body-mind is forever negated. Transcending as it does space and time, the *purusha* is without body, and its identification with a body-mind is merely an inexplicable self-inflicted illusion of dire consequences. That misidentification can be compared to a person mistaking his or her mirror image for the real "I."

Tantra, too, acknowledges that such a misidentification occurs but understands it differently. The mirror (i.e., nature) is as real as the person gazing in it. The mistake is made when the mirror image is taken to be oneself exclusively, when the image is separated from the imaged being. The Tantric authorities never tire of reiterating that Shiva and Shakti are distinct entities only in our conceptualization of them but are identical at the level of absolute Reality. Thus our senses show us not an altogether illusory external world but a half-truth. Likewise, our mind presents us not with an illusory internal universe but something that simply is not entirely true. When we see things as they truly are (*yathā-bhūta*), all opposites—such as inner/outer, subject/object, spirit/matter—melt away. What remains is the finally incomprehensible One, which encompasses all the countless distinctions that the senses and the mind can possibly conjure up.

The *Kula-Arnava-Tantra* (8.109) explains the state of ecstatic transcendence, or *samādhi*, as follows:

> The time at which the union (*samāyoga*) of Shiva and Shakti is accomplished, [which is] the "juncture" (*sandhyā*)[1] of those devoted to the *kula*, is described as ecstasy.

The "juncture" is the paradoxical point of being omnipresent while apparently animating a finite body; of being omniscient while apparently possessing limited knowledge; of being eternal while apparently being manifested as a human being with a finite span of life; of being infinitely blissful while apparently experiencing pleasure and pain. This is the point of liberation, which is no point at all, as it transcends space as well as time. The liberated adept is fully illumined and yet is simultaneously present in the world of darkness, the world of ignorance and suffering.

The *Kula-Arnava-Tantra* (9.14) also gives another, contrasting definition of *samādhi*:

> The mind does not hear, smell, touch, see, experience pleasure and pain, or conceptualize. Like a log, he neither knows nor is aware of anything. The person who is thus absorbed in Shiva is said to abide in ecstasy.

This is a good description of *nirvikalpa-samādhi*, or transconceptual ecstasy, which ensues when there is not the slightest movement in the mind and when Consciousness stands stripped of all false superimpositions. This must not be confused with liberation itself, however, because this elevated state still excludes the external world. The ultimate ecstasy is called *sahaja-samādhi*, which is identical with liberation. It does not require the demise of the body-mind but is realized here and now. This superlative condition is known as living liberation (*jīvan-mukti*).

The *Kula-Arnava-Tantra* (9.23) states that after the supreme Self (*parama-ātman*) has been realized, "wherever the mind may turn, there it is collected (*samādhaya*)." In other words, the enlightened mind is ecstatically centered on whatever object may arise to its attention. Although this scripture does not specifically contrast *nirvikalpa-samādhi* with actual liberation, its descriptive account implies this important distinction. Speaking of the liberated being, the *Kula-Arnava-Tantra* (9.22) declares:

> He who abides in the single state of the Self,[2] his every activity is worship, his every utterance is a true *mantra*, and his every gaze is meditation.

For such a one, the text continues (9.26), nothing remains to be done. And yet precisely because the liberated being is no longer subject to the constraints of karma, as manifesting in the habits of the ego-driven personality, he or she enjoys supreme freedom to pursue any goal and engage in any action without planting anew the karmic seeds of ignorance and suffering. The liberated being is truly a free agent—at least from the ordinary human perspective. From the vantage point of liberation itself, the question of freedom and bondage does not arise at all. It could even be said that the liberated being acts under the constraint of the totality of existing forces.

Thus when the Indic texts claim that the liberated person could annihilate the universe in an instant, this is undoubtedly true but ought not to be understood in a conventional manner. As an individual, the liberated being is completely incapable of such a deed. But since he or she no longer is an individual but the Divine, the destruction of the whole cosmos lies indeed within "his" or "her" range of possibility.[3] In any case, no mental decision or personal impulse would be involved. Omnipotence is not merely personal power multiplied infinitely but is of an entirely different order.

The same can be said of omniscience. The liberated being is by definition omniscient, since he or she *is* all knowledge, but this is true only at the level of absolute existence. Here in our realm of distinct phenomena, the liberated adept may well be ignorant of many things but has access to knowledge as and when needed in the scheme of things. This is another instance of the paradox of liberation. These thoughts take us to the subject of paranormal powers.

PARANORMAL POWERS AND THE POWER
OF PERFECTION

Just as there is ecstasy and ecstasy, there also is power and power. *Samādhis* that are not liberating are nevertheless greatly enjoyable and enriching and in most cases even necessary steps toward full enlightenment. Similarly, the numerous paranormal abilities, called *siddhis*, that naturally come to practitioners in the course of their *sādhanā* can be useful and essential as well. Some verticalists schools, notably Advaita Vedānta, regard them with great suspicion and frequently advise against their cultivation or use. This attitude is a direct product of the Advaitic metaphysics that conceives of nature as *māyā,* or pseudoreality. A philosophy that considers the world itself as dangerous to the spiritual practitioner must be expected to transfer this belief to all conceivable interactions with the illusory world. Thus the paranormal powers that arise within a finite human body can only serve the cause of delusion and bondage to the world. Therefore they must be rejected or at least never used or displayed.

A similar position is expressed in the *Yoga-Tattva-Upanishad* (3.111), which teaches Tantric Hatha Yoga on the basis of Advaita Vedānta and explicitly favors the ideal of *videha-mukti* or disembodied liberation (see 3.142). The full Tantric view is altogether different from this. It is capsulated in another important Hatha Yoga text, the *Yoga-Shikhā-Upanishad* (1.40ff.), which speaks of the divinized body of the *yogin*. This deathless transubstantiated body is lucid like the ether and is said to be invisible even to the deities. It is possessed of all kinds of paranormal powers, especially the ability to assume any shape whatsoever. The shape-shifting ability of great adepts is well known in the Yoga tradition and is a favorite folkloristic motif.

The *Yoga-Shikhā-Upanishad* (1.48–49) mildly pokes fun at the man of knowledge, the intellectual, who is under the spell of the meat body (*māmsa-pinda*) rather than in total control of it. Such a one is born again and again by the power of the karmic merit and demerit created during his lifetime. The true knower (*jnānin*), however, transcends all karma and is liberated while yet alive. He appears to have a physical frame, yet is as insubstantial as empty space and therefore cannot in reality be located, touched, hurt, or killed.

This medieval Yoga scripture (1.152–55) also distinguishes between natural and artificial paranormal powers as follows:

> In this world the powers are twofold: artificial (*kalpita*) and nonartificial (*akalpita*).

The powers that come about through the cultivation of alchemy, herbs, rituals, magic, and such practices as *mantra* [recitation] are called artificial.

The powers arising from such cultivation are temporary and of little energy. However, [those powers] that arise without such cultivation, of their own accord,

through self-reliance in the case of those who are exclusively intent on union (*yoga*) with their own Self are dear to the Lord. Such [spontaneously] arising powers are known as devoid of artifice (*kalpanā*).

[Such spontaneous powers] are accomplished (*siddha*), enduring, of great energy, conforming to the [divine] will (*icchā*), springing from one's own Yoga. They arise after a long time in those who are devoid of [karmic] traits (*vāsanā*).

The fully accomplished Tantric adept (*siddha*) is not merely a liberated being but also a thaumaturgist for whom the laws of the material cosmos are no limitation. Thus, like Shiva, the adept is *shakti-mat*—possessed of power. The paranormal powers (*siddhi*) are simply manifestations of the divine Power, or *shakti*. In contrast to the typical position of Advaita Vedānta, the *Yoga-Shikhā-Upanishad* (1.159–60) unequivocally applauds the possession of paranormal powers:

Even as gold is determined by assaying goldsmiths, one should identify an adept and *jīvan-mukta* by his powers.

Surely a transcendental (*alaukika*) quality will sometimes be evident in him. However, the person lacking powers should be deemed bound.

North India remembers eighty-four great adepts (*mahā-siddha*), some of whom were Hindus, while others were Buddhists. The best-known masters are Mīnapa[4] (a Bengali fisherman who is often identified with Matsyendra Nātha), Luīpa (a born prince who renounced the world at a young age and begged alms from the local fishermen), Virūpa (a Buddhist monk who dined on pigeon and wine until he was asked to leave the monastery; he demonstrated his high spiritual attainment by walking across the surface of a lake merely by stepping

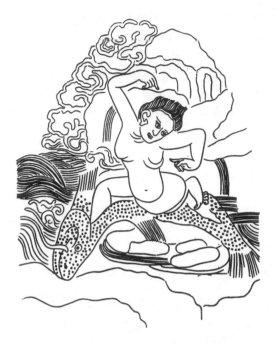

*A Tibetan woodblock print of Matsyendra Natha
(Lord of Fish), considered one of the eighty-four
mahā-siddhas, or great adepts.*

from lotus to lotus), Saraha (a brahmin who enjoyed liquor but pro-
claimed that he never drank and passed several self-designed tests in
proof of his innocence, including swallowing liquid copper), Goraksha
(the illustrious founder of Hatha Yoga), Caurangipa (a prince whose
stepmother accused him of rape, for which he was dismembered,
though by his magical powers he was able to regrow his arms and
legs), Nāgārjuna (one of the greatest Buddhist adepts and scholars),
Tilopa (chief priest of a king, who renounced his official position to
become a wandering mendicant and subsequently acquired all the
powers of body, speech, and mind), Nāropa (chief disciple of Tilopa
and teacher of Marpa, who in turn initiated the famous Tibetan adept
Milarepa), Jālandhara (a brahmin *siddha* who entered the paradise
of the *dākinīs* with three hundred disciples), Kanhapa (a disciple of
Jālandhara, who became a fabled Buddhist master), and Kapālapa (a

low-caste laborer who called himself the *"yogin* of the skull (*kapāla*)" because he always carried a skull).

The South Indian tradition speaks of eighteen *cittars* (the Tamil synonym for *siddhas*). Among them the foremost adepts are Akattiyar (Sanskrit: Agastya, who is thought to have brought Tantra to the south of the subcontinent), Tirumūlar (who possibly as early as the seventh century CE composed the famous Tamil work *Tiru-Mantiram*), Pām-pātti (a popular adept whose name means "he with the dancing snake," a reference to the awakened *kundalinī*; he sought to shock and awaken others by his crude poetry), Akappēy (a late medieval adept who described reality as pure Void, or *shūnya*), Itaikkātar (who, per-haps in the fifteenth century CE, lived in Tiruvannamalai, where five centuries later the great sage Ramana Maharshi settled as well). Other great masters not usually listed among the eighteen *mahā-siddhas* are Civavākkiyar (a great mystic, poet, and critic of conventional society, who may have lived in the ninth century CE), Pattinattār (a tenth-century adept, some of whose mystical poetry was included in the *Tiru-Murai,* the Shaiva canon of the South; there also is a fifteenth-century adept by the same name, whose poetry is among the finest compositions of the *cittars*). In the nineteenth century the great Tamil adept and poet was Rāmalinga (Tamil: Irāmalinka Cuvamikal), who reportedly exited this world in a flash of light. Many of his songs speak of his achievement of a "golden hued" immortal body, which corresponds to the "body of glory" in Gnosticism.

It was among the *siddhas* and *mahā-siddhas* that the closely related arts of alchemy, Tantric medicine, and "body cultivation" (*kāya-sād-hana*) were intensively pursued and developed. Body cultivation meant the exploration of the hidden potential of the human body as a tool for spiritual transformation. The goal was the creation of a bodily vehicle that was immune to the ravages of time—an immortal, ada-mantine (*vajra*) or divine (*divya*) body invested with all the powers of the universe. Around 1000 CE this preoccupation gave rise to Hatha Yoga, especially under the *nātha-siddhas*.

The northern tradition knows of nine *nāthas* (lords), whose feats are remembered in countless legends to this day. Shiva is called the

first lord (*ādi-nātha*), who taught Matsyendra. By far the most venerated *nātha* is Matsyendra's disciple Goraksha, who is the founder of
the Kānphata order, in whose ranks Hatha Yoga was developed into a
fine art.

The declared purpose of Hatha Yoga is to prepare the body first
for the rigors of intensive meditation, as practiced in Rāja Yoga, and
then for the onslaught of enlightenment, which inevitably leads to
significant subtle energetic and biochemical changes. In the unprepared body, the descent of divine energy (*shakti*) can cause havoc and
premature death, and therefore the system must be thoroughly purified through the various ingenious means of Hatha Yoga. Beyond a
superhealthy body, the *hatha-yogins* also aspire to create for themselves
an indestructible body that can assume any form whatsoever and is
endowed with all kinds of paranormal powers.

Tantra and Yoga in general recognize eight great paranormal
powers, called *mahā-siddhis*:

1. *Animā* (atomization), the ability to make oneself as small as
   an atom (*anu*), implying invisibility.

2. *Mahimā* (magnification), the ability to make oneself infinitely
   large.

3. *Laghimā* (levitation), the ability to defy the law of gravity, or
   in the words of Vijnāna Bhikshu's *Yoga-Vārttika* (3.45), "to
   become as light as a cotton tuft on a painter's brush."

4. *Prāpti* (extension), in the words of the *Yoga-Bhāshya* (3.45),
   the ability to "touch the moon with one's fingertips."

5. *Prākāmya* (will), the ability to exert one's will without obstruction. For instance, the *yogin* who possesses this power
   can, according to the *Yoga-Bhāshya* (3.45), dive into the earth
   as if it were water.

6. *Vashitva* (mastery), the ability to control the five material elements (*bhūta*) and their subtle templates (i.e., the five *tanmātra*).

7. *Īshitritva* (lordship), the ability to completely control the
   manifestation, arrangement, and destruction of the elements
   and the objects composed of them.

8. *Kāmāvasāyitva* (from *kāma*, "desire," and *avasāyitva*, "fulfillment"), the ability to have all one's desires fulfilled by con-
   trolling the very nature of the elements. Thus the adept can
   call into existence a particular being for a particular purpose,
   and this being will persist until it has met its designated end.
   For instance, the traditional literature knows of artificially
   created minds (*nirmāna-citta*) that can perform specific tasks,
   notably the consumption of *karmas* either for the adept personally or someone else.

The texts also mention or describe numerous minor paranormal
powers. This shows that they are by no means incidental to the great
process of spiritual transformation undertaken by the *sādhaka*. Western parapsychology, which is a comparatively young scientific discipline and badly underfunded, has so far not systematically studied this
aspect of Tantra and the Yoga tradition in general. Few *yogins* would
be willing to subject themselves to lab testing, which they would presumably consider a pointless and perhaps even ridiculous endeavor.
However, those who have done so, like Swami Rama, have demonstrated highly unusual abilities that support some of the claims of
Tantra and Yoga.

If the Tantric path of Self-realization can be described as white
magic, there is a whole other side to Tantra, which corresponds to
our notion of black magic. Certainly Tantra as a whole does not ex-
clude the deliberate cultivation and use of "artificial" powers, and at
times the texts describe practices that can only be of interest to someone pursuing egotistical and even morally reprehensible ends. In fact,
there are entire *Tantras* specializing in black magic.[5] The *Damara-Tantra*
is an example of this unfortunate trend within Tantra.

Even such a highly respected Tantra as the *Vāmakā-Īshvarī-Mata*
mentions a number of questionable practices. For instance, it recommends (2.1ff.) a magical practice that excites and subjugates young
women everywhere. Like Krishna's flute play, the prescribed *mantra*
draws women to the practitioner, and when he touches them they
become completely compliant. They behave, as the text states, as
if (*iva*) they were deluded, confused, unconscious, agitated, or in-
toxicated.

This power belongs to the well-known Tantric set of "six actions" (*shat-karma*) by which enemies can be brought under one's
control. According to the *Damara-Tantra,* these are:

1. *Vashīkarana* (subjugation), the ability to control other human
   beings, deities, and spirits from the lower realms

2. *Stambhana* (stoppage), the ability to effectively block other's
   actions or prevent their actions from bearing fruit

3. *Vidveshana* (engendering enmity), the ability to create dissatis-
   faction and strife between people

4. *Uccātana* (causing flight), the ability to drive off enemies, but
   also the ability to explode things merely through the power
   of thought

5. *Mārana* (causing death), the ability to kill by sheer mental
   intent

6. *Shānti* (pacification), the ability to ward off evil influences,
   whether they be due to *karma*, the stars, or curses

It was presumably for financial gain that some Tantric practitioners adopted destructive practices in their works, even though
the very exercise of black magic not only precludes the practitioner
from transcending his or her karmic baggage but adds to it. It is easy
enough to understand why the adepts have developed various rituals
of protection, which involve the use of paranormal abilities. The sacred work that is performed in the magical circle (*mandala*) and that
ultimately benefits everyone must be safeguarded against outside interference on the material but especially the subtle planes of existence. But to employ paranormal powers or even conduct rituals in
order to deliberately harm another being violates the high ethical
principles of Tantra. We must therefore regard any such manifestations of Tantra as a degeneration.

At the same time, we must be careful not to judge a spiritual
tradition by its failures. At its best, Tantra is a unique heritage created
by high-souled adepts whose wisdom teachings have lost none of their
relevance. We need not share the pessimism expressed by Carl Jung

in the 1934 seminar on *kundalinī-yoga* that the symbolism of the East is basically inaccessible to us.[6] Much of it is accessible, and through personal practice of the Tantric or yogic disciplines a great deal more can open up for us. But we must be as diligent in our study and practice of the spiritual heritage of India as we would be with any scientific experiment. Of course, in practicing Tantra or other forms of Yoga far more is at stake for us, because we are both the experimenter and the subject of the experiment. Yet the potential gain is considerable. At the very least it will enhance our self-understanding, and at best it will lead us to the great liberating bliss extolled in the *Tantras*. The great power (*siddhi*) is liberation, which is the utterly blissful union of the all-powerful Shiva and Shakti.

We are free to choose which path to tread. And our choice will determine our future, both individually and collectively. May we choose wisdom!

Epilogue

 Tantra Yesterday, Today, and Tomorrow

The Lord stands waiting for those who seek Him.
—*Tiru-Mantiram* (vs. 1889)

Tantra has produced thousands of adepts and many more thousands of scriptures in various languages. Only a few of the truly great names of Tantric heroes are known to us and still fewer biographical details. Also, our knowledge of the literature of Tantra is quite fragmentary, not to mention Tantric practice and experience. What little understanding we have acquired, however, thanks to the labors of a small number of dedicated scholars, is sufficient to appreciate the enormous significance of the Tantric heritage within the world's spiritual traditions.

Tantra originated and flourished at the margins of Hindu society and gradually helped shape it. Tantra provided a home for all those who longed for direct spiritual experience but found orthodox Hinduism (Smārta Brāhmanism) far too restrictive and exclusivist. The Tantric circles were open to members of all castes, and at least for the duration of the rituals brahmins and untouchables drank from the same cup, ate from the same plate, and freely mingled their bodily juices, for during the *cakra-pūjā* all were transformed into sacred beings—gods and goddesses—free from all cultural stereotyping and societal constraints. A brahmin could have a *shūdra* teacher and vice versa. No one was barred from receiving the precious teachings or excluded from the possibility of attaining enlightenment in this lifetime. Regrettably, the embracing spirit of Tantra did not succeed in eliminating ethnic prejudice in the larger society.

Tantra did, however, change the life of its practitioners. And perhaps to the degree that they were able to live out of the Tantric wisdom they also benignly influenced their immediate environment—family, friends, and neighbors. As Patanjali stated in his *Yoga-Sūtra* (2.35), the person firmly grounded in the virtue of nonharming (*ahimsā*) reduces feelings of enmity in others. In this way he or she contributes to the greater good, which is the ideal of *loka-samgraha*, as first announced in the *Bhagavad-Gītā* (3.20) well over two millennia ago. This ideal came to form the foundation stone of Mahāyāna and Vajrayāna Buddhism, where it is known as the *bodhisattva* path. The *bodhisattva* is the being (*sattva*) who strives for enlightenment (*bodhi*) in order to help others more effectively. This great ideal has often been misunderstood by Westerners, who assume that the *bodhisattva* defers his or her enlightenment so as to continue to serve others. But the Buddhist teachers were wiser than that. They realized that other beings can best be helped on all levels, especially in their spiritual growth, by someone who has conquered his or her personal problems and has in fact attained enlightenment. What the *bodhisattva* vows to do is remain, as an enlightened being, in the manifest realms until *all* others are liberated as well. Only then will he or she abandon all bodily vehicles and become one with the formless Reality. The *bodhisattva* is perfectly willing to fulfill this task lifetime after lifetime—

forever if necessary. What nobler ideal could there be to inspire a person?

Without such a long-term perspective, which takes the suffering of others into account, any form of spirituality risks degenerating into mere narcissism. In that case the practitioner succumbs to exactly the very aspect of the psyche that he or she set out to overcome, namely, the illusion of being an isolated self (ego). Philosophically, Tantra is thoroughly ecological. It recognizes the ultimate unity, even identity, of all beings and things. Otherness is a mental artifact. Translated into social action, Tantric practitioners must not erect intellectual or emotional walls between themselves and other beings or between themselves and inanimate things. Since everything participates in the ultimate Reality, which is pure Consciousness, there is nothing that is not Consciousness. To view life in this way does not have to blur necessary distinctions but can be a stimulus for doing away with artificial barriers.

The great Tantric adept-scholar Gopinath Kaviraj (1887–1976) believed in the collective liberation of humanity and even maintained that a single advanced adept could accomplish this goal by his own *sādhanā* in one lifetime. He called his teaching *akhanda-mahāyoga,* or Great Integral Yoga. He had received it from his *guru,* Vishuddhananda, an adept who is associated with the mysterious Jnānaganj hermitage somewhere in Tibet—a place of great masters not unlike Shambhala. Kaviraj himself did not succeed in reaching the highest stage of this extraordinary *sādhanā.* Thus far no one individual has been able to lift the *karma* of the world, or we would see indubitable signs of a global spiritual awakening. Perhaps, after all, collective liberation is an asymptotic ideal, which great masters can approach but never completely realize.

With the arrival of Tantra in the Western hemisphere, this ancient tradition is experiencing new challenges. There still are great teachers, but, as ever, qualified students are few. All too often students transfer Western competitiveness to their spiritual practice, where it has no place. They want to be masters overnight and have their own students before they are ready for the tremendous responsibility this entails. This attitude has led to a mushrooming of Neo-Tantric schools, many of which are little more than caricatures of traditional Tantra. The same criticism applies to numerous Yoga teachers and schools, but where Tantric or Tantra-style teachings are involved, the danger of self-delusion and abuse of power is particularly great. Unless the Tantric teacher is of high moral caliber, he or she can do considerable damage to students.

Many are attracted to Neo-Tantrism because it promises sexual excitement or fulfillment while clothing purely genital impulses or neurotic emotional needs in an aura of spirituality. If we knew more about the history of Tantra in India, we would no doubt find a comparable situation for every generation. In other words, the attitude that characterizes many Neo-Tantrics today also characterized a number of those who in bygone centuries flocked to Tantric circles for the wrong reasons. The *Tantras* would not contain so many warnings if genuine seekers alone had found their way to Tantra. Thrill seekers have lived in every age, and the sacred teachings were not spared their prying intrusions. Today translations of several major *Tantras* are readily available in book form, and many formerly secret practices are now, in the language of the texts, "like common harlots." This gives would-be Tantrics the opportunity to concoct their own idiosyncratic ceremonies and philosophies, which they can then promote as Tantra.

Yet the real substance of the Tantric teachings is as hidden as ever and is disclosed only to those who have received proper initiation from a qualified *guru*. This is why genuine adepts continue to be vitally important on the spiritual path. Without initiation and oral transmission the teachings will not come alive. When *guru* and disciple sit face to face, the special process of transmission can occur, which opens gates in the disciple's mind that allow him or her to pass to the next level of spiritual growth.

Many Western seekers have been struggling with the function of the *guru*, which is so alien to our culture, a culture in which we do not even respect our elders any longer. Unquestionably, there have been a number of saddening instances in recent years wherein well-known *gurus* from the East have failed to live up to the highest standards of their tradition. There also have been many cases in which Eastern teachers have not understood the psychology of their Western students, causing consternation and frustration, or worse. Some Western seekers have abandoned the idea of a traditional discipleship altogether, opting for a more "democratic" style of teaching and learning. For them, the traditional *guru*-disciple relationship is too asymmetrical, with the disciple adopting the role of the "underdog." They prefer to learn and grow from their interaction with peers.

While this position is understandable, it also has a built-in limitation. If our peers were fully accomplished Tantra or Yoga adepts, we could most certainly benefit from interacting with them. This is, however, not the case. It is still largely a matter of the blind leading the blind. Our peers can prove helpful facilitators, but if our sight is fixed on the supreme goal of Tantra, which is liberation, yogic induction by a qualified *guru* is absolutely essential. Such induction, or transmission, will unlikely be given outside the well-tested traditional framework of discipleship, for the *guru* is responsible for the disciple's further evolution. Discipleship involves a constant monitoring of the *shishya*'s spiritual and moral growth.

Tantra in particular awakens latent abilities that must be managed wisely and in the spirit of compassion and kindness toward others. Any misuse of these abilities or powers will have severe karmic consequences, both for the disciple and for the teacher who granted initiation and transmitted the teachings and the energy supporting them. Tantra is a powerful tool, calling for maturity, self-knowledge, and good-heartedness in its handling. The fact that Tantra has never been easily accessible protects both the Tantric tradition and would-be disciples. This is as true today as it was a hundred or a thousand years ago. Those who are truly ready to receive initiation and transmission are sooner or later bound to come in contact with the right teacher and tradition. If the law of karma holds true at all, we certainly must expect it to apply to this situation. We are drawn to teachers and teachings because of our inner resonance with them. So long as we look at our disappointments on the path as learning experiences, we will continue to grow. Honesty and integrity are our best protection whether or not we have found a teacher.

Despite the growing popularity of Hatha Yoga (which is a Tantric Yoga), Tantra in the strict sense will presumably not attract large numbers of people in the foreseeable future. Even the current surge of interest in Vajrayāna Buddhism (Tibetan Tantra), desirable as it is, must not mislead us into assuming that therefore there are thousands of qualified aspirants who in our lifetime will become masters in their own right. However, Tantra, like Yoga, definitely has entered our Western civilization and is here to stay. It can be expected to be a transformative force through the agency of its genuine practitioners, though who can tell what form and degree this influence will take? Nor can one predict how the Tantric heritage itself will be shaped by its encounter with the West.

As Western initiates achieve adeptship, we should not be surprised to see all kinds of adaptations take place, just as Indic Tantra changed form when it entered Tibet. Perhaps the transformation of Tantra will be even more far-reaching, because the cultural differences between the Tantric legacy and Western culture are vastly more significant than the differences between the cultures of India and Tibet. It is safe to say that Tantra has embarked on a whole new pathway, whose future is highly uncertain.

If Tantra can recruit enough authentic Western practitioners, it could have an important role to play in the birthing of a civilization that is dedicated to the welfare of all people, whatever their nationality or ethnic background may be. The Tantric tradition now has the opportunity to extend its philosophical egalitarianism beyond the narrow confines of the ritual clan to society at large across all national borders. This will be its ultimate test and possible fulfillment.

Notes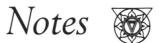

PREFACE

1. Herbert V. Guenther, *Yuganaddha: The Tantric View of Life* (Varanasi, India: Chowkhamba Sanskrit Series Office, 1969), p. 3.

2. Robert Beer, "Autobiographical Note by the Illustrator," in Keith Dowman and Robert Beer, *Masters of Enchantment: The Lives and Legends of the Mahasiddhas* (Rochester, Vt.: Inner Traditions International, 1988), p. 27.

3. See Arthur Avalon [Sir John Woodroffe], *Shakti and Shākta*, 6th ed., reprint (New York: Dover, 1978).

4. Avalon, *Shakti and Shākta*, pp. 78–79.

5. In his preface to the first edition of *Shakti and Shākta* (1918), Woodroffe explained the reason for his using the pseudonym Arthur Avalon: he wished to indicate that his various works on Tantra "have been written with the direct cooperation of others and in particular with the assistance of one of my friends who will not permit me to mention his name."

6. See, e.g., His Holiness the Dalai Lama, Tsong-ka-pa, and Jeffrey Hopkins, *Deity Yoga In Action and Performance Tantra* (Ithaca, N.Y.: Snow Lion, 1987); D. Cozort, *Highest Yoga Tantra: An Introduction to the Esoteric Buddhism of*

Tibet (Ithaca, N.Y.: Snow Lion, 1986); Khetsun Sangpo Rinbochay, *Tantric Practice in Nying-Ma* (Ithaca, N.Y.: Snow Lion, 1982).

7. See John Hughes, *Self-Realization in Kashmir Shaivism: The Oral Teachings of Swami Lakshmanjoo* (Albany: SUNY Press, 1994).

8. See Georg Feuerstein, "Tantra vs. Neo-Tantrism," posted on the web site of the Yoga Research Center at *http://members.aol.com/yogaresrch/tantra1.htm.*

9. See Georg Feuerstein, *The Shambhala Guide to Yoga* (Boston: Shambhala Publications, 1996).

INTRODUCTION

1. Related terms are *tantra-vāya* ("weaver"), *tanu* ("slender" or "delicate," which is something that is spread thin, occasionally used as a synonym for "body"), *tanutra* ("armor"), and *tantrin* ("soldier").

2. See Agehananda Bharati, *The Tantric Tradition* (London: Rider, 1965), p. 16.

3. To the confusion of nonspecialists, the *Tantras* are also often called *Āgamas,* meaning specifically *Shākta-Āgamas* as opposed to *Shaiva-Āgamas.* Other related literary categories are the *Nigamas* and the *Yāmalas.* As a general rule, in the *Tantras* the feminine aspect of the Divine—in the form of Shakti (Power) or individual goddesses—is more prominent than it is in the *Shaiva-Āgamas,* which revolve around the worship of Shiva as the supreme Being. According to the *Rudra-Yāmala,* a twelfth-century text, the *Nigamas* are those *Tantras* that are revealed by the Goddess (Devī) to Shiva. The *Yāmalas* are typically revealed by the male deity, be it Rudra, Vishnu, Brahma, or Ganesha. All these labels are somewhat fluid, however. According to the *Parama-Ānanda-Tantra,* there are 6,000 Vaishnava, 7,000 Bhairava, 10,000 Shaiva, and 100,000 Shākta *Tantras.*

4. Even such a knowledgeable writer as Richard Lannoy commits this mistake in his excellent book *The Speaking Tree: A Study of Indian Culture and Society* (London: Oxford University Press, 1971), p. 288.

5. The chronology of ancient India is one of the great problem areas of Indic studies. Western scholars are generally distrustful of the native histories (such as lists of kings and sages) provided in the *Purānas* and other literary genres. However, with the recent redating of the *Rig-Veda* and the debunk-

ing of the scholarly myth of an Aryan invasion into India around 1200–1500 BCE, more and more scholars are inclined to take native Indic traditions more seriously than before. See Georg Feuerstein, Subhash Kak, and David Frawley, *In Search of the Cradle of Civilization: New Light on Ancient India* (Wheaton, Ill.: Quest Books, 1995).

6. A notable exception is Sri Yukteswar, the *guru* of Paramahamsa Yogananda. He maintained that we are in a *dvāpara-yuga* (which supposedly started in 1699 CE). This is based on a precessional cycle of 24,000 years rather than the customary cycle of 25,900 years.

7. Some authorities give the duration of the *kali-yuga* as being 432,000 years, but this includes the period of latency between the *kali-yuga* and the next *krita-yuga*. For the duration of the four *yugas* and an explanation of their large spans see chapter 2.

8. The English adjective "Vedic" corresponds to the Sanskrit *vaidika,* meaning "that which relates to the *Vedas,*" or the sacred revelation. It is contrasted with "traditional" (*smārta,* derived from *smriti*) or nonrevelatory knowledge.

9. Feuerstein, Kak, and Frawley, *In Search of the Cradle of Civilization,* offer a complete reappraisal of the Vedic civilization and early Indic chronology. The proposed new model is being vigorously discussed, especially by India's scholars, many of whom have long been skeptical about the Aryan invasion theory inherited from the nineteenth century. While some Western scholars are beginning to accept the available evidence calling for a revision of ancient Indic chronology, many are resistant to the simultaneously proposed notion that the Vedic civilization is more or less identical with the so-called Harappan (Indus) civilization.

10. Manoranjan Basu, *Fundamentals of the Philosophy of Tantras* (Calcutta: Mira Basu, 1986), p. 63.

11. According to Lopon Tenzin Namdak, the head of the Yung-drung Bon school of the Bonpo tradition of Tibet, the Buddha Tenpa Shenrab lived eighteen thousand years ago. See Namkhai Norbu, *Dream Yoga and the Practice of Natural Light,* edited and introduced by M. Katz (Ithaca, N.Y.: Snow Lion, 1992), p. 35.

12. See Swāmī Mādhavānanda, *The Bṛhadāraṇyaka Upaniṣad,* 4th ed. (Calcutta: Advaita Ashrama, 1965).

CHAPTER 1: SAMSĀRA

1. Some other Sanskrit words for "world" are *bhava, jagat, vishva,* and *loka.*

2. See Robert E. Svoboda, *Aghora: At the Left Hand of God* (Albuquerque, N.M.:
    Brotherhood of Life, 1986), p. 111. The same idea was expressed by the
    great modern gnostic Omraam Mikhaël Aïvanhov, a master of "Solar
    Yoga"; see his *Toward a Solar Civilisation* (Los Angeles: Prosveta, 1982).

3. The expression "cheating time" (*kāla-vancana*) is a typical Tantric expres-
    sion, but the idea goes back to early Vedic times.

4. Tradition speaks of 18 primary and 18 secondary *Purānas* (created by reli-
    gious communities worshiping the Divine in the form of Shiva, Vishnu,
    Krishna, Kālī, and other deities), 28 *Āgamas* (of the Shiva-worshiping com-
    munity), 108 *Samhitās* (of the Vishnu-worshiping community), and 64
    Tantras. The *Mahābhārata* epic shares many features with the Purānas and
    in fact calls itself a *Purāna.* The *Rāmāyana* epic is traditionally considered
    the original poem (*ādi-kāvya*). Although its present Sanskrit version is un-
    doubtedly later than the *Mahābhārata,* its story goes further back in time.

5. The expression "brahmic egg" relates to an archaic mythological motif
    found in the *Chāndogya-Upanishad* (3.19.1) according to which the world
    was created out of nothing and was at first an egg, which after a period of
    one year burst open. From it emerged a silver part and a gold part, repre-
    senting earth and sky respectively.

6. In the *Tantra-Rāja-Tantra* (28.7), the size of *bhū-loka* is given as being only
    five thousand yojanas.

7. We must not make too much of such coincidences, however. The ancients
    apparently did not know of Pluto's existence and also included in the
    brahmic egg the stars, which they did not regard as suns. Besides, the
    scriptures are very clear that their descriptions apply not merely to the
    physical dimension but also include the subtle realms of existence.

8. The word *pātāla* is also often used as a generic term for the underworld.

9. According to some traditions, Brahma's lifespan is only 100 brahmic years,
    which translates into 311,040,000,000,000 human years.

10. Joseph Chilton Pearce, *The Crack in the Cosmic Egg: Challenging Constructs of
    Mind and Reality* (New York: Pocket Books, 1977), p. xiv.

CHAPTER 2: TIME, BONDAGE, AND THE GODDESS KĀLĪ

1. Savitri (written Savitṛ in the scholarly literature) must not be confused with Savitrī, the goddess of learning and the arts.

2. The word *kāla* is used only once in the *Rig-Veda* (10.42.9), in a portion that Western scholars consider as belonging to a late stratum, but this does not mean that the Vedic seers ignored time in their philosophical musings. We find their thoughts epitomized in the key concept of *rita*, or cosmic order, which is closely connected with the sun as the engine of time. The sun (*sūrya*) was of enormous importance in Vedic spirituality, which can be characterized as a Solar Yoga. This aspect of the Vedic teachings has barely been studied and would make one of the most fascinating and instructive chapters in ancient history.

3. In the early Vedic literature, *brahman* does not have the philosophical meaning of "Absolute," as in Vedānta metaphysics.

4. The *gandharvas* (from *gandh*, "to adhere" or "to smell") are spirits associated particularly with music. The *apsarases* (singular *apsaras*, from *apas*, "water") are generally described as celestial nymphs.

5. In the *Tantra-Rāja-Tantra* (18.9), the "wheel of time" is said to move perpetually in a clockwise direction around the various levels of the cosmic egg. In this context, the *kāla-cakra* is part of the manifest universe. It specifically refers here to the movement of the sun, which is pictured as a wagon wheel rolling on the most distant mountain range encompassing the layers of the cosmic egg. The wheel's axle is fixed to the top of Mount Meru, the cosmic mountain. The *kāla-cakra* is fundamental to the symbolism of the *shrī-cakra*, also known as the *shrī-yantra*. This geometric design is explained in chapter 13.

6. The *nāgas* are ophidian spirits, who are custodians of underground treasure and esoteric wisdom.

7. *The Gospel of Sri Ramakrishna*, trans. Swami Nikhilananda (New York: Ramakrishna-Vivekananda Center, 1952), p. 271.

8. Mahānirvāna is here Shiva.

9. *Samādhi* is ecstasy, the unitive state in which the meditator becomes one with the object of meditation.

10. *The Gospel of Sri Ramakrishna,* p. 692.

11. Ibid., p. 579.

12. Interestingly, according to a South Indian myth associated with the Shiva temple at Citamparam (often spelled Chidambaram) fifty miles south of Pondicherry, two of Shiva's devotees witnessed his dance of bliss. Their names were Vyāghrapāda (meaning "tiger-footed") and Patanjali, who is venerated as an incarnation of the cosmic serpent Shesha, serving as Vishnu's couch. Some native scholars identify this Patanjali with the author of the well-known *Yoga-Sūtra.*

CHAPTER 3: THIS IS THE OTHER WORLD

1. See, e.g., Morris Berman, *The Reenchantment of the World* (New York: Bantam Books, 1984); Jean Gebser, *The Ever-Present Origin* (Athens: Ohio University Press, 1985); Ken Wilber, *Sex, Ecology, Spirituality: The Spirit of Evolution* (Boston: Shambhala Publications, 1995).

2. See the *Yoga-Sūtra* (2.15), which contains the phrase *duhkham eva sarvam vivekinah.*

3. The phrase "This is the 'other' world" was coined by Adi Da (a.k.a. Franklin Jones, Da Free John, etc.), who occasionally has declared his teaching to be a form of Tantra. See his *Knee of Listening* (Middletown, Calif.: Dawn Horse Press, 1995), p. 499.

4. Anagarika Govinda, *Foundations of Tibetan Mysticism* (London: Rider, 1969), pp. 107–8.

5. The Sanskrit runs: *sarvam khalvidam (= khalu idam) brahma.*

6. Herbert V. Guenther, *The Royal Song of Saraha* (Berkeley, Calif.: Shambhala Publications, 1973), pp. 63–70, stanzas 3, 14, and 35.

7. Cited in Surendranath Dasgupta, *Obscure Religious Cults* (Calcutta: Firma KLM, 1976), p. 145n (*Ratna-Sāra,* manuscript, p. 19).

8. See Georg Feuerstein, *Wholeness or Transcendence? Ancient Lessons for the Emerging Global Civilization* (Burdett, N.Y.: Larson, 1992).

9. See *Viveka-Cūḍāmani,* verses 77 and 87.

10. *Kula-Arnava-Tantra* 1.75–76, 79–80, 84.

CHAPTER 4: THE SECRET OF EMBODIMENT

1. The Sanskrit text reads *tam yathā yathā upāsate tad eva bhavati* (whatever one attends to/worships, that one becomes).

2. For an abbreviated English rendering of the *Yoga-Vāsishtha,* see Swami Venkatesananda, The *Concise Yoga-Vāsishtha* (Albany: SUNY Press, 1984). This translation, though not literal, is faithful to the spirit of the Sanskrit original.

3. Gerald Heard, *Pain, Sex, and Time: A New Hypothesis of Evolution* (London: Cassell, 1939), pp. 50–51.

4. In Sanskrit the statement reads: *yad ihāsti* [= *iha asti*] *tad anyatra yan nehāsti* [= *na iha asti*] *na tat kvacit.*

5. For a clear popular account of this seminal idea, see Michael Talbot, *The Holographic Universe* (New York: HarperCollins, 1991). For a classic scientific presentation, see David Bohm, *Wholeness and the Implicate Order* (London: Routledge & Kegan Paul, 1980).

6. Knows not merely intellectually but experientially.

7. According to the renowned Shaiva adept and scholar Abhinava Gupta, *Parama-Shiva* is the thirty-seventh principle or *tattva.* However, according to Utpalācārya, another well-known learned adept of Kashmiri Shaivism, Shiva should be understood as being the ultimate Reality rather than an emergent ontological principle.

8. *Sac-cid-ānanda* is composed of *sat* (being), *cit* (consciousness), and *ānanda* (bliss).

9. *Chāndogya-Upanishad* 6.2.1–2.

10. In recent years, a number of excellent publications on the Pratyabhijnā system and other closely related schools of Kashmiri Shaivism have been published. See, e.g., Deba Brata SenSharma, *The Philosophy of Sādhanā* (Albany: SUNY Press, 1990); Kamalakav Mishra, *Kashmir Śaivism: The Central Philosophy of Tantrism* (Cambridge, Mass.: Rudra Press, 1993); André Pa-

doux, *Vāc: The Concept of the Word in Selected Hindu Tantras* (Albany: SUNY Press, 1990); and Paul Eduardo Müller-Ortega, *The Triadic Heart of Śiva: Kaula Tantricism of Abhinava Gupta in the Non-Dual Shaivism of Kashmir* (Albany: SUNY Press, 1989).

Chapter 5: The Divine Play of Shiva and Shakti

1. The term *kaivalya* means literally "aloneness" and is also used in Patanjali's *Yoga-Sūtra* as the supreme state aspired to by *yogins*.

2. The Sanskrit word *parama* means "supreme" or "ultimate."

3. For euphonic reasons, the word *sat* is changed to *sac* and *cit* is changed to *cid* in the phrase *sac-cid-ananda*.

4. David Bohm, *Wholeness and the Implicate Order* (London: Routledge & Kegan Paul, 1980), p. 203.

5. Jaideva Singh, *The Yoga of Vibration and Divine Pulsation* (Albany: SUNY Press, 1992), p. 33.

6. The name Ardhanārīshvara is composed of *ardha* (half), *nārī* (woman), and *īshvara* ("lord," here meaning "man").

7. Some texts mention eight coils.

8. In Tantric Buddhism, the active principle (*upāya*, "means") is considered masculine; the passive principle (*prajnā*, "wisdom") is deemed feminine.

9. Carl Gustav Jung, *Memories, Dreams, Reflections* (New York: Vintage Books, 1965), p. 276.

Chapter 6: The Guru Principle

1. Swami Muktananda, *Secret of the Siddhas* (South Fallsburg, N.Y.: SYDA Foundation, 1980), p. 13.

2. See, e.g., C. G. Jung, *Psychology and the East* (Princeton, N.J.: Princeton University Press, 1978), p. 85. While it is true that exceedingly few Western students of Eastern spiritual teachings ever experience a stable breakthrough, this may not necessarily be due to some psychological incompatibility with Eastern teachings. More likely the failure relates to a

certain lack of self-discipline and understanding on the part of the Western students. Curiously, despite his critical stance toward Yoga, Jung admits in his autobiography that he used "certain yoga exercises" to calm his mind whenever the unconscious assaulted him; see C. G. Jung, *Memories, Dreams, Reflections* (New York: Vintage Books, 1965), p. 177.

3. See His Holiness the Dalai Lama, *The Path to Enlightenment* (Ithaca, N.Y.: Snow Lion, 1995), p. 72: "The teachings on seeing the guru's actions as perfect should largely be left for the practice of Highest Tantra, wherein they take on a new meaning. One of the principal yogas in the tantric vehicle is to see the world as a mandala of great bliss and to see oneself and all others as Buddhas. Under these circumstances it becomes absurd to think that you and everyone else are Buddhas, but your guru is not!"

4. The first member of the compound *sad-guru* is *sat,* meaning "true," "real," or "authentic," which changes its terminal *t* to a *d* when followed by a soft consonant. The *sad-guru* is a genuine teacher but also one who has realized that which is true or real, and is therefore qualified to transmit Reality. The *Tantras* understandably place such a one above all other teachers.

5. This statement was made by Adi Da (a.k.a. Franklin Jones, Da Free John, etc.).

6. Swami Muktananda, *Secret of the Siddhas,* p. 65.

7. Ibid., p. 68.

CHAPTER 7: INITIATION

1. The term *pashu* (beast) refers to the ordinary person, who is unenlightened and uninitiated.

2. The Sanskrit word *vedha* (piercing) is a technical term in Tantra that refers to the *guru*'s ability to penetrate the body-mind of the disciple during initiation and to pierce the subtle energy centers (*cakra*) so as to awaken and raise the disciple's *kundalinī*.

3. This appears to be the earliest known version of the Matsyendra legend.

4. For more information about the Kaula school of Tantra, see chapter 9.

5. See, e.g., the *Kula-Arnava-Tantra* (14.12).

6. This explanation is based on the two syllables of the term *dīkshā. Dī* is associated with *divya* (divine), and *kshā* with *kshālana* (wiping away).

7. The Buddha himself is said to have stayed in a cemetery during his early years of fierce asceticism, using charred bones for a pillow; see the *Majjhima-Nikāya* (1.79).

8. Mircea Eliade, *Yoga: Immortality and Freedom* (Princeton, N.J.: Princeton University Press, 1970), p. 296.

9. The word *aghora,* "nonterrible," is one of the epithets of Shiva, who is the object of worship for the *aghorins.*

10. See Brajamadhava Bhattacharya, *The World of Tantra* (New Delhi: Munshiram Manoharlal, 1988), pp. 202–5.

11. See Brajamadhava Bhattacharya, *Śaivism and the Phallic World,* 2 vols. (New Delhi: Oxford & IBH, 1975).

12. Written *kulākula-cakra.*

13. See Agehananda Bharati, *The Tantric Tradition* (London: Rider, 1965), p. 190.

14. The seven modes of initiation described in the *Kula-Arnava-Tantra* (14.39ff.) are the following: (1) *kriyā-dīkshā,* or initiation by means of ritual; (2) *varna-dīkshā,* which is the same as *varna-mayī-dīkshā;* (3) *kalā-dīkshā,* which is identical to *kalā-ātma-dīkshā;* (4) *sparsha-dīkshā,* or initiation by touch, a form of *shāmbhavī-dīkshā* (as described earlier in this chapter); (5) *vāg-dīkshā,* or initiation by speech (*vāc*), another form of *shāmbhavī-dīkshā;* (6) *drig-dīkshā,* or initiation by the mere glance (*drik*) of the *guru,* again a form of *shāmbhavī-dīkshā;* (7) *māna-dīkshā,* or initiation by mere thought (*manas*), which has been described under *anupāya-dīkshā.*

    The Kashmiri Shaiva schools distinguish between the following four modes of initiation: (1) *anupāya-dīkshā,* or initiation without external means, which is possible in the case of highly evolved practitioners who can attain enlightenment simply by proximity to an enlightened adept; this appears to be identical with the *vedha-mayī-dīkshā;* (2) *shāmbhavī-dīkshā,* which has been described; (3) *shakti-dīkshā,* or initiation by means of the innate power; this seems to be identical with the *shākteyī-dīkshā* referred to earlier; (4) *āṇavī-dīkshā,* or "atomic" initiation, which refers to the individual self called *anu* in Kashmir's form of Shaivism; this type of initiation comprises various ritual means and conscious cultivation through Yoga.

15. The Sanskrit term *dhāman* can denote both "light" and "dwelling place" and thus could be rendered as "lustrous abode."

CHAPTER 8: DISCIPLESHIP

1. The Sanskrit term *kulīna,* here translated as "noble," can also mean "of good family."

2. The word *āstikya* (from *asti,* meaning "it is") denotes affirmation of the Vedic revelation.

3. I have addressed this important issue in my book *Holy Madness* (New York: Paragon House, 1990).

4. For an explanation of the words *kula, kaula,* and *kaulika,* see chapter 9.

5. This Sanskrit passage is defective. Fire probably means here the sacred fire lit during rituals.

6. C. C. Chang, trans., *The Hundred Thousand Songs of Milarepa* (Boulder, Colo.: Shambhala Publications, 1962), vol. 1, p. 273.

7. *Kula-Arnava-Tantra* (17.25). Here the word *vīra* is associated with *vīta-rāga* ("free from passion") and *rajas-tamo-vidhūra* ("far removed from *rajas* and *tamas*").

CHAPTER 9: THE TANTRIC PATH

1. See Abhinava Gupta's monumental *Tantra-Āloka* (chapter 1, p. 25).

2. John Blofeld, *The Tantric Mysticism of Tibet: A Practical Guide* (New York: Dutton, 1970), p. 217.

3. This computation was made by Helene Brunner, "Jñāna and Kriyā: Relation between Theory and Practice in the *Śaivāgamas,*" in *Ritual and Speculation in Early Tantrism: Studies in Honor of Andre Padoux,* ed. Teun Goudriaan (Albany: SUNY Press, 1992), p. 25. Agehananda Bharati analyzed the contents of twenty-five Hindu and Buddhist *Tantras* and came up with the following average percentages for various subject matters discussed: 60 percent *mantra;* 10 percent *mandala;* 10 percent *dhyāna* (including often lengthy descriptions of the graphic representations of deities); 7 percent teachings on liberation; 5 percent preparation of ritual substances; 3 per-

cent amulets and charms. Other minor themes addressed in the Tantras are paranormal powers, magical spells and incantations, and alchemical and astrological matters; see Agehananda Bharati, *The Tantric Tradition* (London: Rider, 1965).

4. The Sanskrit names for these postures are *padma-, svastika-, vajra-, bhadra-,* and *vīra-āsana* respectively.

5. The *Brihan-Nīla-Tantra* adds the ritual act of bathing (*snāna*).

6. See Arthur Avalon, *Greatness of Shiva,* 2nd ed. (Madras: Ganesh, 1925).

7. For this and many other fine stavas, see Arthur and Ellen Avalon, *Hymns to the Goddess* (London: Luzac, 1913).

8. See W. N. Brown, ed. and trans., *Saundaryalaharī,* Harvard Oriental Series, vol. 43 (Cambridge, Mass.: Harvard University Press, 1958).

9. See the rendering and yogic commentary on this text by Gopi Krishna, *Secrets of Kundalini in Panchastavi* (New Delhi: Kundalini Research & Publication Trust, 1978).

10. Anagarika Govinda, *Foundations of Tibetan Mysticism* (London: Rider, 1969), p. 53.

11. See Mircea Eliade, *Yoga: Immortality and Freedom* (Princeton, N.J.: Princeton University Press, 1970), p. 253.

12. Ibid., p. 249.

13. In addition to the seven hierarchically arranged modes of Tantric practice, the *Tantras* also know of several other classifications, such as lineage traditions (*āmnāya*), "currents" (*srota*), and the four directional "seats" (*pītha*). It would go beyond the scope of this introductory volume to describe these various arrangements of the Tantric literature and teachings, which have their own subdivisions and are quite complicated.

14. The five "faces" of the eternal Shiva are Sadyojāta (west), Vāmadeva (north), Aghora (south), Tatpurusha (east), and Īshāna (upward-facing). Often the twenty-eight *Āgamas* of the Siddhānta tradition of South India are associated with Shiva's upper face, but according to the Kaula scriptures, so is the Kaula system.

15. According to Abhinava Gupta, who lived in the tenth century CE, there were ten early Kaula teachers (see *Tantra-Āloka,* chapter 28), not counting his own immediate lineage or the sons of Macchanda, who, since they are remembered by tradition, in all probability were his successors.

16. The most important Kaula scriptures are the *Kula-Arnava-Tantra, Kaula-Jnāna-Nirnaya, Samketa-Paddhati, Kaula-Avalī-Nirnaya, Kaula-Cūdāmani-Tantra, Akula-Vīra-Tantra* (existing in two versions), *Kubjikā-Tantra, Siddha-Yogīshvara-Tantra* (a voluminous but no longer extant work that is often referred to as the first Kaula Tantra).

17. M. Rabe, "Sexual Imagery on the 'Phantasmagorical Castles' at Khajuraho," *International Journal of Tantric Studies* 2, no. 2 (November 1996). This is an online journal located at *http://www.shore.net/~india/ijts/* or *ftp://ftp.shore.net/india/members/.*

18. The wordplay here is on the first syllable of the words *kaumāra* and *laya.*

CHAPTER 10: THE SUBTLE BODY AND ITS ENVIRONMENT

1. The term *ātivāhika* is used, for instance, in the *Yoga-Vāsishtha,* a remarkable Shaiva work authored in the tenth century CE.

2. See Eleanor Criswell, *How Yoga Works* (Novato, Calif.: Freeperson Press, 1989) and *Biofeedback and Somatics* (Novato, Calif.: Freeperson Press, 1996).

3. *Cittar* is the Tamil synonym for the Sanskrit term *siddha* and must not be confused with the Sanskrit word *citta,* meaning "mind" or "consciousness."

4. See, e.g., Richard Gerber, *Vibrational Medicine: New Choices for Healing Ourselves* (Santa Fe, N.M.: Bear & Co., 1988). The author, who is an internist, makes some very insightful observations about the *cakras.*

5. See Vasant G. Rele, *The Mysterious Kundalini: The Physical Basis of the "Kundalini (Hatha Yoga)" in Terms of Western Anatomy and Physiology,* foreword by Sir John Woodroffe (1927; 7th ed., Bombay: D. B. Taraporevala Sons, [1950?]).

6. *Cakra* is popularly spelled *chakra* in English.

7. According to the *Yoga-Vishaya,* a short text attributed to Matsyendra, there are nine psychoenergetic centers beyond the *ājnā-cakra,* namely, *tri-kuta*

(triple peak), *tri-hatha* (triple force), *golhāta* (perhaps from *gola-hātaka,* "golden bull"), *shikhara* (summit), *tri-shikha* (triple crest), *vajra* (thunderbolt), *om-kāra* (*om-*maker), *ūrdhva-nākha* (probably for *ūrdhva-nāka,* "upper vault"), and *bhrūvor-mukha* (opening between the brows).

8. See Hiroshi Motoyama, "Functions of Ki and Psi Energy," *Research for Religion and Parapsychology,* no. 15 (August 1985): 1–83.

9. Swami Rama, Rudolph Ballantine, and Swami Ajaya (A. Weinstock), *Yoga and Psychotherapy: The Evolution of Consciousness* (Glenview, Ill.: Himalayan Institute, 1976), p. 223.

10. The term *sahasrāra* is composed of *sahasra* (thousand) and *ara* (spoke).

11. The term *svādhishthāna* consists of *sva* (own) and *adhishthāna* (base or foundation).

12. See Swami Sivananda Radha, *Kundalini Yoga for the West* (Spokane, Wash.: Timeless Books, 1978).

13. The term *mūlādhāra* is composed of *mūla* (root) and *adhāra* (base or prop), reminding one of the archaic word *fundament* for buttocks.

14. Because of the male-orientedness of the *Tantras* and Yoga scriptures, the vagina is not listed as a separate "gate."

15. See David Gordon White, *The Alchemical Body: Siddha Traditions in Medieval India* (Chicago: University of Chicago Press, 1996).

CHAPTER 11: AWAKENING THE SERPENT POWER

1. Gopi Krishna, *Kundalini: The Evolutionary Energy in Man* (Boston & London: Shambhala Publications, 1997), p. 54. This edition has an excellent psychological commentary by James Hillman.

2. Ibid., p. 64.

3. Ibid., p. 64–65.

4. Lee Sannella, *The Kundalini Experience* (Lower Lake, Calif.: Integral Publishing, 1992), p. 31.

5. *Hatha-Yoga-Pradīpikā* 3.107.

6. This is the practice of *nyāsa,* which is discussed in chapter 13.

7. B. K. S. Iyengar, *The Tree of Yoga* (Boston: Shambhala Publications, 1989), p. 127.

8. This alternation can easily be tested, because it opens the left and the right nostril respectively, with a short period of free flow through both nostrils. It is possible to change the flow simply by putting pressure on the armpit of the side that one wants to activate. The flow of vital energy is also used for diagnostic and divinatory purposes, and this craft is known as *svarodaya-vijnāna* (knowledge of the rising of the sound [of the breath]).

9. See Arthur Avalon (Sir John Woodroffe), *Shakti and Shākta* (New York: Dover, 1978), pp. 694ff; this volume was first published sixty years earlier.

10. See, e.g., the *Shārada-Tilaka-Tantra* (25.78). The three *gunas* are *sattva* (principle of lucidity), *rajas* (dynamic principle), and *tamas* (principle of inertia). These are fundamental constituents of nature (*prakriti*). Some-times eight coils are spoken of, and various explanations have been given for them.

11. Interestingly, the common Sanskrit name for the ultimate Reality is *brahman,* which is derived from the verbal root *brih,* meaning "to grow." In the *Upanishads,* the world is described as emerging out of the indescribable, unqualified *brahman,* which affords a parallel to the Big Bang model of creation. The original quantum vacuum or foam is also indescribable, since—like the *brahman*—it transcends space and time, yet out of it sprang in logical sequence the entire universe.

12. *Buddhi-yoga* can mean "mental discipline" or, more specifically, "unitive discipline by means of the higher mind."

13. See Robert E. Svoboda, *Aghora II: Kundalini* (Albuquerque, N.M.: Brother-hood of Life, 1993), p. 72.

14. The use of the term *paridhāna* in the present context is curious. It means "putting on" or "surrounding" and here is meant to convey the idea of agitation. Some commentators understand it as a synonym for *naulī,* which is performed by rolling the abdominal rectus muscles clockwise and coun-terclockwise.

15. This is poem 31 in the edition by B. N. Parimoo, *The Ascent of Self* (Delhi: Motilal Banarsidass, 1978).

16. This is poem 42 in ibid.

17. This is poem 53 in ibid.

18. See David Bohm, *Wholeness and the Implicate Order* (London: Routledge & Kegan Paul, 1980), pp. 150ff.

CHAPTER 12: MANTRA

1. John Woodroffe, *The Garland of Letters: Studies in the Mantra-Śāstra,* 6th ed. (Madras: Ganesh, 1974), p. 230.

2. Gopi Krishna, *Kundalini: The Evolutionary Energy in Man* (London: Robinson & Watkins, 1971), p. 88.

3. The word *vānī* suggests speech that is musical and beautiful.

4. The *Tantras* distinguish between a Vedic, Shaiva, and Shākta *pranava.* The first mentioned is the *om* sound, the second is *hum,* and the third is *hrīm.*

5. Other subtle distinctions are known as well. See Georg Feuerstein, "The Sacred Syllable Om," *Yoga Research Center Studies Series,* no. 2 (Lower Lake, Calif.: Yoga Research Center, 1997).

6. The terms *ūrdhva-* and *adhah-kundalinī* are also used to refer to the ascending and descending movement of the serpent power respectively.

7. In North India the autumnal skies are brilliant and largely free from clouds. When a cloud does appear, it will not produce rain.

8. The *mantrin* is a practitioner reciting a *mantra.*

9. Swami Chetanananda, *Dynamic Stillness,* vol. 1, *The Practice of Trika Yoga* (Cambridge, Mass.: Rudra Press, 1990), p. 145.

10. Some Tantric texts explain *yoni-mudrā* differently in the present context.

11. See Subhash Kak, "The Astronomy of the Vedic Altars and the Ṛgveda," *Mankind Quarterly* 33, no. 1 (1992): 43–55.

12. Swami Sivananda Radha, *Mantras: Words of Power* (Porthill, Id.: Timeless Books, 1980), p. 8.

CHAPTER 13: CREATING SACRED SPACE

1. The Ganeshas and Yoginīs mentioned in this verse are masculine and feminine energies respectively. The former are various manifestations of the elephant-headed deity Ganesha (from *gana,* meaning "host," and *īsha,* meaning "lord"). They are male companions of Shiva. The Yoginīs, as the word suggests, are female adepts of Yoga who have gained the status of deities. For further details, see chapter 14.

2. The best-known "seals" of this type are the *mahā-mudrā* (great seal), *vajrolī-mudrā* (adamantine seal), and *viparīta-karanī-mudrā* (seal of reversed action). These are described in manuals such as the *Gheranda-Samhitā, Shiva-Samhitā,* and *Hatha-Yoga-Pradīpikā.*

3. The wordplay is around the terms *modana* (delighting) and *drāvana* (chasing away, removing).

4. Douglas Renfrew Brooks, *The Secret of the Three Cities: An Introduction to Hindu Śākta Tantrism* (Chicago: University of Chicago Press, 1990), p. 59.

5. Ibid.

6. For an informative article on therapeutic hand gestures, see Richard C. Miller, "The Power of Mudra," *Yoga Journal,* September/October 1996, pp. 81–89.

7. This and the following therapeutic hand gestures have been described by Acharya Kesav Dev in a number of articles in the *Times of India* (1980 and 1981), as mentioned in P. R. Shah, *Tantra: Its Therapeutic Aspect* (Calcutta: Punthi Pustak, 1987), pp. 133–34.

8. Here the pun revolves around the words *yama* (= *yan*) and *trāyate* (= *tra*).

9. Mircea Eliade, *Yoga: Immortality and Freedom* (Princeton, N.J.: Princeton University Press, 1970), p. 219.

10. See C. G. Jung, *Mandala Symbolism* (Princeton, N.J.: Princeton University Press, 1972), p. 4.

11. The title of this text is written *Yantroddhāra-Sarvasva,* meaning "All about Constructing *Yantras.*"

12. This is *stotra* 8 (verse 3) in the edition of the *Shiva-Stotra-Avalī* by N. K. Kotru, *Śivastotravalī of Utpaladeva* (Delhi: Motilal Banarsidass, 1985), p. 188.

13. Translation by B. N. Parimoo, *The Ascent of Self* (Delhi: Motilal Banarsidass, 1978), p. 161.

CHAPTER 14: THE TRANSMUTATION OF DESIRE

1. *Tiru-Mantiram* (704–5), trans. by Kamil V. Zvelebil, in *The Siddha Quest for Immortality* (Oxford: Mandrake, 1996), p. 30.

2. See, e.g., the *Amrita-Bindu-Upanishad* (2): "The mind alone is the cause of bondage or liberation for humans. Attached to objects, [it moves toward] bondage; devoid of objects, it is said to be liberated."

3. Sigmund Freud, *Civilization and Its Discontents* (1930; New York: Norton, 1961).

4. See Georg Feuerstein, *Sacred Sexuality: Living the Vision of the Erotic Spirit* (Los Angeles: Tarcher, 1993).

5. See Ken Wilber, *The Atman Project* (Wheaton, Ill.: Theosophical Publishing House, 1980).

6. See Wendy Doniger O'Flaherty, *Asceticism and Eroticism in the Mythology of Śiva* (Delhi: Oxford University Press, 1975).

7. See, e.g., *Skanda-Purāna* (6.257.11).

8. O'Flaherty, *Asceticism and Eroticism,* p. 315.

9. See S. A. Dange, *Sexual Symbolism from the Vedic Ritual* (Delhi: Ajanta, 1979).

10. David Gordon White, *The Alchemical Body: Siddha Traditions in Medieval India* (Chicago: University of Chicago Press, 1996), p. 7: "Following Abhinava-gupta, tantrism became transformed into an elite mystic path that was all too complicated, refined, and cerebralized for common people to grasp. . . . The thirty-six or thirty-seven metaphysical levels of being were incomprehensible to India's masses and held few answers to their human concerns and aspirations."

11. Although the female sexual fluid is described as being red, we need not necessarily understand the term *rakta* as menstrual blood only. It could encompass vaginal secretions in general, especially the hormone-rich secretion produced through sexual stimulation. This is also known as *yoni-tattva* or "womb's substance/principle."

12. *The Gospel of Sri Ramakrishna,* trans. Swami Nikhilananda (1942; New York: Ramakrishna-Vedanta Center, 1952), p. 603.

13 Ibid., p. 491.

14. Ibid., p. 134.

15. Ibid., p. 331.

16. Glen A. Hayes, "The Vaiṣṇava Sahajiyā Traditions of Medieval Bengal," in *Religions of India in Practice,* ed. D. S. Lopez, Jr. (Princeton, N.J.: Princeton University Press, 1995).

17. See, e.g., the *Spanda-Kārikā* (1.22) and *Vijñāna-Bhairava* (118).

18. In Hindu society, drinking alcohol is traditionally considered a cardinal sin.

19. For euphonic reasons *cit* (consciousness) is changed to *cic* in the compound *cic-candra.*

20. A fairly detailed description can be found in the *Mahānirvāṇa-Tantra* (chapter 6).

21. Bhagwan Shree Rajneesh, *Tantra Spirituality and Sex,* 2nd ed. (Rajneeshpuram, Ore.: Rajneesh Foundation International, 1983), p. 2.

22. Ibid., p. 114.

23. Brajamadhava Bhattacharya, *The World of Tantra* (New Delhi: Munshiram Manoharlal, 1988), p. 42.

24. Ibid., p. 44.

25. Ibid. p. 448.

26. See the *Kula-Arnava-Tantra* (5.74).

27. See the *Bhagavad-Gītā* (6.32).

CHAPTER 15: ENLIGHTENMENT AND THE HIDDEN POWERS OF
THE MIND

1. *Sandhyā* refers to the transition between light and darkness at dawn and at dusk.

2. The Sanskrit phrase is *ātma-eka-bhāva-nishtha* (written *ātmaika-*).

3. Christopher Chapple, in a personal communication to the author, made the interesting suggestion that the yogic notion of dissolution of the cosmos could be specific to the subjective world of the *yogin* (i.e. the mind).

4. The Tibetan honorific *-pa* corresponds to the Sanskrit *-pāda,* meaning something like "honorable" or "worshipful" when appended to a personal name.

5. The *Netra-Tantra* distinguishes between *Vāma-Tantras* (dealing with paranormal powers), *Garuda-Tantras* (dealing with poisons), and *Bhūta-Tantras* (dealing with ghosts and exorcism).

6. See Sonu Shamdasani, ed., *The Psychology of Kundalini Yoga: Notes of the Seminar Given in 1932 by C. G. Jung* (Princeton, N.J.: Princeton University Press, 1996), p. 94.

Select Bibliography

Alper, Harvey, ed. *Mantra*. Albany: SUNY Press, 1989.

————, ed. *Understanding Mantras*. Albany: SUNY Press, 1989.

Arya, Usharbudh. *Mantra and Meditation*. Honesdale, Pa.: Himalayan International Institute, 1981.

Avalon, Arthur [Sir John Woodroffe]. *Principles of Tantra: The Tantratattva of Śri-yukta Śiva Candra Vidyārnava Bhattacharya*. 3d ed. Madras: Ganesh, 1960.

————. *The Serpent Power, Being the Ṣaṭcakranirūpaṇa and the Pādukāpanchaka*. 1913. 10th ed. Madras: Ganesh, 1974.

Avalon, Arthur, and Ellen Avalon. *Hymns to the Goddess*. 1952. Reprint. Madras: Ganesh, 1973.

Bailly, Constantina Rhodes. *Shaiva Devotional Songs of Kashmir: A Translation and Study of Utpaladeva's Shivastotravali*. Albany: SUNY Press, 1987.

Banerjea, Akshaya Kumar. *Philosophy of Gorakhnath with Goraksha-Vacana-San-graha*. Gorakhpur, India: Mahant Dig Vijai Nath Trust, [1961].

Banerji, Sures Chandra. *New Light on Tantra*. Calcutta: Punthi Pustak, 1992.

Basu, Manoranjan. *Fundamentals of the Philosophy of Tantras*. Calcutta: Mira Basu, 1986.

Bharati, Agehananda. *The Tantric Tradition*. London: Rider, 1965. Rev. ed. New York: Samuel Weiser, 1975.

Bhattacharya, Brajamadhava. *The World of Tantra*. New Delhi: Munshiram Mano-harlal, 1988.

————. *Śaivism and the Phallic World*. 2 vols. New Delhi: Oxford & IBH, 1975.

Bhattacharyya, Narendra Nath. *History of Indian Erotic Literature*. New Delhi: Munshiram Manoharlal, 1975.

Brooks, Douglas Renfrew. *Auspicious Wisdom: The Texts and Traditions of Śrīvidyā Śākta Tantrism in South India*. Albany: SUNY Press, 1992.

————. *The Secret of the Three Cities*. Chicago: University of Chicago Press, 1990.

Brown, C. Mackenzie. *The Triumph of the Goddess: The Canonical Models and Theological Visions of the Devī-Bhāgavata Purāṇa*. Albany: SUNY Press, 1990.

Chattopadhyaya, Sudhakar. *Reflections on the Tantras*. Delhi: Motilal Banarsidass, 1978.

Chetanananda, Swami. *Dynamic Stillness*. Vol. 1. *The Practice of Trika Yoga*. Vol. 2. *The Fulfillment of Trika Yoga*. Cambridge, Mass.: Rudra Press, 1983, 1991.

Coburn, Thomas B. *Devī Māhātmya: The Crystallization of the Goddess Tradition*. Columbia, Miss.: South Asia Books, 1985.

Daniélou, Alain. *The Complete Kāma-Sūtra*. Rochester, Vt.: Park Street Press, 1994.

Das Gupta, Shashibhusan. *Obscure Religious Cults as Background of Bengali Literature*. 3d. ed. Calcutta: Firma KLM, 1969.

Dimock, E. C. *The Place of the Hidden Moon: Erotic Mysticism in the Vaiṣṇava Sahajiyā Cult of Bengal*. Chicago: University of Chicago Press, 1966.

Douglas, Nik, and Penny Slinger. *Sexual Secrets*. New York: Destiny Books, 1979.

Dyczkowski, Mark S. G. *The Canon of the Śaivāgama and the Kubjikā Tantras of the Western Kaula Tradition*. Albany: SUNY Press, 1988.

————. *The Doctrine of Vibration: An Analysis of the Doctrines and Practices of Kashmir Śaivism*. Albany: SUNY Press, 1987.

Eliade, Mircea. *Yoga: Immortality and Freedom*. Princeton, N.J.: Princeton University Press, 1969.

Evola, Julius. *The Metaphysics of Sex*. New York: Inner Traditions International, 1983.

Feuerstein, Georg. *The Shambhala Encyclopedia of Yoga*. Boston: Shambhala Publications, 1997.

————. *The Shambhala Guide to Yoga*. Boston: Shambhala Publications, 1996.

————. *The Yoga-Sūtra of Patañjali: A New Translation and Commentary*. Reprint. Rochester, Vt.: Inner Traditions International, 1989.

Feuerstein, Georg, Subhash Kak, and David Frawley. *In Search of the Cradle of Civilization: New Light on Ancient India*. Wheaton, Ill.: Quest Books, 1995.

Frawley, David. *Tantric Yoga and the Wisdom Goddesses.* Salt Lake City, Utah: Passage Press, 1994.

Govinda, Anagarika. *Foundations of Tibetan Mysticism.* London: Rider, 1969.

Goudriaan, Teun. The *Vīṇāśikhatantra: A Śaiva Tantra of the Left Current.* Delhi: Motilal Banarsidass, 1985.

Goudriaan, Teun, and Sanjukta Gupta. *Hindu Tantric and Śākta Literature.* Wiesbaden, Germany: Otto Harrassowitz, 1981.

Guenther, Herbert V. *The Tantric View of Life.* Berkeley, Calif.: Shambhala Publications, 1972.

Gupta, Sanjukta. *Lakshmi Tantra.* Leiden: E. J. Brill, 1972.

Gupta, Sanjukta, Dirk Jan Hoens, and Teun Goudriaan. *Hindu Tantrism.* Leiden: E. J. Brill, 1979.

Hayes, Glen. "The Vaiṣṇava Sahajiyā Traditions of Medieval Bengal." In D. S. Lopez, Jr., ed., *Religions of India in Practice,* pp. 333–51. Princeton, N.J.: Princeton University Press.

Hughes, John. *Self Realization in Kashmir Shaivism: The Oral Teachings of Swami Laksmanjoo.* Albany: SUNY Press, 1994.

Johari, Harish. *Tools for Tantra.* Rochester, Vt.: Destiny Books, 1986.

Kaulajnana-nirnaya of the School of Matsyendranatha. Edited by P. C. Bagchi, translated by Michael Magee. Varanasi, India: Prachya Prakashan, 1986.

Khanna, Madhu. *Yantra: The Tantric Symbol of Cosmic Unity.* London: Thames and Hudson, 1979.

Kleen, Tyra de. *Mudrās: The Ritual Hand-Poses of the Buddha Priests and the Shiva Priests of Bali.* London: Kegan Paul, 1924.

Kotru, N. K. *Śivastotrāvalī of Utpaladeva.* Delhi: Motilal Banarsidass, 1985. Sanskrit text with English translation.

Kramrisch, Stella. *The Presence of Śiva.* Princeton, N.J.: Princeton University Press, 1981.

Krishna, Gopi. *Kundalini: The Evolutionary Energy in Man.* Revised edition. Boston & London: Shambhala Publications, 1997.

Kulārṇava Tantra. Introduction by Arthur Avalon, readings by M. P. Pandit, Sanskrit text edited by Tārānātha Vidyāratna. Reprint. Delhi: Motilal Banarsidass, 1984.

Kulārṇava Tantra. Text with English translation by Ram Kumar Rai. Varanasi, India: Prachya Prakashan, 1983.

Lorenzen, D. N. *The Kāpālikas and Kālāmukhas, Two Lost Śaivite Sects.* Reprint. New Delhi: Motilal Banarsidass, 1972.

Mantramahodadhi of Mahidhara. Translated by a Board of Scholars. Delhi: Sri Satguru, 1984.

Mantra-Yoga Saṃhitā. Edited Sanskrit text with English translation by Ramkumar Rai. Varanasi, India: Chaukhambha Orientalia, 1982.

Meyer, Johann Jakob. *Sexual Life in Ancient India: A Study in the Comparative History of Indian Culture.* Delhi: Motilal Banarsidass, 1971.

Mookerjee, Ajit. *Kali: The Feminine Force.* New York: Destiny Books, 1988.

————. *Tantra Art: Its Philosophy and Physics.* Basel: Ravi Kumar, 1971.

Mookerjee, Ajit, and Madhu Khanna. *The Tantric Way: Art, Science, Ritual.* London: Thames and Hudson, 1977.

Muktananda, Swami. *Secret of the Siddhas.* South Fallsburg, N.Y.: SYDA Foundation, 1983.

Müller-Ortega, Paul Eduardo. *The Triadic Heart of Śiva: Kaula Tantricism of Abhinavagupta in the Non-Dual Shaivism of Kashmir.* Albany: SUNY Press, 1989.

O'Flaherty, Wendy Doniger. *Asceticism and Eroticism in the Mythology of Śiva.* Delhi: Oxford University Press, 1973.

Padoux, André. "A Survey of Tantric Hinduism for the Historian of Religions." *History of Religions* 20 (1981): 345–60.

————. *Vāc: The Concept of the Word in Selected Hindu Tantras.* Translated By Jacques Gontier. Albany: SUNY Press, 1990.

Pandey, Kanti Chandra, *Abhinavagupta: An Historical and Philosophical Study.* Varanasi, India: Chowkhamba Sanskrit Series Office, 1963.

Pott, P. H. *Yoga and Yantra: Their Interrelation and Their Significance for Indian Archeology.* The Hague: E. J. Brill, 1966.

Rao, S. K. R. *The Yantras.* Delhi: Sri Satguru, 1988.

Rastogi, N. *Krama Tantricism of Kashmir: Historical and General Sources.* Vol. 1. Delhi: Motilal Banarsidass, 1981.

Rawson, Phillip. *The Art of Tantra.* London: Thames and Hudson, 1978.

————. *Tantra: The Indian Cult of Ecstasy.* New York: Avon Books, 1973.

Sanderson, Alexis. "Śaivism and the Tantric Traditions." In S. Sutherland et al., eds., *The World's Religions,* pp. 660–704. London: Routledge, 1988.

Sannella, Lee. *The Kundalini Experience: Psychosis or Transcendence?* Rev. ed. Lower Lake, Calif.: Integral Publishing, 1992.

Saunders, E. Dale. *Mudrā: A Study of Symbolic Gestures in Japanese Buddhist Sculpture.* Princeton, N.J.: Princeton University Press, 1985.

Schoterman, J. A. *The Yonitantra.* New Delhi: Manohar, 1980. Sanskrit text with English translation.

SenSharma, Deba Brata. *The Philosophy of Sādhanā, with Special Reference to the Trika Philosophy of Kashmir.* Albany: SUNY Press, 1990.

Shamdasani, Sonu, ed. *The Psychology of Kundalini Yoga: Notes of the Seminar Given in 1932 by C. G. Jung.* Princeton, N.J.: Princeton University Press, 1996.

Silburn, Lilian. *Kuṇḍalinī: The Energy of the Depths.* Albany: SUNY Press, 1988.

Singh, Jaideva. *Pratyabhijñāhṛdayam: The Secret of Self-Recognition.* Rev. ed. Delhi: Motilal Banarsidass, 1980.

————. *Śiva Sūtras: The Yoga of Supreme Identity.* Delhi: Motilal Banarsidass, 1979.

————. *Spanda-Kārikās: The Divine Creative Pulsation.* Delhi: Motilal Banarsidass, 1980.

————. *The Yoga of Delight, Wonder, and Astonishment.* Albany: SUNY Press, 1991.

————. *The Yoga of Vibration and Divine Pulsation.* Albany: SUNY Press, 1992.

Singh, Jaideva, Swami Lashmanjee, and Bettina Bäumer. *Abhinavagupta, Parātrītriśikā-Vivarana: The Secret of Tantric Mysticism.* Delhi: Motilal Banarsidass, 1988.

Strickmann, M., ed. *Tantric and Taoist Studies in Honor of R. A. Stein.* Brussels: Institut Belge des Hautes Études Chinoises, 1981.

Svoboda, Robert E. *Aghora: At the Left Hand of God.* Albuquerque, N.M.: Brotherhood of Life, 1986.

Tigunait, Rajmani. *Śakti Sādhanā: Steps to Samādhi—A Translation of the Tripura Rahasya.* Honesdale, Penn.: The Himalayan International Institute, 1993.

————. *Saktism: The Power in Tantra.* Honesdale, Penn.: The Himalayan International Institute, 1998.

Van Lysebeth, André. *Tantra: The Cult of the Feminine.* York Beach, Me.: Samuel Weiser, 1995.

White, David Gordon. *The Alchemical Body: Siddha Traditions in Medieval India.* Chicago: University of Chicago Press, 1996.

Woodroffe, Sir John. *The Garland of Letters.* 7th ed. Madras: Ganesh, 1979.

————. *Introduction to Tantra Śāstra.* 6th ed. Madras: Ganesh, 1973.

————. *Shakti and Shakta: Essays and Addresses on the Shakta Tantrashastra.* 8th ed. Madras: Ganesh, 1975.

————. *Tantrarāja Tantra: A Short Analysis.* 3d ed. Madras: Ganesh, 1971.

————. *See also* Avalon, Arthur.

Zvelebil, Kamil V. *The Poets of the Powers.* Lower Lake, Calif.: Integral Publishing, 1993.

————. *The Siddha Quest for Immortality.* Oxford: Mandrake, 1996.

Index

Abhinava Gupta, x, xii, 77–78, 95, 100, 122–123, 138, 175, 178, 218, 231, 255–256, 281 n. 7, 287 n. 15, 292 n. 10
ācāras, 4, 135, 137
adhikāra, 89, 100, 110–111
Advaita Vedānta. *See* Vedānta
Āgamas, xi, 14, 26, 72, 96, 126, 276 n. 3, 278 n. 4, 286 n. 14
Agastya, 146–147, 263
Aghorī sect, 9, 101–102, 176–177, 284 n. 9
Agni, 15, 66, 237
aham, 77, 183
ahamkāra. *See* ego-personality
ahimsā, 113, 124, 125, 269
air element. *See* elements
Aitareya-Brāhmana, 16
ākāsha. *See* elements
akula, 137, 183
Akula-Vīra-Tantra, 45–46, 287 n. 16
alchemy, 145, 163, 181, 233, 234, 238, 261, 263, 285–6 n. 3
alcohol, 9, 119, 231, 232, 239, 240–241, 247, 248, 261, 262, 293 n. 18
āmnāyas. *See* lineage
amrita. *See* nectar
Amrita-Bindu-Upanishad, 292 n. 2
amulets, 130, 218, 285–6 n. 3
ānanda. *See* bliss; Bliss
Ānanda-Laharī, 131, 149–150
angas, 124–125, 203, 205
anger, 79, 125, 158, 239, 251
antahkarana, 64–65, 141

antar-yāga, 50–51, 124
anu. *See* purusha
anupāya, 122, 284 n. 14
apāna, 148, 174, 177, 255
Āranyakas, 16, 26, 48
ardha-indu, 187
Ardhanārīshvara, 79–80, 282 n. 6
Aryan invasion theory, 276–277 n. 5, 277 n. 9
āsanas, 124, 125, 169–170, 217
Asanga, 97
asceticism, 50, 58, 102, 108, 115, 147, 224–225, 226, 229–230
astrology, 60–61, 103, 286 n. 3
Atharva-Veda, 10, 11, 15, 16, 33–34, 148, 237–238
ātman, 30, 55, 115, 141. *See also* Self
Atman Project, 229
attachment, 60, 63, 64, 116–117, 159, 182, 229, 230, 245
avadhūtas, 8–9, 133
Avalon, A. *See* Woodroffe, Sir John
avidyā, 22, 66, 115–116, 223, 251
awareness, 76, 143–144, 192, 253. *See also* consciousness
Āyurveda, 145, 146, 163, 182–183, 216, 233, 237

balance, 145, 150, 154–155, 163–164
Basu, Manoranjan, 14
beasts. *See* pashus
Beer, Robert, x
Being: deities and, 71–72

Being-Consciousness, 22, 62, 188, 196
Being-Consciousness-Bliss, 66, 74, 75–77,
 78–79, 89, 94, 117, 253, 281 n. 8,
 282 n. 3
Bhagavad-Gītā, 20, 34, 48, 49, 67, 71, 121,
 201, 223, 229, 269
Bhāgavata-Purāna, 27, 48, 56, 236
Bhairava, 72, 137, 249
Bhairavī-Stotra, ix
bhakti, 72, 93, 121–122, 123–124, 234
Bhārata war, 5, 6
Bharati, Agehananda, 2, 106, 286–287 n. 3
Bhāskara, 87
Bhatta, Rāghava, 108
Bhattacharya, Brajamadhava, 102–103,
 243–245
bhāvas, 118–119
bhoga, 222, 226–227, 234
Bhoja, King, 256
bhū-mandala, 26–27
bhūr-loka, 27, 278 n. 6
bhūtas. See elementals; elements
bhūta-shuddhi, 127, 179–180, 202, 203
bījas, 16, 170–171, 187–188, 195–197, 247
bindu, 187–188, 219, 220
bliss, xiv, 59–60, 80, 141–142, 178, 182,
 183, 220, 222, 227, 230, 240, 250–256.
 See also ecstasy
Bliss, 183, 226, 256. *See also* Being-Consciousness-Bliss
bodhisattva path, 269–270
body: bliss and, 230, 240, 252; causal (higher),
 142; consecrating the, 201–207; cultivation
 of, 263; divine, 83, 180, 181, 206, 260,
 263; Divine and, 50, 53, 180, 181, 185,
 224–226, 236; as energy, 184–190; Hatha
 Yoga and, 264; healing and, 144–147; *karma*
 and, 53, 54, 55, 142, 144; liberation and,
 53–57, 60, 142, 185, 226–227; mind-body
 split, 143, 185; Reality and, 53, 141, 226;
 Self and, 53, 54, 55; sheaths of, 28–29,
 140–144; *shrī-yantra* and, 220–221; subtle,
 28–29, 139–164, 166; Tantra and, 50, 52–
 69, 144, 224–229; verticalism and, 49, 52–
 53, 224–225; world as, 60. *See also* desire
Bohm, David, 75, 180
bondage, 30, 49, 158, 169, 227, 259, 260
book learning, 85–86, 123, 132–133
Brahma, 9, 27–28, 85, 257, 276 n. 3, 278 n. 9
brahmacarya. See chastity
brahman, 2, 116–117, 151, 187, 195–196,

 230, 236, 240, 242, 255, 279 n. 3,
 289 n. 11
Brāhmanas, 11, 15–16, 19, 26, 48, 202. *See also
 specific Brāhmanas*
brahma-randhra, 150–152
brahmic egg, 26, 27–28, 29–30, 35, 39,
 278 n. 5, 278 n. 7, 279 n. 5
brahmins (*brāhmanas*), 7, 9–10, 13, 14, 15–
 16, 99, 269
breath. *See prāna*
breath control, 105, 124, 125, 144–145,
 170–172, 174, 176, 177, 183
Brihad-Āranyaka-Upanishad, 17, 49, 160, 230,
 246
Brihad-Yoni-Tantra, 246
Brooks, Douglas Renfrew, 207–208
Buddha, Gautama the, 14, 44, 50
buddhi, 34, 64, 141, 151–152, 153, 176, 181
Buddhist Tantra (Vajrayāna Buddhism): Hindu
 Tantra vs., xi–xii, xiv, 10; history of, x, xii,
 10, 14; *mahā-siddhas* of, 261–262; nature
 of, 34, 44, 71, 100, 128, 208, 218, 240,
 269–270, 282 n. 8. *See also* Mahāyāna Buddhism

cakra-pūjā, 241, 242, 248, 269
cakras, 15, 16, 130, 148–164; *ājnā-cakra*, 152–
 154, 181, 182, 189, 190; *anāhata-cakra*,
 155–156, 181, 190; higher, 287–8 n. 7;
 kāla-cakra, 4, 34, 279 n. 5; *kundalinī-shakti*
 and, 151, 156, 159, 160, 181–182, 190;
 manipūra (nābhi)-cakra, 156–157, 181, 190;
 mūlādhāra-cakra, 81–82, 158–159, 160,
 174–175, 181, 190, 228; nature of, 149–
 159, 180; *sahasrāra-cakra*, 150–152, 158,
 160, 181, 183; *svādhishthāna-cakra*, 156,
 157–158, 181, 190, 228; *vishuddha-cakra*,
 154–155, 181
Candī, 34
candra. See moon
caste system, 99, 247, 269
Caurangipa, 262
cause and effect: law of, 22
celibacy, 102, 103
cemeteries, 9–10, 81, 101–102, 103, 178,
 218, 284 n. 7
central channel. *See sushumnā-nādī*
Chāndogya-Upanishad, 16–17, 45, 49, 173–
 174, 278 n. 5
change, 31, 32, 44, 115, 166, 180
channels. *See nādīs*
chanting, 234, 245

Chapple, Christopher, 294 n. 3
chastity, 124, 125, 237–238
Chetanananda, Swami, 192
Chinnamastā, 3
cid. *See* Consciousness
cid-ānanda, 183, 256
Cidghanānanda Nātha, 145
cit-kundalinī, 182
cit-shakti, 77
cittars, 146–147, 263, 287 n. 3
citta-vaittiyam, 146–147
Civavākkiyar, 263
clairvoyance, 25, 149, 150, 153
compassion, 125, 156, 272
confusion, 143, 144, 231
consciousness, 62, 163, 192–193. *See also* awareness
Consciousness, 22, 175, 182, 185–186, 187–188, 208, 240–242, 270; Consciousness-Bliss, 183, 256; Shiva as principle of, 62, 63, 68–69, 77–78, 81, 82, 188. *See also* Being-Consciousness; Being-Consciousness-Bliss
cosmic egg. *See* brahmic egg
cosmology, 25–29, 60–62, 175–176
creation, 66–67, 142, 157, 187, 219, 257
creativity, 78, 208, 228–229
Creator, 27–28, 62, 64
Criswell, Eleanor, 143–144
currents. *See* *nādīs*; *srotas*

daiva, 21–22
dakshina, 129
dakshina-mārga, 134, 135
Dalai Lama, His Holiness the, 90, 283 n. 3
Damara-Tantra, 265, 266
Dattātreya, 8–9
deafness, 216–217
death, 31, 35, 38, 44, 55, 115, 178, 217, 233, 257, 260, 266
deha, 141. *See also* body
deities, 70–74, 97, 104–106, 186–187, 193, 206–208, 215, 217–220, 222, 240, 246; worshiping, 70, 128–129, 130–131, 144, 179, 202, 205–206. *See also specific deities*
delusion, 79, 118, 125, 158, 223, 227, 254–255, 260, 271
desire, 56, 125, 141, 156, 196, 223, 224–249, 265. *See also kāma*
devatās. *See* deities
deva-vānī, 186–187
Devī, 72, 129, 246, 276 n. 3

Devī-Māhātmya, 34
devotion, 72, 93, 121–122, 123–124, 234
dhāranā, 124, 126
dharma, 6, 7, 47
dharma-shāstras, 47
dhauti, 170
dhvani, 187
dhyāna. *See* meditation; visualization
Dhyāna-Bindu-Upanishad, 155–156
diet, 125, 145
dīkshā. *See* initiation
discernment, 125, 151–152, 256
discipleship, 91, 93, 110–119, 121–124, 130–131, 132; initiation/transmission and, 85–89, 95–109, 117, 121, 123, 231, 272; process of, 112–119, 121–122, 127–138, 286 n. 13; purification and, 89, 103, 106–107, 115–117, 122, 127, 130; qualifications for, 89, 90, 98–99, 100, 110–112, 114, 118–119, 121–122, 123–124, 283 n. 3. *See also gurus*; Westerners
disease, 115, 144, 145, 183, 200. *See also* therapy
dispassion, 116–117, 156, 256
Divine, 28–30, 43–46, 56–57, 72–73, 126–127, 131, 201–202, 259; body and, 50, 53, 180, 181, 185, 224–226, 236; *gurus* and, 85–91, 94, 283 n. 3; liberation and, 28–30, 56–57, 259. *See also* One, the; Parama-Shiva; Reality; Self; Shiva and Shakti and
divine body, 180, 181, 206, 260, 263
divine speech, 188–190
divya-deha. *See* divine body
doubt, 143, 144
dreams, 103–104, 188
drugs, 33, 247
duality, 126–127, 143, 185, 270
duhkha, 22–24, 30, 114, 226, 250. *See also* pain; suffering
dūra-darshana. *See* clairvoyance
Durgā, 40, 72, 130, 209
dvandvas, 82, 124
dynamism, 76, 77, 82, 87, 164, 187, 239, 252. *See also rajas*

earth element. *See* elements
ecstasy, 58–59, 107, 122–123, 125, 126, 234, 245, 248, 253–255, 257–258, 279 n. 9. *See also* bliss; *samādhi*
ego-personality, 22, 38, 63, 64, 77, 89, 93–94, 115, 116, 158, 183, 223, 231, 237, 270
eight limbs, 124–125, 127–130

eka, 51, 115. *See also* One, the
elementals, 140
elements, 63, 66, 104, 105, 127, 130, 137,
    154, 157, 158–159, 171, 172, 175, 178–
    181, 197, 208, 216–217, 264–265
Eliade, Mircea, 101, 134, 218
emotions, 141–142, 158, 226, 227, 234, 238,
    245–246. *See also specific emotions*
enemies, 113–114, 264, 266
energy, 59, 144–145, 184–190, 238, 239,
    245. *See also kundalinī-shakti*; *prāna*; *shakti*;
    Shakti, as Energy principle; *tapas*
enlightenment. *See* liberation
envy, 125, 158
ether element. *See* elements
evil, 133, 159, 266
evolution, 59, 62, 78, 175–176

faith, 91, 93, 121, 141
fasting, 103, 130, 145
fear, 60, 101, 114–115, 118, 217, 223
fire element. *See* elements
fire sacrifice, 129, 130–131
fish, 118–119, 210, 213, 239, 241
five *m*'s (five "substances"), 118–119, 134,
    207, 231, 232, 239–241, 248–249
freedom, 158, 232, 251, 259
Freud, Sigmund, 228

gandharvas, 33, 34, 131, 279 n. 4
Ganesha, 72, 195, 209, 219, 276 n. 3,
    291 n. 1
Ganges, 101, 102, 130
Gautamīya-Tantra, 157
gāyatrī-mantra, 195
genitals, 26, 230, 236, 245–246, 247. *See also
    linga*; *yoni*
Gheranda-Samhitā, 170–171, 178, 291 n. 2
Goddess, the. *See* Shakti (goddess)
gods/goddesses. *See* deities
Goraksha Nātha, 137, 262, 264
Goraksha-Paddhati, 176
Govinda, Lama Anagarika, 44, 133
grace, 87–88, 93, 107, 108, 117, 122, 189.
    See also transmission
grain, 118–119, 207, 239–240
granthi, 182–183
Great Integral Yoga, 270
greed, 79, 125, 158
greedlessness, 124, 125
Guenther, Herbert V., x
gunas, 87, 175, 257. *See also rajas*; *sattva*; *tamas*

guru-bhakti, 121–122
Guru-Gītā, 87
guru-pūjā, 129
gurus, 85–91; approaching, 95–100, 129, 201;
    choosing, 91–93, 95–97; defined, 4,
    86–87; devotion to, 72, 121–122, 123–
    124; as divine agency, 85–89, 90–91, 94,
    283 n. 3; failed, 88, 271–272; as function,
    90, 91, 93–94, 116; grace of, 87–88, 93,
    107, 117; importance of, xv, 86, 88, 99,
    100–101, 108–109, 123–124; initiation/
    transmission and, 85–89, 95–109, 117,
    121, 123, 231, 271, 272; liberation and,
    87–88, 96–97, 106; lineage and, 97–98;
    maithunā and, 241, 242, 248; monitoring,
    272; *nyāsas* and, 206–207; obedience to,
    111; responsibility of, 98, 111–112, 272;
    sad-gurus, 91–93, 283 n. 4; Shiva and Shakti
    and, 85, 108, 109. *See also* discipleship;
    mahā-siddhas; *siddhas*; Westerners
guru-yoga, 90–94

habits, 116, 166, 254
hamsa, 154, 197
happiness, 43–44, 57, 76, 124, 143, 172,
    222, 242
harmonization, 145, 150, 156, 164, 172–173
Hatha Yoga, xv, 137, 144, 145, 163, 170, 173,
    175, 178, 183, 194, 207, 233–234, 236,
    239, 260, 262, 263–264, 273
Hatha-Yoga-Pradīpikā, 165, 169, 173, 177, 179,
    233–234, 291 n. 2
hatred, 239
Hayes, Glen, 237
healing. *See* medicine; therapy
health, 144–147, 163, 172, 263
Heard, Gerald, 59
hearing, 65, 154, 216–217
heart, 75, 127, 155–156, 170, 181, 190, 216
hells, 27, 232
Hemalekhā and Hemacūda, 253–255
heroes, 119, 285 n. 7
higher mind. *See buddhi*
Hindu Tantra. *See* Tantra (Hindu)
Hiranyakashipu, King, 57
history. *See* Tantra: history of
holograms, 61, 80, 180
homa, 129, 131
horizontalism, 46–47, 48
householders, 47
hridaya. *See* heart

hrit-padma, 155–156
humor, 60

icchā, 62, 76, 77
idā-nādī, 125, 130, 153–154, 162–163, 164,
    166, 171, 172, 174
ignorance. *See avidyā*
illusion. *See māyā*
imagination, 25, 29, 57, 141
imitatio Dei, 201–202
immortality, 28, 60, 160, 163, 171, 210, 232,
    237, 238, 263
impermanence, 31, 44
indriyas. See senses
Indus civilization, 11–13, 277 n. 9
inertia. *See tamas*
initiation, 85–89, 93, 95–109, 117, 123, 132,
    190–192, 206–207, 231, 271–272,
    284 n. 14
inner sacrifice, 50–51, 124
inner sound. *See dhvani; nāda*
integralism, 46, 47–48, 49–51, 229–230
interconnectedness, 143, 206, 270
ishta-devatā, 144, 202
īshvara, 62, 63
Īshvara Krishna, 67–68
Itaikkātar, 263
Iyengar, B. K. S., 172

Jainism: Tantra and, xi, 208
Jālandhara, 129, 262
jālandhara-bandha, 177
japa, 197–200, 207
Jayākhya-Samhitā, 208
Jayaratha, 178, 218
jealousy. *See* envy
jīva. See ego-personality
jīvan-mukti, 258, 261
jnāna, 76, 109, 217, 223. *See also* wisdom
joy, 60, 76–77, 222, 226–227, 234, 254–255
Jung, Carl Gustav, 82–83, 90, 218, 266–267,
    282–283 n. 2

Kailāsa, Mount, 73, 183
kaivalya, 73, 256, 257, 282 n. 1
Kak, Subhash, 198
kalā, 63, 64, 137, 219
kāla, 31, 33–34, 63, 64, 279 n. 2. *See also* time
Kālī, 5, 32, 35–41, 80–81, 186
Kālikā-Purāna, 129
kali-yuga, x, xvi, 4–5, 6–8, 13–14, 21, 26,
    118, 119, 132, 277 n. 7

kalpas, 28
kāma, 47, 158, 224, 230, 251, 265. *See also*
    desire
Kāmākhyā-Tantra, 247
Kāmarūpa, 129
Kāma-Sūtra, 61, 237, 242
kancukas, 63, 64, 142
kanda, 162, 176
Kanhapa, 262
Kankāla-Mālinī-Tantra, 87, 128
Kānphata order, 175, 207, 264
Kapālapa/Kāpālikas, 102, 262–263
karma, 60, 88, 108, 144, 145, 166, 218, 265,
    266, 272; body and, 53, 54, 55, 142, 144;
    kundalinī and, 178, 179, 183; liberation and,
    30, 46, 259, 260; *samsāra* and, 21–22, 24,
    51, 79
Kashmiri Shaivism, 77, 78–79, 103, 108, 131,
    177, 180, 183, 223, 251–252, 263, 281–
    2 n. 10, 284 n. 14
Kaula-Avalī-Nirnaya, 99, 118, 119, 132, 247,
    287 n. 16
Kaula-Jnāna-Nirnaya, 97–98, 111–112, 139,
    232, 237, 287 n. 16
Kaula path, 101–103, 119, 130, 135–138,
    221, 226–228, 286 n. 14, 287 n.16; history
    of, 97–98, 135–136, 287 n. 15; sexuality
    and, 16–17, 227–228, 230–231, 233,
    239–249, 252–253
kavacas, 130
Kaviraj, Gopinath, 270
kāya-sādhana, 263
Khajuraho: temple at, 136–137
Kirana-Tantra, 130
knowledge, 1–2, 43, 48, 62, 64, 76, 122, 223
koshas, 28–29, 140–144
Krama tradition, 136
Krishna (Dark Lord), 6, 34, 186, 195, 234–
    236, 238, 249
Krishna, Gopi, 166–168, 185–186
Krishnadāsa, 238
kriyā, 76, 77, 223
krodha. See anger
Kshemarāja, 94, 191, 208
Kubjikā, 72, 136. *See also kundalinī-shakti*
kula, 14, 111, 137–138, 231, 242, 249
kula-āgama, 97–98
kula-akula-cakra, 104–105, 130
Kula-Arnava-Tantra, 14, 24, 50, 53–55, 92–93,
    96–97, 98–99, 100, 107, 108, 112–113,
    117, 118, 123–124, 126, 127–128, 135,
    138, 181, 192–193, 194–195, 197, 199,

202–203, 205–206, 217, 226–227, 230,
   231–232, 240–241, 242, 245, 248, 249,
   250, 257–259, 286 n. 7, 287 n. 16
kula-kundalinī, 183
Kula path. *See* Kaula path
kumbhaka, 177, 183
kunamnamā, 15
kundalinī-shakti, 15, 165–183; ascent of, 181–
   183, 255; blockages of, 164, 166–169,
   182–183; *cakras* and, 151, 156, 159, 160,
   181–182, 190; dangers of, 156, 166–169,
   178; initiation and, 107, 108; Kālī and, 38;
   Kaula path and, 136; liberation and, 169,
   176, 178, 183, 190; *mantras* and, 190–192;
   nādīs and, 162, 164, 166, 186; nature of,
   173–186; nectar and, 171, 178, 183, 240–
   241; *prāna* and, 169, 173, 174–175, 176,
   177, 185; Sanskrit alphabet and, 38, 186,
   190; sexuality and, 228–229, 245; Shakti
   and, 173, 175, 179–180, 182, 183, 185,
   190; types of, 175, 182, 183, 190

Lakshmanjoo, Swami, xii, xiii
Lakshmī, 72, 196, 209
Lallā, 177, 223
latā-sādhanā, 130
law. *See* dharma; *dharma-shāstras*
laya-yoga, 178–179, 181, 183, 294 n. 3
left-hand path, 9, 81, 101–102, 103–104,
   130, 132, 134–135, 228; sexuality and, 9,
   16–17, 81, 228, 230–231, 233, 239–249,
   252–253
levitation, 264
liberated beings, 47–48, 258–259, 261–265.
   See also siddhas
liberation: as aloneness, 73, 256, 257,
   282 n. 1; *bodhisattvas* and, 269–270; body
   and, 53–57, 60, 142, 185, 226–227; *cakras*
   and, 150–151, 159; collective, 270; death
   and, 257; defined, 29–30, 55, 115, 223,
   256–259; of deities, 70–71; desire and, 56,
   114, 116, 117, 229; Divine and, 28–29, 30,
   56–57, 259; grace and, 93; *gunas* and, 87;
   gurus and, 87–88, 96–97, 106; initiation
   and, 89, 95, 100, 109; *karma* and, 30, 46,
   259, 260; *kundalinī-shakti* and, 169, 176,
   178, 183, 190; literature of, 48–49, 74;
   mantras and, 193, 196; materialism and, 48;
   mind and, 115–116, 227, 257; paradox of,
   258, 259; purification and, 89; *sahaja-
   samādhi* and, 253–255, 258; Self and, 29, 30,
   55, 94, 223, 255–256; sexuality and, 242,

246; verticalism and, 48–49, 256, 257;
   wisdom and, 10, 22, 29–30, 122; *yantras*
   and, 218, 219; yogic practice and, 122–123
life, 47–48, 52, 57, 216
life force. *See prāna*
Light, 76, 183, 256
līlā, 234
lineage, 97–98, 134, 286 n. 13
linga, 81–82, 133, 139, 158, 175, 236, 247
lobha. See greed
lokas, 27, 28, 99, 278 n. 6
longevity, 145, 163
Lopāmudrā, 147
love, 93, 121–122, 127, 229–249. *See also*
   bhakti
lucidity. *See sattva*
Luīpa, 261
lunar channel. *See idā-nādī*
lust. *See kāma*

Macchanda, 138, 287 n. 15
macrocosm. *See* microcosm
mada. See pride
madya, 239. *See also* wine
magic, 4, 9–10, 15, 60, 122, 130, 134, 194,
   207, 261, 265–266, 286 n. 3
Mahābhārata, 5, 19, 23–24, 48, 61, 86,
   278 n. 4
Mahācīna-Ācāra-Krama-Tantra, 247
Mahākāla, 35, 39
Mahānirvāna-Tantra, xi, 5, 6–7, 13–14, 32, 35,
   38, 39, 73–74, 94, 99–100, 105–106, 116,
   119, 122, 126, 128, 132, 137, 191, 196,
   198, 203, 241, 242, 247
mahā-siddhas, 2, 24, 45, 140, 261–263. *See also*
   liberated beings
mahā-siddhis, 264–265. *See also* siddhis
mahā-sukha, xiv, 60, 222
Mahāyāna Buddhism, 10, 97, 269
Mahimnā-Stava, 131
maithunā, 9, 16–17, 230–231, 232, 234, 239,
   241–249
Maitrāyanī-Upanishad, 32, 52–53
Maitreya, 97
mālās, 198
māmsa, 239, 241
manas, 63, 65, 141, 153, 181, 284 n. 14
Mānava-Dharma-Shāstra, 47
mandalas, 105, 128, 131, 140, 218, 266,
   285 n. 3
Māndūkya-Upanishad, 188
Manjushrī-Mūla-Kalpa, 208

Mantra-Mahodadhi, 219

mantras, 13, 15, 16, 19, 122, 127–128, 184–200, 258, 261; *bīja-* (*see bījas*); breath control and, 125, 170–171; deities and, 70, 104–105, 106, 193, 206–207; ear to impart, 105–106; examples of, 195–196; *gurus* and, 86, 93, 96, 103, 104–105; importance of, 128, 181, 285 n. 3; initiation and, 86, 93, 102, 103, 104–105, 107, 191, 206–207; liberation and, 193, 194, 196; *maithunā* and, 245, 247, 248; mantric consciousness, 192; meditation and, 200; *mudrās* and, 207; nature of, 187–188, 190–197, 222–223; *nyāsas* and, 197, 202–207; purification and, 127, 202, 240; reciting, 194–195, 197–200; secrecy of, 105, 195; Shakti and, 187–188, 190, 193; for Shiva, 77, 105; sound and energy and, 184–190; as spiritual discipline, 114, 125, 131; uses for, 13, 130, 193–194

Mantra-Shiro-Bhairava, 117

Mantra-Yoga-Samhitā, 86, 101, 103, 104, 114, 187, 193–194, 195, 196–197, 198, 199, 203–207, 209

Manu, 47–48

marmans, 182–183

Marpa, 100, 113, 122, 262

materialism, 48, 75

Mātrikās, 219

mātsarya. See envy

matsya, 210, 213, 239, 241

Matsyendra Nātha, 97–98, 137, 138, 261, 262, 264, 287 n. 7

Matsyendra-Samhitā, 1

matter: as energy, 184–190

māyā, 22, 30, 62–64, 66–67, 68, 83, 108, 109, 142, 226, 260

meat, 9, 118–119, 231, 232, 239, 240, 241

medicine, Tantric, 144–147, 263. See also therapy

meditation, 29, 101, 105, 127, 144, 149, 200, 207, 217, 245, 258; defined, 125, 126; importance of, 181, 223, 285 n. 3. See also visualization

memory, 22, 217

menstrual blood, 233, 241, 247, 292 n. 11

Meru, Mount, 27, 61, 151, 198, 279 n. 5

microcosm, macrocosm and, 60–69, 78, 84, 163, 178, 179, 186, 206, 222

Milarepa, 100, 113, 122, 262

mind: advanced practice and, 75; artificially created, 265; enlightened, 258–259; healing and, 144, 145, 146–147; higher (*see buddhi*); initiation by thought, 284 n. 14; liberation and, 115–116, 117, 227, 257; lower (*see manas*); mind-body split, 60, 143, 185; purification of, 144, 145, 217, 223; semen and, 234; Shakti and, 186; sheaths composed of, 141, 142; suffering and, 227, 251; as timeless, 60; Westerners and, 87, 123. See also avidyā; body

modesty, 125

moha. See delusion

moksha-mārga. See sushumnā-nādī

moksha-shāstras, 48, 256

moon, 163, 171, 187, 198, 219, 240–241, 248

moral restraints, 124, 125

Mother Goddess, 72, 276 n. 3

Motoyama, Hiroshi, 149

mudrā (parched grain), 207, 239

Mudrā-Avadhi, 208

mudrās, 207–217, 222–223; *anjali-mudrā*, 209; *āvāhani-mudrā*, 209–210; defined, 128, 207–215, 239–240; deities and, 207–208; *dhenu-mudrā*, 127, 210, 212; *dhyāna-mudrā*, 217; *jnāna-mudrā* (*cin-mudrā*), 217; *kūrma-mudrā*, 213, 214; *mahā-mudrā*, 291 n. 2; *maithunā* and, 245; *matsya-mudrā*, 210, 213; *padma-mudrā*, 213, 214; *prāna-mudrā*, 216; purification and, 127, 202; *samnidhāpanī-mudrā*, 210, 211; *samnirodhanī-mudrā*, 210, 212; *shūnya-mudrā*, 216–217; *sthāpana-karmanī-mudrā*, 210, 211; *sūrya-mudrā*, 217; therapeutic uses for, 215–217, 291 nn. 6, 7; *vajrolī-mudrā*, 233–234, 248, 291 n. 2; *viparīta-karanī-mudrā*, 293; whole-body, 215; *yoni-mudrā*, 194, 213, 215

Muktananda, Swami, 89, 93

mumukshutva, 114

Mundaka-Upanishad, 28

Murphy, Michael, 59

music, 131, 279 n. 4

Muyalaka, 39–40

mystical experiences, 152, 156

nāda, 156, 173, 182, 184, 187–188, 191

Nāda-Bindu-Upanishad, 184

nādīs, 16, 126, 148, 160–164, 166–173, 176, 186. See also idā-nādī; pingalā-nādī; sushumnā-nādī

Nāgārjuna, 262

nāgas, 34, 279 n. 6

narakas, 27

Nārāyana. *See* Vishnu
Nārāyanīya-Tantra, 14
narcissism, 270
Naropa, 100, 262
Natarāja, 39, 40
nāthas, 106, 263–264
nature, 63, 64, 68, 83, 87, 175, 179, 181, 226, 256, 257. *See also* gunas; *samsāra*
necromancy, 9–10
nectar, 163, 171, 178, 183, 203, 210, 219, 232, 240–241, 252
Neo-Tantrism, xiii–xiv, xv, 80, 85–86, 98, 237, 270–271
nervous system, 148–149, 162–163, 186
Netra-Tantra, 294 n. 5
New Age, 6, 48
Nigamas, 72, 276 n. 3
nihsanga. See nonattachment
nirdvandva, 82–83
Nirriti, 15
nirvāna: samsāra and, 2, 42–51, 222, 255
nirvikalpa-samādhi, 107, 258
Nityananda, Bhagavan, 93
Nityās, 219
nivritti-mārga, 46, 163
niyamas, 124
niyati, 63, 64
nonattachment, 117, 229, 230
nonbeing, 66–67
nondualism, 51, 60, 62, 66–68, 126. *See also* Vedānta
numbers, 137, 198
nyāsas, 128, 130, 197, 202–207, 222–223

Oddiyāna, 129
O'Flaherty, Wendy Doniger, 229–230
ojas, 237–238
om, 150, 156, 177, 188, 191, 195, 200, 203, 290 n. 4. *See also nāda*
om-kāra, 187, 288 n. 7
omnipotence, 77, 259
omnipresence, 143, 158
omniscience, 77, 143, 259
One, the, 51, 60, 62, 66–68, 115. *See also* Divine; Whole, the
ontology, 62–69, 83–84
orgasm, xiv, 233–234, 237, 252–253

padma, 213, 214, 217. *See also cakras*
pādukās, 129
pain, 58–60, 114–115, 166–168, 183, 250–251. *See also* suffering

Pāmpātti, 263
panca-anga-upāsana, 128
panca-ma-kāras. See five m's
Panca-Stavi, 131
panca-tattva. See five m's
para-bindu, 181
paradox, 28, 258, 259
parā-kundalinī, 190
Parama-Ānanda-Tantra, 276 n. 3
Parama-Shiva, 62, 63, 68, 72, 74–77, 97, 206, 281 n. 7
paramparā. See lineage
paranormal powers, 4, 9–10, 25, 83, 130, 134, 152–153, 157, 165, 237, 259–266, 286 n. 3. *See also* clairvoyance; magic; *siddhis*
parā-samvid, 75
para-sharīra, 142
Parashu-Rāma, 209
Parā-Trīshikhā-Laghu-Vritti, 100
Parā-Trīshikhā-Vivarana, 95
paridhāna, 177, 289 n. 14
Pārvatī, 72, 73, 230
Pashupatas, 175
pashus, 96, 108, 118–119, 242, 283 n. 1
pātāla, 27, 278 n. 8
Patanjali, 44, 124–125, 127, 146, 238, 256, 257, 269, 280 n. 12, 282 n. 1. *See also Yoga-Sūtra*
pathless path, 122–123
patience, 125, 144
Pattinattār, 263
peace, 164, 197, 200, 229, 266
Pearce, Joseph Chilton, 29
perception, 165–166, 227
pilgrimage, 129–130, 246
pinda, 142–143, 175, 183
pingalā-nādī, 125, 130, 133, 153–154, 162–163, 164, 166, 171, 172, 174
pīthas, 129, 134, 205, 286 n. 13
placement. *See nyāsa*
pleasure, xiv, 48, 56, 80, 183, 222, 226–227, 230, 250–256
poetry, 234, 238, 263
polarity, 80, 82, 126–127, 173, 230, 234
polytheism. *See* deities
postures. *See āsanas*
Power. *See shakti*; Shakti
powers: of Reality, 76. *See also* paranormal powers
Prahlāda, 56–57
prajnā. See wisdom
prakāsha, 76, 181

prakriti. See nature
prakriti-laya, 83
pralaya, 142
prāna, 141, 142, 144–145, 146, 148–149, 169, 172–177, 180, 185–186, 228, 237, 253
prāna-danda-prayoga, 178
prāna-kundalinī, 175
prāna-pratishthā, 222
Prāna-Toshanī, 135, 241
prānāyāma. See breath control
Pratyabhijnā-Hridaya, 42
Pratyabhijnā school, 62–66, 68, 281–2 n. 10
pratyāhāra, 124, 125
pravritti-mārga, 46
prāyashcitta, 131
prayer, 70, 114
pride, 125, 158
protection, 133, 140, 197, 218, 266
pūjā, 13, 15–16, 50, 128–129, 130, 131, 207. *See also cakra-pūjā*; ritual; *yoni-pūjā*
punishment, 113
Purānas, 7, 8–9, 26–29, 48, 61, 229–230, 246, 276 n. 5, 278 n. 4
purashcarana, 127–128, 192–193
purification, 115–117, 126, 127, 144–145, 164, 166–173, 176–180, 202–203, 223, 240, 245. *See also* discipleship, purification and
purity, 116–117, 124, 154–155, 227
pūrna. See Whole, the
pūrna-mārga, 46
Pūrnānanda, 85, 157
purusha, 63, 64, 68, 221, 226, 256, 257
purusha-artha, 47, 193
puryashtaka, 141, 142
Pushpadanta, 131

Rabe, Michael, 136–137
Rādhā, 234–236
Radha, Swami Sivananda, 157–158, 200
rāga. See attachment
Rāghava, 125
rajas: as energy, 87, 118, 119, 133, 141, 164, 175, 187, 239, 252. *See also* dynamism; menstrual blood
Rāja Yoga, 233, 264
Rajneesh, Bhagwan Shree (Osho), 243
Raktabīja, 40
Rāma, 103, 209
Rama, Swami, 150, 265
Ramakrishna, Sri, 35, 37, 38, 107, 236

Rāmalinga, 263
Rāmāyana, 278 n. 4
Rang Avadhoot, 9
rasa, 232–239, 248, 292 n. 11; as taste, 65, 75, 157–158, 181
rasa-cakra, 241, 242
Ratna-Sāra, 45
Reality: body and, 53, 141, 226; deities and, 72; liberation and, 30, 56–57; nature of, 28, 34, 43, 45, 46, 50, 62, 66–69, 75, 77, 109, 115, 223, 257, 279 n. 5. *See also* brahman; Divine; Parama-Shiva; Self
reincarnation, 55
relativity, 42–43
Rele, Vasant G., 148
renunciation, 24, 47, 56, 102, 163, 178, 234
retas, 232, 233, 237
retirement, 48
reversal, 8–9, 234, 237
right-hand path, 134, 135
Rig-Veda, 6, 11, 15, 67, 147, 148, 155, 188–189, 191, 230, 276–277 n. 5, 279 n. 2
rishis, 19, 147, 191, 203, 205
rita, 279 n. 2
ritual, 13, 15–16, 50, 100–108, 120–134, 140, 179–181, 223, 261, 284 n. 14, 285 n. 3. *See also* deities, worshiping; five *m*'s; *mai-thunā*; *mantras*; *mudrās*; *nyāsas*; *yantras*
rosaries, 198–199
Rudra, 15, 276 n. 3
rudra-aksha, 198
Rudra-Yāmala, 158, 169, 242

sabīja, 170–171
sac-cid-ānanda. See Being-Consciousness-Bliss
sacrifice, 15, 16, 50–51, 115, 121, 124, 129, 131, 241
sadākhyā, 62, 63
Sadā-Shiva, 62, 63
sad-gurus, 91–93, 283 n. 4
sādhakas/sādhikas, 2, 131
sādhanā. See spiritual discipline
Sādhanā-Mālā, 124
Sādhu-Samkalinī-Tantra, 130
sad-vidyā, 62, 63
sahaja, 10, 45–46, 234, 251
sahaja-samādhi, 253–255, 258
Sahajiyā tradition, 45, 234–239
sakala-kriti, 215
sakalī-karana, 206
samādhi, 35, 107, 125, 126, 253–255, 257–258, 279 n. 9. *See also* ecstasy

samāna, 174, 255
samanu, 170–171
samarasa, 133
Sāma-Veda, 11, 191
samaya, 130, 221
sambhoga, 234
Samhitās, 6, 26, 278 n. 4. See also specific Sam-
    hitās
samkalpa, 55
Sāmkhya school, 67–68
samsāra, 2, 20–41, 46–47, 75, 114, 141, 142,
    159, 229; nirvāna and, 2, 42–51, 222, 255.
    See also change; nature
sandhyā, 257, 258, 293 n. 1
sandhyā-bhāshā, 133–134
sanga. See attachment
Sannella, Lee, 168–169
Sanskrit alphabet, 38, 104, 107, 186–187,
    190, 191, 194, 198, 203–205, 218
Saraha, 45, 262
Sarasvatī, 129–130, 186, 209
sat, 62
Sat-Karma-Samgraha, 145
sat-kārya-vāda, 67
sattva, 87, 118, 119, 141, 164, 175, 187, 252
satya-loka, 27, 28
Saundarya-Laharī, 131, 219
Savitri, 32, 195, 279 n. 1
seals. See mudrās
seats, 129, 134, 286 n. 13
secrecy, 74, 105, 132–134, 195, 271, 272
seed syllables. See bījas
seers. See rishis
Self, 49, 53–56, 64, 68, 96, 115, 141–142,
    193, 229, 253–256; liberation and, 29, 30,
    55, 94, 223, 255–256. See also Divine; Re-
    ality
self-awareness, 76
self-purification. See purification
Self-realization. See liberation
self-restraint, 124, 125
self-sacrifice, 115
semen, 232, 233–234, 237, 248
senses, 63, 65, 75, 157–158, 178–179, 180,
    222–223, 226–227, 245, 251, 257
sensory inhibition, 124, 125
separation. See duality
serpent power. See kundalinī-shakti
sexuality: bliss and, 252–253; cakra-pūjā, 241,
    242, 248, 269; cakras and, 156, 157–158;
    ecstasy and, 234, 245, 248; five m's and (see
    five m's); hostility toward Tantric, 230–231,

242–243; Krishna and Rādhā and, 234–
    236; left-hand path and, 9, 16, 228; mai-
    thunā (see maithunā); menstrual blood and,
    233, 241, 247, 292 n. 11; Neo-Tantrism
    and, xiii–xiv, 237, 271; orgasm and, xiv,
    233–234, 237, 252–253; rajas and, 233,
    241; rasa and, 232–239, 248, 292 n. 11; Sa-
    hajiyā and, 234–239; scriptures and, 16–
    17, 147; self-indulgence and, 231–232;
    sublimation and, 228–229; Tantra and,
    226, 227, 229–249, 252–253; universe
    and, 233, 234; yoni-pūjā, 245–248. See also
    genitals; Kāma-Sūtra; Shakti, sexuality and;
    Shiva, sexuality and
shabda, 65, 181, 187
shabda-brahman, 187
Shaiva-Āgamas, 276 n. 3
Shākta-Āgamas, 276 n. 3
shakti (power), 14, 68, 72, 76, 78, 136, 143,
    148, 261, 276 n. 3. See also energy; kun-
    dalinī-shakti
Shakti (goddess), 34, 108–109, 116, 121,
    137–138, 178, 180–190, 191, 193, 196,
    208, 219, 226–228, 240, 241–249; as En-
    ergy principle, 62, 63, 78–79, 81, 82, 173,
    175, 179–180, 182, 183, 185, 188; kun-
    dalinī-shakti and, 173, 175, 179–180, 182,
    183, 185, 190; Sanskrit alphabet and, 38,
    186, 190, 203; sexuality and, 80, 228, 232,
    233, 234, 241–242, 245. See also Kālī;
    Shiva, Shakti and
shakti-cālana, 177
shaktimat, 76, 261
shakti-pāta, 108, 123
Shakti-Sangama-Tantra, 240
Shaktism, 68–69
Shambhala, 270
shāmbhavī-dīkshā, 107, 284 n. 14
Shāndilya-Upanishad, 183
Shankara, 30, 49, 66, 68, 127, 131, 149–150,
    219
shānti. See peace
shape-shifting, 260
Shāradā-Tilaka-Tantra, 96, 107–108, 110–111,
    113, 125–126, 175, 187–188, 190, 194,
    208, 289 n. 10
sharīra, 141. See also body
shāstras, 47. See also specific shāstras
Shata-Patha-Brāhmanas, 16, 57
Shata-Ratna-Samgraha, 120
shat-cakra-bhedana, 182
Shat-Cakra-Nirūpana, 154, 156–157, 162

shat-karmas, 266
sheaths, 28–29, 140–144
Shenrab, Buddha Tenpa, 14, 277n. 11
shishyas, 110–111, 112–113. See also discipleship
Shiva: 27, 53–55, 116, 129, 131, 209, 218, 219, 229–230, 240, 264; 286n.14; as Consciousness principle, 62, 63, 68–69, 77–78, 81, 82, 188; gurus and, 85, 92, 108; initiation and, 86, 103, 105, 107, 108, 109; Kaula path and, 97–98, 135, 137–138; kundalinī-shakti and, 173, 175, 182, 183; mantra for, 77, 105, 195; sexuality and, 227, 229–230, 233, 234, 236, 241, 245; Shakti and, 28, 35, 38, 40–41, 50, 62, 63, 68–69, 78–84, 109, 151, 154, 173, 182, 183, 189, 206, 227, 230, 233, 234, 241, 245, 256–258, 267; Tantras and, 15, 68, 72–74, 276n. 3; yugas and, 6, 7, 9, 14. See also Kashmiri Shaivism; Mahākāla; Natarāja; Parama-Shiva; Sadā-Shiva
Shiva-Jnāna-Upanishad, 251–252
shiva-linga, 82
Shiva-Samhitā, 61, 88, 90, 121, 160, 172–173, 291n. 2
Shiva-Sūtra, 191, 208
Shiva-Sūtra-Vārttika, 87
Shiva-Sūtra-Vimarshinī, 94
Shiva-Svarodaya, 160
shmashāna. See cemeteries
shraddhā, 91, 93, 121
shravana. See hearing
Shrī, 219
shrī-cakra. See shrī-yantra
Shrī-Kanthīya-Samhitā, 191–192
Shrī-Tattva-Cintāmani, 85, 96, 99, 107, 192–193
Shrī-Vidyā, x, 131, 136, 206, 207, 213, 215, 219, 221, 253–255
shrī-yantra, 82, 213, 215, 219–221, 279n. 5
shruti, 48
shuddha-vidyā, 62
shuddha-vikalpa, 123
shuddhi, 116–117
Shukla-Yajur-Veda, 188
shūnya, 133, 216–217
Shvetaketu, 67
siddha-anganās, 2
Siddhānta tradition, 72, 135, 136, 286n. 14
siddhas, 2, 96, 112, 261–264. See also cittars; liberated beings; mahā-siddhas
Siddha-Siddhānta-Paddhati, 15, 142–143

siddhis, 4, 83, 112, 134, 206, 264–265. See also paranormal powers
sin, 8, 87, 99, 226, 227, 240
Singh, Jaideva, 78–79
Skanda, 97
skulls, 101–102
sleep, 188, 217
smriti, 48
Smritis, 6, 7
solar channel. See pingalā-nādī
solar plexus, 156–157, 181
Solar Yoga, 279n. 2. See also sun
soma, 17, 18, 232, 248
Somānanda, 108
Somatic Yoga, 143–144
sorrow. See duhkha
sound, 65, 150, 154, 181, 184–190. See also bījas; mantras; nāda
spanda, 75, 78, 188
Spanda-Kārikā, 52, 78–79
Spanda school, 180
sparsha, 65, 181, 284n. 14
speech, 65, 107, 154, 155, 174, 188–190, 284n. 14
spells, 130, 285n. 3
Spirit, 22, 148, 226. See also Self
spiritual competence, 89, 100, 110–111
spiritual discipline, 55–56, 87, 89, 93, 109, 112–119, 120–138, 282–283n. 2
spontaneity, 10, 45, 47, 120, 132, 234
srotas, 134, 286n. 13
stavas, 131
stress, 172, 217
study, 124
subjugation, 247, 265–266
sublimation, 228–229
subtle body, 28–29, 139–164, 166
subtle elements, 63, 65
subtle realms, 139–140
subtle sounds. See dhvani; nāda; om; vāc
suffering, 22–24, 30, 31, 44, 58–60, 183, 226, 251–252, 254. See also pain
sukha. See pleasure
sūkshma-prakriti, 181
sūkshma-sharīra. See subtle body
sun, 163, 171, 198, 217, 279nn. 2, 5
sūrya, 133, 217, 279nn. 2, 5
Sūrya, 16
sushumnā-nādī, 125, 129, 133, 149, 153–154, 160–162, 163–164, 166, 174, 176, 178, 186, 198
Sūtras, 48. See also Yoga-Sūtra

Svātmarāma, 169, 179
Svāyambhūva-Sūtra-Samgraha, 109

Taittirīya-Upanishad, 110, 141
tamas, 87, 118, 119, 141, 164, 175, 187, 252
Tamils, 146–147, 263, 287 n. 3
tanmātras, 63, 65, 181, 264
Tantra (Hindu): antinomianism of, x, 7–10;
    body and, 50, 52–69, 144, 224–229; Brāh-
    manas and, 11, 15–16, 19, 26; Buddhist
    Tantra vs., xi–xii, xiv, 10; cosmology of,
    25–29, 60–62, 175–176; cyclic existence
    and, 2, 20–31, 32–51; dangers of, xv–xvi,
    74, 98–99, 132–133, 156, 166–169, 178,
    200, 271; defined, 1–3, 18–19, 51, 55–56;
    egalitarianism of, 99, 247, 269, 273; future
    of, 273; goal of, 29–31; heroic nature of,
    119, 285 n. 7; history of, ix–x, 2, 10–18,
    34, 224, 268–269; integralism and, 49–51;
    interconnectedness and, 143, 206, 270;
    Jainism and, xi; kali-yuga and, x, xvi, 4–5,
    6–8, 13–14, 118; lack of research on, xii–
    xiii; liberation concept in, 256–259; micro-
    cosm and macrocosm and, 60–69, 78, 84,
    163, 178, 179, 206, 222, 287; misconcep-
    tions about, ix–xii, xiii–xiv, xv–xvi, 10, 80;
    nondualism and, 51, 60, 62, 66–68, 126;
    ontology of, 62–69, 83–84; optimism of,
    7, 74; path of, 120–138, 286 n. 13; plea-
    sure and pain and, 250–256; practical na-
    ture of, 14, 19, 46; Purānas and, 7, 8–9,
    26–29; radical nature of, x, 7–10, 16;
    right-hand path, 134, 135; secrecy and, 74,
    105, 132–134, 271, 272; sexuality and (see
    sexuality); significance of, x–xi; Trika
    school, 142; Upanishads and, 16–17, 19;
    Vedānta and, x, 66, 68; Vedas and, 5, 7,
    10–19; verticalism and (see verticalism). See
    also Buddhist Tantra; initiation; Kashmiri
    Shaivism; Kaula path; kundalinī-shakti; left-
    hand path; magic; mantras; meditation;
    Neo-Tantrism; ritual; Shakti; Shiva; Shrī-
    Vidyā; visualization
Tantra-Āloka, 77–78, 138, 175, 178, 218, 255–
    256, 287 n. 15
Tantra-Rāja-Tantra, 208, 278 n. 6, 279 n. 5
Tantras, xi, 2, 13, 18, 24, 46, 48, 73, 74, 134,
    148, 271, 276 n. 3, 287 n. 16. See also specific
    Tantras
Tantra-Sadbhāva, 191
Tantra-Sāra, 70, 106–107
Tantra Yoga. See Tantra (Hindu)

tāntrikas, 2
tapas, 33, 58, 115, 230
Tārā, 209
Tattva-Vaishāradī, 121
tattvas, 62–69, 77–79, 179–180. See also ele-
    ments
teachers. See gurus
telepathy, 152–153
temperaments, 118–119
therapy, 144–147, 183, 215–218, 263,
    291 nn. 6, 7
Tilopa, 100, 262
time, 24, 31, 32–41, 64, 279 n. 5
Tiru-Mantiram, 263, 268
Tirumūlar, 225–226, 263
Tiru-Murai, 263
touch, 65, 107, 181, 284 n. 14
transcendence, 24, 29, 30, 80, 87, 158, 229,
    237, 257–258
transmission, 85, 87, 89, 98, 117, 121, 231,
    271, 272. See also grace
Trika-Sāra, 208
Trika school, 142
tri-mūrti, 8–9
Tri-Pura-Rahasya, 253–255
Tripurā Sundarī, 131, 209, 213, 215, 216, 220
Tri-Shikhi-Brāhmana-Upanishad, 160
Truth, 30, 43, 96–97, 256
truthfulness, 124, 125
turīya, 188
twilight language, 133–134
tyāga, 24

udāna, 174, 256
ullāsa, 248
Umā, 72
Umāpati Shivācārya, 120
understanding, 34, 43, 63, 64
underworld, 27, 278 n. 8
universe: as energy, 184–190; as erotic, 233,
    234
Upanishads, 16–17, 19, 26, 48, 49, 53, 126,
    148, 188, 256, 289 n. 11. See also specific
    Upanishads
upaprāna, 174
upāya, 282 n. 8
Utpalācārya, 281 n. 7
Utpaladeva, 108, 223

vāc, 65, 188–190
Vāc, 188–189
Vācaspati Mishra, 121

vaginal secretions, 232, 233, 234, 239, 248, 292 n. 11
vairāgya, 116, 256
Vaishnava Sahajiyā, 45, 234–239
vajra, 133, 162
Vajrasattva: *mantra* of, 128
Vajrayāna Buddhism. *See* Buddhist Tantra
Vāmakā-Īshvara-Tantra, 224
Vāmakā-Īshvarī-Mata-Tantra, 206, 246–247, 265
vāma-mārga. *See* left-hand path
Vasishtha, 57–58
vastu, 238
Vasubandhu, 97
Vatsyayana, 242
vāyu, 16, 66
Vedānta, x, 49, 51, 66, 68, 223, 260
Vedas, 5, 7, 10–19, 26, 48, 61, 96, 110–111, 140–141, 148, 186, 191, 196, 232. *See also specific Vedas*
vegetarianism, 9, 239
verticalism, 46, 47, 48–49, 50, 52–53, 83, 224–225, 226, 251, 256, 257, 260
vibration, 75, 180–181, 184–190. *See also mantras*
videha-mukti, 256, 257, 260
vidyā, 63, 64, 203. *See also* knowledge
Vijnāna-Bhairava, 251–252
Vijnāna Bhikshu, 264
Vimalananda, 22, 176–177
vimarsha, 76
Vimarshinī, 191, 208
vīnā-danda, 186
Vīnā-Shikha-Tantra, 86, 103, 104, 105, 128, 203
vīras, 119, 285 n. 7
virgins, 246
Virūpa, 261–262
vīrya, 237
Vishnu, 9, 16, 27, 34, 56–57, 72, 85, 87, 175, 195, 209, 219, 234, 246, 276 n. 3
Vishuddhananda, 270
Vishva-Sāra-Tantra, 61
vishva-uttīrna, 75
visualization, 15, 19, 70, 105, 114, 126, 127, 131, 144–145, 149–150, 180, 202, 245. *See also yantras*
viveka. *See* discernment
Viveka-Cūdāmani, 30, 49
Vivekananda, Swami, 107
vows, 130
vratas, 130

Vyāghrapāda, 280 n. 12
vyāna, 148, 174, 256

waking state, 188
water element. *See* elements
Westerners, 90–91, 111, 113, 114–115, 122–123, 270–272, 273, 282–283 n. 2. *See also* Neo-Tantrism
White, David Gordon, 163, 231, 232, 292 n. 10
White, Rhea A., 59
Whitehead, Alfred North, 22
Whole, the, 51, 74, 254–255
Wilber, Ken, 229
will, 62, 76, 77, 144, 264
wine, 118–119, 231, 232, 239, 240, 247, 248, 261
wisdom: action vs., 223; body of, 203; Buddhist Tantra and, 282 n. 8; knowledge vs., 1–2, 43, 48; liberation and, 10, 22, 29–30, 122; *mandalas* and, 218; passive principle and, 282 n. 8; Reality and, 109; *sandhyā-bhāshā* and, 133; seal of, 217; sheaths and, 141; Tantric, 14
Wisdom Goddesses, 246
witnessing, 60, 87
womb. *See* yoni
women, 2, 102–103, 136–137, 219, 226–227, 241–249, 265–266. *See also* menstrual blood; vaginal secretions
Woodroffe, Sir John, xi–xii, 174–175, 275 n. 5
world, 2, 60
world ages. *See* yugas

Yajur-Veda, 11, 191
Yama, 217
Yāmalas, 276 n. 3
yamas, 124
Yamī, 15
Yantra-Prakāsha, 219
Yantra-Pūjana-Prakāra, 219
Yantra-Uddhāra-Sarvasva, 219
yantras, 15, 96, 128, 131, 217–223. *See also shrī-yantra*
yātrā, 129–130
Yoga: defined, 18, 55–56, 121, 124–125, 127–130, 256; *kundalinī* and, 169; *marmans* and, 183; Tantra vs., 243; types of, xi, 18–19, 90–94, 143–144, 233, 264, 270, 279 n. 2. *See also* Hatha Yoga; *laya-yoga*
Yoga-Bhāshya, 116, 121, 264

Yoga-Bīja, 86
yoga-darshana, 256
Yoga-Shikhā-Upanishad, 86, 233, 260–261
Yoga-Sūtra, 44, 48, 117, 124–125, 146, 238,
    251, 269, 280 n. 12, 282 n. 1
Yoga-Tattva-Upanishad, 260
Yoga-Vārttika, 264
Yoga-Vāsishtha, 57–58
Yoga-Vishaya, 287–288 n. 7
Yoginīs, 136–137, 206, 215, 291 n. 1
yogins/yoginīs, 2, 9–10, 19, 59, 61, 114–115

yoni, 219, 244, 246, 247, 248
yoni-linga, 81–82
yoni-mudrā, 194, 213, 215
yoni-pūjā, 245–248
Yoni-Tantra, 245–246
yoni-tattva, 247–248, 292 n. 11
yugas, 4–7, 8, 13, 20–21, 277 n. 6. *See also*
    kali-yuga
Yukteswar, Sri, 277 n. 6

Zen, 162

About the Author

Georg Feuerstein, Ph.D., is internationally known for his many interpretative studies of the Yoga tradition. Since the early 1970s, he has made significant contributions to the East-West dialogue and is particularly concerned with preserving the authentic teachings of Yoga in its various forms. His interest in India's spirituality was awakened when he was thirteen years old, and he has followed the yogic path in various forms since that time. He is the founder and director of the Yoga Research Center and editor of the Center's bimonthly newsletter, *Yoga World*. He serves on the directorial board of the Healing Buddha Foundation in Sebastopol, California, and also is a contributing editor of *Yoga Journal*, *Inner Directions*, and *Intuition*. His thirty books include *The Shambhala Encyclopedia of Yoga, The Shambhala Guide to Yoga*, and *Teachings of Yoga*. Among his forthcoming works are *The Yoga Tradition* and *Yoga and Health*.

If you would like to see his current work, he periodically posts new articles on his website at:

http://members.aol.com/yogaresrch/index

He may be contacted at: Dr. Georg Feuerstein
Yoga Research Center
P. O. Box 1386
Lower Lake, CA 95457

or by e-mail at: *yogaresrch@aol.com*